Drug-Herb-Vitamin Interactions Bible

Other Books in THE NATURAL PHARMACIST™ LIBRARY

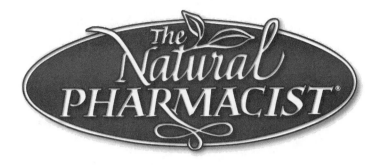

Drug-Herb-Vitamin Interactions Bible

From A–Z, Know the Dangers and Benefits of Combining Drugs, Herbs, and Vitamins

Richard Harkness, Pharm., FASCP
Steven Bratman, M.D.

Prima Publishing

Published by Prima Publishing, Roseville, California. Member of the Crown Publishing Group, a division of Random House, Inc.

THE NATURAL PHARMACIST is a trademark of Random House, Inc. PRIMA PUBLISHING and colophon and THE NATURAL PHARMACIST logo are registered trademarks of Random House, Inc., registered with the United States Patent and Trademark Office.

Certain trade names and brands for drugs are mentioned in this book. These trade names and brands may be trademarks of the respective manufacturers of those products and are listed herein for referential purposes only. This book is not affiliated with or sponsored by any of these manufacturers.

Disclaimer

This book is intended to provide general information, and not medical advice. As with all medical conditions, you should consult your physician or medical professional to determine what treatment is appropriate for any individual case. This book is sold with the understanding that the publisher and the authors are not liable for the misconception or misuse of information provided. Neither the authors nor the publisher shall have liability or responsibility to any person or entity with respect to any loss, damage, or injury caused or alleged to be caused directly or indirectly by the information contained in this book or the use of any products mentioned.

The Food and Drug Administration has not approved the use of any of the natural treatments discussed in this book. This book, and the information contained herein, has not been approved by the Food and Drug Administration.

Library of Congress Cataloging-in-Publication Data
Harkness, Richard.
      The natural pharmacist : drug-herb-vitamin interactions bible / Richard Harkness,
Steven Bratman.
      p. cm. — (The natural pharmacist series)
      Includes bibliographical references and index.
      ISBN 0-7615-3013-4 (pbk.)
      1. Drug-herb interactions. 2. Drug-nutrient interactions. I. Bratman, Steven. II.
      Title. III. Natural pharmacist.
RM302.H3675 2000
615'.7045—dc21   00-066908

02 03 04 DD 10 9 8 7 6 5 4 3 2
Printed in the United States of America
First Edition

Visit us online at www.primapublishing.com

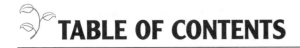

TABLE OF CONTENTS

PART TWO:
APPENDICES

PART THREE:
NOTES

WHAT MAKES THIS BOOK DIFFERENT?

The interest in natural medicine has never been greater. According to the National Association of Chain Drug Stores, 65 million Americans are using natural supplements, and the number is growing! Yet it is hard for the consumer to find trustworthy sources for balanced information about this emerging field. Why? Frankly, natural medicine has had a checkered history. From snake oil potions sold at the turn of the century to those books, magazines, and product catalogs that hype miracle cures today, this is a field where exaggerated claims have been the norm. Proponents of natural medicine have tended to abuse science, treating it more as a marketing tool than a means of discovering the truth.

But there is truth to be found. Studies of vitamins, minerals, and other food supplements have been with us since these nutritional substances were first discovered, and the level and quality of this science has grown dramatically in the last 20 years. Herbal medicine has been neglected in the United States, but in Europe, this, the oldest of all healing arts, has been the subject of tremendous and ongoing scientific interest.

At present, for a number of herbs and supplements, it is possible to give reasonably scientific answers to the following questions: How well does this work? How safe is it? What types of conditions is it best used for?

THE NATURAL PHARMACIST series is designed to cut through the hype and tell you what we know and what remains to be researched regarding popular natural treatments. These books are more conservative than any others available, more honest about the weaknesses of natural approaches, more fair in their comparisons of natural and conventional treatments. You won't find any miracle cures here, but you will discover useful options that can help you become healthier.

WHY CHOOSE NATURAL TREATMENTS?

Although the science behind natural medicine continues to grow, this is still a much less scientifically validated field than conventional medicine. You might ask, "Why should I resort to an herb that is only partly proven, when I could take a drug with solid science behind it?" There are at least three good reasons to consider natural alternatives.

First, some herbs and supplements offer benefits that are not matched by any conventional drug. Echinacea is a good example. If you have a cold and take echinacea, you'll recover faster. No standard medication can do the same.

Another example is glucosamine sulfate for arthritis. Glucosamine seems to slow the progression of arthritis, meaning that it protects your joints from getting worse over time. There is no pill or tablet your doctor can prescribe that offers the same benefit.

In many cases, the science behind natural treatments is very strong. For example, there is more evidence for the herb St. John's wort than there was for Prozac when it was first approved as a drug. The science behind other natural treatments is less than perfect, but when the risks are low and the possible benefit high, a natural treatment may be worth trying. It is a little-known fact that for many conventional treatments the science is less than perfect as well, and physicians must balance uncertain benefits against incompletely understood risks.

A second reason to consider natural therapies is that some may offer benefits comparable to those of drugs with fewer side effects. Again, the herb St. John's wort is a good example. Scientific evidence suggests that this herb is just as effective for mild to moderate depression as standard drugs, while producing fewer side effects. Saw palmetto for benign enlargement of the prostate, ginkgo for relieving symptoms and perhaps slowing the progression of Alzheimer's disease, and chondroitin for osteoarthritis are other examples. This is not to say that herbs and supplements are completely harmless—they're not—but for most the level of risk is quite low. The biggest potential problems are interactions between drugs and herbs, and we cover these thoroughly in our books.

Finally, there is a philosophical point to consider. For many people, it "feels" better to use a treatment that comes from nature instead of from a laboratory. Just as you might rather wear all-cotton clothing than polyester or look at a mountain landscape rather than the skyscrapers of a downtown city, natural treatments may simply feel more compatible with your view of life. We can quibble endlessly about just what "natural" means and whether a certain treatment is "actually" natural or not, but such arguments are beside the point. The difference is in the feeling, and feelings matter. In fact, having a good feeling about taking an herb may lead you to use it more consistently than you would a prescription drug.

Of course, at times synthetic drugs may be necessary and even lifesaving. But on many other occasions it may be quite reasonable to turn to an herb or supplement instead of a drug.

To make good decisions you need good information. Unfortunately, while hundreds of books on alternative medicine are published every year, many are highly misleading. The phrase "studies prove" is often used when the studies in question are so small or so badly conducted that they prove nothing at all. You may even find that the "data" from other books comes from studies with petri dishes and not real people!

You can't even assume that books written by well-known authors are scientifically sound. Many of these authors rely on secondary writers, leading to a game of "telephone," where misconceptions are passed around from book to book. And there's a strong tendency to exaggerate the power of natural remedies, whitewashing them with selective reporting.

THE NATURAL PHARMACIST series gives you the balanced information you need to make informed decisions about your health needs. Setting a new, high standard of accuracy and objectivity, these books take a realistic look at the herbs and supplements you read about in the news. You will encounter both favorable and unfavorable studies in these pages and will learn about both the benefits and the risks of natural treatments.

THE NATURAL PHARMACIST series is the source you can trust.

Steven Bratman, M.D.
David Kroll, Ph.D.
Series Editors

INTRODUCTION

Natural medicines, including herbs, vitamins, minerals, and various other supplements, have surged to enormous popularity in recent years. Unfortunately, sources of trustworthy, balanced information on the effects of taking dietary supplements has not kept pace with the increased use of these products.

Perhaps the greatest unmet need has been access to reliable information on interactions between supplements and drugs. As with drug-drug interactions, drug-supplement interactions can present significant health risks. For example, supplements that increase the effects of a drug can amplify drug side effects. Conversely, those that decrease drug effects might prevent the drug from working properly.

Being unaware of such interactions can seriously complicate matters. For instance, the adverse consequences of an interaction might mistakenly be blamed on some unknown cause or on the illness itself, resulting in faulty treatment decisions and further complications. With the realization that an interaction is the most likely cause, your physician can, in many cases, simply adjust the dose or time of administration of the drug or supplement to alleviate the problem.

For these reasons, it is vitally important that both you and your doctor be aware of potential harmful drug-supplement interactions.

There's another side to the issue, too. Some drugs can impair your body's absorption or utilization of essential nutrients. In these cases, you might be able to improve your general health or reduce specific side effects by taking supplemental nutrients.

With all this in mind, we set out to fill the need for a single source of accurate and comprehensive information on this "new wave" of potential drug-supplement interactions. The result of our efforts is the *Drug-Herb-Vitamin Interactions Bible*, a "big" book written in a concise, easy-to-read style especially for consumers. It is the product of exhaustive research—hundreds of published original studies were pored over and their findings carefully analyzed, with the relevant information serving as the foundation for this evidence-based guide. The information provided in the book is extensively referenced and the original study citations are listed in the Notes section. We used double-blinded studies in humans whenever available; if the findings discussed came from studies in test tubes or animals, that is specified.

During the development of this text, a few surprises were in store for the authors. Some "accepted" drug-supplement interactions, widely promulgated and considered to be important, were found not to be as significant as thought, while a number of important interactions were uncovered that had been generally unknown. Additionally, some nutrients routinely recommended to be taken along with certain drugs proved to present risks along with benefits.

Clearly, there is no substitute for having the right information to guide you in your decision-making. The *Drug-Herb-Vitamin Interactions Bible* is simply the best and most reliable source of up-to-date information on drug-supplement interactions available. Keeping the book handy and referring to it before mixing supplements and drugs can help you and your family avoid unnecessary health risks—and perhaps even save a life.

SPECIAL FEATURES OF THIS BOOK

In addition to an easy-to-use table of contents and comprehensive index, the *Drug-Herb-Vitamin Interactions Bible* provides the following valuable features:

Rating Key

Each interaction is rated on a numerical scale of 1 to 4 according to its significance:

1	Significant interaction
2	Possibly significant interaction
3	Interaction of relatively little significance
4	Reported interaction that does not in fact exist or is insignificant

Helpful Organization

In the text, interactions are arranged alphabetically by drug or drug family. Within each drug topic, interacting supplements are listed alphabetically according to interaction type: Negative, Mixed, and Positive.

Negative interactions are potentially harmful. *Positive* interactions include nutrient and drug combinations that may be helpful. *Mixed* interactions are a "benefits and risks" issue—the combination may be beneficial and potentially harmful at the same time.

Table of Interactions

Located at the beginning of each drug topic, this table presents a brief preview of the supplement interactions discussed, including rating and interaction type: Negative, Mixed, or Positive.

Appendices

Four appendices provide important information in concise form:

Appendix A: Interactions by Herb or Supplement is arranged by supplement name rather than by drug name. This makes it easy to find out which drugs may interact with a particular supplement. For each supplement entry, interacting drugs or drug families are listed alphabetically according to interaction type: Negative, Mixed, and Positive.

Appendix B: Nutrient Depletions lets you see at a glance which drugs may deplete nutrients or impair the body's ability to absorb or use them, effects which may lead to nutrient deficiencies. The respective nutrients are listed alphabetically along with interaction ratings. Supplemental intake of nutrients may be helpful in many of these cases.

Appendix C: Herb and Drug Interactions That Might Cause Excess Sedation lists herbs and drugs known to cause sedation and central nervous system depression. If you combine any of these herbs and drugs, you may be subjecting yourself to "add-on" depressant effects such as excessive drowsiness, dizziness, and loss of muscle coordination and alertness, and, in some cases, more serious consequences. Checking this appendix before combining herbs and drugs can help prevent this type of problem.

Appendix D: Safety Issues covers safety issues for herbs and supplements given positive or mixed interaction ratings. If you are considering using one of those substances, you can find relevant safety considerations here.

USING THE *DRUG-HERB-VITAMIN INTERACTIONS BIBLE*

There are several ways to find information in the book. The drug topics are arranged alphabetically in the text so that you can look up a particular drug name by paging through the book. A quicker way is to find the drug name in the table of contents and go directly to the page number shown. Use the index to look up interactions by drug/generic name, trade name, or supplement name. And remember to check the appendices for specialized information in concise format.

Because much of this interaction information is not generally known or has not been readily available in one place until now, you can use the book as an educational source for both yourself and your physician. Please note, however, that a book cannot take the place of advice from a qualified healthcare professional, and that it is not possible to list every potential drug-supplement interaction. Finally, you should not adjust medication doses or stop taking a prescribed drug without the advice of your physician.

Drug-Herb-Vitamin Interactions

ACE INHIBITORS

Interactions	Rating*
Negative Interactions	
Arginine	3
Iron	2
Licorice	2
Potassium	1
St. John's Wort, Dong Quai	3
Positive Interaction	
Zinc	2

*Rating Key

1 Significant interaction

2 Possibly significant interaction

3 Interaction of relatively little significance

4 Reported interaction that does not in fact exist or is insignificant

ACE inhibitors block the conversion of a naturally occurring substance, angiotensin, to a more active form. These medications are widely used to treat hypertension as well as congestive heart failure and other conditions. Drugs in this category include

- benazepril hydrochloride (Lotensin, Lotrel)
- captopril (Capoten)
- enalapril maleate (Lexxel, Teczem, Vaseretic, Vasotec)
- fosinopril (Monopril)
- lisinopril (Prinivil, Prinzide, Zestril, Zestoretic)
- moexipril hydrochloride (Uniretic, Univasc)
- quinapril hydrochloride (Accupril)
- ramipril (Altace)
- trandolapril (Mavik, Tarka)
- and others

NEGATIVE INTERACTIONS

Arginine: Possible Harmful Interaction

 Arginine is an amino acid that has been used to improve immunity in hospitalized patients as well as for many other conditions.

Based on experience with intravenous arginine, it is possible that the use of high-dose oral arginine might alter potassium levels in the body, especially in people with severe liver disease.[1] This is a potential concern for individuals who take ACE inhibitors.

Iron: Take at a Different Time of Day

2 NEGATIVE Iron supplements can interfere with the absorption of captopril and perhaps other ACE inhibitors.[2] Iron appears to bind with captopril, resulting in a compound that the body cannot absorb. This, of course, also impairs iron absorption. To minimize any potential problems, take iron supplements and ACE inhibitors 2 to 3 hours apart.

Licorice: Possible Harmful Interaction

2 NEGATIVE Licorice root, a member of the pea family, has been used since ancient times as both food and medicine.

Whole licorice (*Glycyrrhiza glabra*, or *G. uralensis*) can cause sodium retention and increase blood pressure, thus counteracting the intended effects of ACE inhibitors.[3,4] An often unrecognized source of licorice is chewing tobacco.[5]

A special form of licorice known as DGL (deglycyrrhizinated licorice) is a deliberately altered form of the herb that should not cause these problems.

Potassium: Possible Harmful Interaction

1 NEGATIVE ACE inhibitors cause the body to retain more potassium than usual. This could raise your blood levels of potassium too high, a condition called hyperkalemia, which can be dangerous.[6–10] Depending on how high your potassium levels are, the symptoms you might experience include irregular heart rhythm, muscle weakness, nausea, vomiting, irritability, and diarrhea. If you are on one of these medications, do not take potassium supplements except on medical advice.

Because ingesting more potassium makes the problem worse, it is important to be aware of the various sources of extra potassium. Besides potassium supplements, sources include high-potassium diets, salt substitutes containing potassium, and potassium-sparing diuretics (diuretics that cause your body to retain potassium).

Your physician will want to keep an eye on the levels of potassium in your blood and let you know if you need to adjust your potassium intake.

St. John's Wort, Dong Quai: Possible Harmful Interaction

 St. John's wort (*Hypericum perforatum*) is primarily used to treat mild to moderate depression.

The herb dong quai (*Angelica sinensis*) is often recommended for menstrual disorders such as dysmenorrhea, PMS, and irregular menstruation.

ACE inhibitors have been reported to cause increased sensitivity to the sun, amplifying the risk of sunburn or skin rash. Because St. John's wort and dong quai may also cause this problem, taking these herbal supplements during treatment with ACE inhibitors might add to this risk.

It may be a good idea to wear a sunscreen or protective clothing during sun exposure if you take one of these herbs while using an ACE inhibitor.

POSITIVE INTERACTIONS

Zinc: Supplementation Possibly Helpful

2 POSITIVE ACE inhibitors may cause zinc depletion.[11,12] The ACE inhibitors captopril and enalapril attach to the trace mineral zinc. Because zinc in this bound form cannot replace the zinc that the body uses to meet its normal needs, a gradual loss of zinc from body tissues may result. Continued drug therapy could lead to zinc deficiency.

It has been suggested, though not proven, that zinc deficiency might account for some of the side effects seen with ACE inhibitors, such as taste disturbances, poor appetite, and skin numbness or tingling.

Whether zinc supplementation will prevent ACE inhibitor–induced zinc deficiency has not been examined, but it seems reasonable to think that taking extra zinc might help. Generally, zinc supplements should also contain copper to prevent zinc-induced copper deficiency.

Please see Appendix D, Safety Issues, for more information.

ACETAMINOPHEN (APAP)

Trade Names: Abenol, Acephen, Aceta, Amaphen, Anoquan, Apacet, Arthritis Foundation, Aspirin Free, Arthritis Foundation Nighttime, Aspirin Free Anacin, Aspirin Free Excedrin, Bayer Select, Dapacin, Dynafed, Endolor, Esgic, Excedrin PM, Fem-Etts, Femcet, Feverall, Fioricet, Fiorpap, Genapap, Genebs, Halenol, Isocet, Liquiprin, Mapap, Maranox, Meda, Medigesic, Midol, Multi-Symptom Pamprin, Neopap, Nighttime Pamprin, Oraphen-PD, Panadol, Phrenilin, Repan, Ridenol, Sedapap, Silapap, Sominex Pain Relief, Tapanol, Tempra, Tylenol, Uni-Ace, Unisom with Pain Relief

Interactions	*Rating**
Negative Interactions	
Chaparral, Comfrey, Coltsfoot	2
Vitamin C	3
Positive Interactions	
Coenzyme Q_{10} (CoQ_{10})	3
Methionine	3
Milk Thistle	3

*Rating Key

1   Significant interaction

2   Possibly significant interaction

3   Interaction of relatively little significance

4   Reported interaction that does not in fact exist or is insignificant

Acetaminophen is a widely used alternative to aspirin and other non-steroidal anti-inflammatory drugs (NSAIDs), such as ibuprofen, for pain and fever. Acetaminophen is easier on the stomach than these other drugs, but does not possess their anti-inflammatory effects. For this reason, acetaminophen has limited benefit for conditions associated with inflammation, such as rheumatoid arthritis. However, acetaminophen may be the drug of first choice for painful conditions not associated with inflammation, such as osteoarthritis.

The major concern with acetaminophen is its potential to damage the liver. This risk, however, is low if you stay within the recommended dosage range: up to 1 g (1,000 mg) every 4 hours, with a maximum of 4 g a day (equal to 8 "extra strength" tablets, for example). The risk of liver damage increases if you take acetaminophen at doses greater than the highest recommended daily dose, either at one time or in multiple doses that exceed the total of 4 g daily. Excessive doses may damage the kidneys in a similar manner.

NEGATIVE INTERACTIONS

Chaparral, Comfrey, Coltsfoot: Possible Harmful Interaction

 The herb chaparral (*Larrea tridentata*, or *L. mexicana*) has been promoted for use in arthritis, cancer, and various other conditions, but there is insufficient evidence supporting its effectiveness. In addition, there are concerns about its apparent liver toxicity.

Several cases of chaparral-induced liver damage have been reported, some of them severe enough to require liver transplantation.[1–6]

Based on these reports, combining chaparral with other agents hard on the liver, such as acetaminophen, may amplify the risk of potential liver problems. Other herbs that are toxic to the liver include comfrey (*Symphytum officinale*) and coltsfoot (*Tussilago farfara*).

Vitamin C: Possible Harmful Interaction

3 NEGATIVE A small study in humans found that high doses of vitamin C (3 g daily) interfered with the normal breakdown of acetaminophen in the body.[7] This could possibly allow the drug to accumulate to levels that may damage the liver.

You probably don't need to be overly concerned if you take acetaminophen in recommended doses now and then for pain or fever. However, a problem might occur if you take higher-than-recommended doses or if you take high doses of acetaminophen on a regular basis, such as for osteoarthritis. The risk increases if you have liver or kidney impairment or if you drink alcoholic beverages regularly, which taxes the liver even more.

POSITIVE INTERACTIONS

Coenzyme Q_{10} (CoQ_{10}): Supplementation Possibly Helpful

3 POSITIVE Coenzyme Q_{10} is a vitamin-like substance that plays a fundamental role in the body's energy production.[8,9]

A study in mice found that coenzyme Q_{10} (ubiquinone) may help prevent the liver damage caused by excessive doses of acetaminophen.[10] It's speculated that CoQ_{10} might have a protective effect on liver membranes.

Warning: Acetaminophen overdose can be fatal! Do not count on CoQ_{10} to protect you from the effects of excessive acetaminophen intake.

Please see Appendix D, Safety Issues, for more information.

Methionine: Supplementation Possibly Helpful

3 POSITIVE Methionine is an essential amino acid. A study in mice found that methionine helps prevent the liver damage caused by excessive doses of acetaminophen.[11] The body uses methionine to manufacture glutathione, a protein-like substance the liver uses to neutralize a toxic byproduct formed in the normal breakdown of acetaminophen. If the liver's supply of glutathione is spent, which may occur from overuse of acetaminophen, this breakdown product is free to damage the liver. Taking extra methionine may offer some protection.

Warning: Acetaminophen overdose can be fatal! Do not count on methionine to protect you from the effects of excessive acetaminophen intake.

Please see Appendix D, Safety Issues, for more information.

Milk Thistle: Supplementation Possibly Helpful

3
POSITIVE   The herbal product silymarin, or milk thistle (*Silybum marianum*), has been used for hepatitis and various other liver-related disorders.

Supplementation with milk thistle may help prevent acetaminophen toxicity, as well as poisoning from other substances that are toxic to the liver, including the *Amanita* "deathcap" mushroom.[12,13,14]

In one study, rats were divided into three groups and treated with acetaminophen alone, acetaminophen and silymarin combined, or placebo.[15] Rats getting only acetaminophen showed significant increases in lipid peroxidation (a known liver-damaging process) as well as several measurable markers of liver damage. In contrast, rats receiving silymarin and acetaminophen showed normal lipid peroxidation and normal levels of most markers for liver damage. These findings suggest that silymarin may protect against acetaminophen liver toxicity through its antioxidant properties, possibly by acting as a free radical scavenger.

Warning: Acetaminophen overdose can be fatal! Do not count on milk thistle to protect you from the effects of excessive acetaminophen intake.

Please see Appendix D, Safety Issues, for more information.

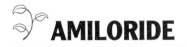

AMILORIDE

Trade Names: Midamor, Moduretic

Interactions	Rating*
Negative Interactions	
Arginine	3
Licorice	1
Magnesium	3
Potassium	1
Zinc	3

*Rating Key

1 Significant interaction

2 Possibly significant interaction

3 Interaction of relatively little significance

4 Reported interaction that does not in fact exist or is insignificant

Amiloride is a diuretic (an agent that reduces fluid accumulation in the body). It is a member of the potassium-sparing family of diuretics, which were developed to avoid the potassium loss that is common with **loop** (see page 102) and **thiazide diuretics** (see page 174). Potassium-sparing diuretics, though not very powerful by themselves, cause the body to retain potassium and may be used in combination with these other diuretics when needed. Other drugs in this family include **spironolactone** (Aldactone; see page 161) and **triamterene** (Dyrenium, Maxzide; see page 181).

NEGATIVE INTERACTIONS

Arginine: Possible Harmful Interaction

3 NEGATIVE Arginine is an amino acid found in many foods, including dairy products, meat, poultry, and fish. Supplemental arginine has been proposed as a treatment for various conditions, including heart problems.

Based on experience with arginine given intravenously (into a vein), it is possible that the use of high-dose oral arginine might alter potassium levels in the body, especially in people with severe liver disease.[1] This is a potential concern for individuals who take amiloride or other potassium-sparing diuretics.

Unless your doctor advises otherwise, it might be best to avoid arginine supplementation if you take amiloride.

Licorice: Possible Harmful Interaction

| **1** **NEGATIVE** | Licorice root (*Glycyrrhiza glabra* or *G. uralensis*), a member of the pea family, has been used since ancient times as both food and medicine.

Potassium-sparing diuretics such as amiloride cause the body to retain potassium and are ordinarily prescribed to take advantage of this effect. Licorice has the opposite effect, causing the body to lose potassium,[2–5] and thus directly counteracts the effect of these drugs. In fact, the potassium-sparing diuretic **spironolactone** has been found to correct the low potassium levels brought about by excessive licorice ingestion.[6]

Based on these findings, licorice should not be combined with potassium-sparing diuretics except to treat licorice toxicity, which must be supervised by a physician.

Magnesium: Possible Harmful Interaction

| **3** **NEGATIVE** | Preliminary evidence from animal studies suggests that amiloride and other potassium-sparing diuretics might cause the body to retain magnesium along with potassium.[7]

Therefore, taking magnesium supplements might conceivably increase the risk of magnesium levels climbing too high and producing toxic effects such as weakness, low blood pressure, and impaired breathing. As a precaution, it may be best to avoid magnesium supplementation while taking amiloride except under medical supervision.

Potassium: Possible Harmful Interaction

| **1** **NEGATIVE** | When taking potassium-sparing diuretics such as amiloride, you generally should not take potassium supplements, since this could raise your potassium levels too high.

Besides potassium supplementation, potassium levels may be raised by high-potassium diets and salt substitutes containing potassium. Symptoms of potassium toxicity include nausea, vomiting, irritability, diarrhea, and changes in heart function.

Treatments that combine **thiazide diuretics** (which cause potassium loss; see page 174) and potassium-sparing diuretics can affect potassium levels unpredictably.

If you are taking amiloride alone or in combination with other diuretics, do not increase your intake of potassium except on the advice of your physician.

Zinc: Possible Harmful Interaction

3 NEGATIVE Amiloride may cause the body to retain significant amounts of the trace mineral zinc.[8] Zinc accumulation in the body could lead to toxic side effects.

However, the potassium-sparing diuretic **triamterene** (see page 181) does not seem to cause this problem.[9]

Because ingesting extra zinc may compound a potential problem, zinc supplementation should probably be avoided if you take amiloride unless your physician advises otherwise. Symptoms of excessive zinc levels include a metallic taste sensation, vomiting, and stomach problems.

AMIODARONE

Trade Names: Cordarone, Pacerone

Interactions	Rating*
Negative Interactions	
Chaparral, Comfrey, Coltsfoot	2
St. John's Wort, Dong Quai	3
Positive Interaction	
Vitamin E	2

*Rating Key

1 Significant interaction
2 Possibly significant interaction
3 Interaction of relatively little significance
4 Reported interaction that does not in fact exist or is insignificant

Amiodarone is a drug used for irregular heart rhythm. Problems with using amiodarone, however, can include adverse effects on the liver or damage to the lungs.

NEGATIVE INTERACTIONS

Chaparral, Comfrey, Coltsfoot: Possible Harmful Interaction

2 NEGATIVE The herb chaparral (*Larrea tridentata* or *L. mexicana*) has been promoted for use in arthritis, cancer, and various other conditions, but there is insufficient evidence supporting its effectiveness. In addition, there are concerns about its apparent liver toxicity.

Several cases of chaparral-induced liver damage have been reported, some of them severe enough to require liver transplantation.[1-6]

Based on these reports, combining chaparral with other agents hard on the liver, such as amiodarone, may amplify the risk of potential liver problems.[7] Other herbs that are toxic to the liver include comfrey (*Symphytum officinale*) and coltsfoot (*Tussilago farfara*).

St. John's Wort, Dong Quai: Possible Harmful Interaction

3 NEGATIVE St. John's wort (*Hypericum perforatum*) is primarily used to treat mild to moderate depression. The herb dong quai (*Angelica sinensis*) is often recommended for menstrual disorders such as dysmenorrhea, PMS, and irregular menstruation.

Amiodarone has been reported to cause increased sensitivity to the sun, amplifying the risk of sunburn or skin rash. Because St. John's wort and dong quai may also cause this problem, taking these herbal supplements during amiodarone therapy might add to this risk.

It may be a good idea to wear a sunscreen or protective clothing during sun exposure if you take one of these herbs while using amiodarone.

POSITIVE INTERACTIONS

Vitamin E: Supplementation Possibly Helpful

2 POSITIVE A test tube study suggests that vitamin E supplements might help prevent amiodarone's toxic effects on the lungs. Researchers added amiodarone and vitamin E to cultures of human lung artery cells and found that the vitamin could prevent drug-induced cell damage.[8] The more vitamin E they used, the greater the protection. Several other antioxidants were also tested but found not to be protective, which suggests that this vitamin E benefit may not be primarily related to its well-known antioxidant action.

Vitamin E is also believed to help stabilize cell membranes, and this may be the chief way it helps in this case. Though test tube results may not be applicable to people, vitamin E supplementation might be good precautionary insurance when taking amiodarone. A typical dose of vitamin E is 100 to 400 IU (international units) daily.

Please see Appendix D, Safety Issues, for more information.

AMOXICILLIN

Trade Names: Amoxil, Polymox, PREVPAC, Trimox, Wymox

Interactions	Rating*
Positive Interaction	
Bromelain	2

*Rating Key

1 Significant interaction
2 Possibly significant interaction
3 Interaction of relatively little significance
4 Reported interaction that does not in fact exist or is insignificant

Amoxicillin is a relative of the antibiotic penicillin, but has been modified to have a broader spectrum of effect.

POSITIVE INTERACTIONS

Bromelain: Supplementation Possibly Helpful

2 POSITIVE Bromelain, a supplement derived from pineapple stems (*Ananas comosus*), may improve absorption of the antibiotics amoxicillin and tetracycline. In a double-blind trial involving 127 individuals, bromelain significantly raised amoxicillin blood levels compared to control groups.[1] Additionally, the bromelain groups had significantly higher amoxicillin levels in their body tissues. Similar results were found for both amoxicillin and tetracycline in another placebo-controlled study of 54 patients given bromelain.[2]

Please see Appendix D, Safety Issues, for more information.

ANTACIDS

Interactions	Rating*
Negative Interaction	
Calcium Citrate	3
Positive Interactions	
Folate	3
Minerals	3

*Rating Key

1 Significant interaction

2 Possibly significant interaction

3 Interaction of relatively little significance

4 Reported interaction that does not in fact exist or is insignificant

The term "antacid" is used to describe certain compounds that directly neutralize stomach acid. Tums, Maalox, and Mylanta all fall into this category. The active ingredients in most antacids are various forms of calcium, magnesium, and aluminum. Antacids are useful mostly for symptomatic relief of uncomfortable "acid stomach" and may also be helpful for heartburn. Many antacids are available today, including

- aluminum carbonate (Basaljel)
- aluminum hydroxide (ALternaGEL, Alu-Cap, Alu-Tab, Amphojel, Dialume, Nephrox)
- aluminum hydroxide/magnesium carbonate (Duracid)
- aluminum hydroxide/magnesium hydroxide (Alamag, Almacone, Aludrox, Gaviscon Liquid, Gelusil, Kudrox, Maalox, Magalox, Magnox, Mintox, Mylanta, Rulox)
- aluminum hydroxide/magnesium hydroxide/calcium carbonate (Tempo)
- aluminum hydroxide/magnesium trisilicate (Alenic Alka, Gaviscon, Genaton, Foamicon)
- calcium carbonate (Alkets, Amitone, Chooz, Equilet, Gas-Ban, Maalox Antacid Caplets, Mallamint, Mylanta Lozenges, Titralac, Tums)
- calcium carbonate/magnesium carbonate (Marblen, Mi-Acid Gelcaps, Mylanta Gelcaps, Mylagen Gelcaps)
- magnesium hydroxide (Milk of Magnesia, Phillips' Chewable)
- magaldrate or aluminum magnesium hydroxide sulfate (Iosopan, Riopan)
- magnesium oxide (Mag-Ox, Maox, Uro-Mag)
- sodium bicarbonate (Bell/ans, Bromo Seltzer)
- sodium citrate (Citra pH)

Other drugs work by reducing the stomach's production of acid. These are discussed separately in the articles on H_2 Antagonists (e.g., cimetidine [Tagamet], famotidine [Pepcid], nizatidine [Axid], ranitidine [Zantac]) and Proton Pump Inhibitors (e.g., lansoprazole [Prevacid], omeprazole [Prilosec], rabeprazole [Aciphex]). These drugs produce a more powerful effect than antacids and are used for ulcers as well as for the treatment of esophageal reflux, commonly known as heartburn.

NEGATIVE INTERACTIONS

Calcium Citrate: Possible Harmful Interaction

3 NEGATIVE Concerns have been raised that the aluminum in some antacids may not be good for you. As there is some evidence that calcium citrate supplements might increase the absorption of aluminum,[1–5] it might be a good idea not to take calcium citrate at the same time of day as aluminum-containing antacids. Another option is to use other forms of calcium, or to avoid antacids containing aluminum.

POSITIVE INTERACTIONS

Folate: Supplementation Possibly Helpful

3 POSITIVE Folate (also known as folic acid) is a B vitamin that plays an important role in many vital aspects of health, including preventing neural tube birth defects and possibly reducing the risk of heart disease. Because inadequate intake of folate is widespread, if you are taking any medication that depletes or impairs folate even slightly, you may need supplementation.

Conditions for folate absorption are best in the slightly acidic part of the intestine nearest to the stomach.

Antacids and other substances that reduce the level of stomach acid have been shown to interfere with the body's absorption of folate. Preliminary evidence suggests that antacids containing aluminum hydroxide may attach to folate in the digestive tract.[6] This binding action, rather than acid-lowering ability, appears to be the way these antacids reduce folate absorption. Though the actual reduction in absorption of the vitamin is relatively minor, dietary folate deficiency is common anyway, so individuals who regularly take antacids containing aluminum hydroxide may benefit from folate supplementation in standard nutritional doses.

Please see Appendix D, Safety Issues, for more information.

Minerals: Supplementation Possibly Helpful, but Take at a Different Time of Day

3 POSITIVE Antacids might affect the absorption of zinc, iron, phosphorus, magnesium, chromium, and manganese through various mechanisms.

Please see Appendix D, Safety Issues, for more information.

Antacids in General

By reducing stomach acid levels, any antacid may reduce the absorption of zinc and iron, and possibly other minerals that are absorbed best under acidic conditions.[7] To minimize potential problems when taking antacids, take them 2 to 3 hours apart from meals or mineral supplements.

Aluminum-Containing Antacids

Aluminum-containing antacids can bind with the phosphorus in your diet and interfere with its absorption.[8] This effect on phosphorus can further lead to calcium depletion and bone loss if you regularly take antacids.[9] In general, it might be advisable to avoid long-term use of aluminum-containing antacids due to aluminum's potential toxicity. If you must use them, it's probably good insurance to take supplemental calcium and phosphorus. A convenient way to get more of both minerals is to drink milk (lowfat milk has the same mineral content as regular milk). It may also help to take the antacid 2 to 3 hours apart from meals or mineral supplements.

Calcium-Containing Antacids

The calcium present in some antacids and calcium supplements may reduce the absorption of iron,[10–13] zinc,[14] magnesium,[15,16] chromium,[17] and manganese[18,19] by competing with these minerals for absorption. To minimize any potential problems, take calcium-containing antacids or calcium supplements 2 to 3 hours apart from these mineral supplements.

Antacids containing calcium interfere with iron absorption according to most studies.[20–23] Although one study in postmenopausal women found that calcium supplementation appeared to have no effect on iron absorption,[24] the women had a high dietary intake of vitamin C (215 mg daily), which is known to enhance iron absorption. Thus, it is possible that vitamin C in that amount could have offset the calcium supplement's interference with iron absorption.

Calcium carbonate may be the form least likely to affect the absorption of iron when both are taken on an empty stomach (between meals).[25]

One study found that calcium substantially decreased zinc absorption when the two were taken together as supplements.[26] Another study found no impairment of zinc absorption from a meal.[27] It appears that, in the presence of meals, zinc levels may be unaffected by either dietary calcium or calcium supplements.[28] A possible explanation is that food ingestion is associated with a variety of complex interactions involving nutrients and digestive products that may affect the handling of nutrients by the body.

Although calcium-containing antacids or supplements may alter the absorption of magnesium, this effect apparently has no significant influence on your body's ability to keep magnesium in proper balance.[29,30]

ANTHRACYCLINES

Interactions	Rating*
Positive Interactions	
Coenzyme Q_{10} (CoQ$_{10}$)	2
Vitamin E	3
Other Supplements	3

*Rating Key

1 Significant interaction
2 Possibly significant interaction
3 Interaction of relatively little significance
4 Reported interaction that does not in fact exist or is insignificant

Anthracyclines are a class of drugs with antitumor effects used in chemotherapy for various cancers. A serious potential side effect of these medications is damage to the heart. Along with other factors, this heart damage is thought to involve free radicals, which are naturally occurring dangerous chemicals that can damage many tissues by oxidizing them.

This observation has led to trying various antioxidants as a way to protect the heart in individuals taking anthracyclines. Most such studies have used doxorubicin. However, because of concerns that antioxidants could in some cases interfere with the effectiveness of chemotherapy drugs, people on chemotherapy should not use these (or any other) supplements except on their physician's advice. This family of drugs includes

- daunorubicin (Cerubidine)
- doxorubicin (Adriamycin, Doxil, Rubex)
- epirubicin (Ellence)
- idarubicin (Idamycin)
- valrubicin (Valstar)

POSITIVE INTERACTIONS

Coenzyme Q_{10} (CoQ$_{10}$): Supplementation Possibly Helpful

2 POSITIVE Coenzyme Q_{10} is a vitamin-like substance that plays a fundamental role in the body's energy production, including that of the heart.[1,2] Doxorubicin appears to interfere with the body's manufacture of CoQ$_{10}$[3] as well as the activity of enzymes containing CoQ$_{10}$.[4,5]

It has been hypothesized that these effects on CoQ$_{10}$ might be a factor in doxorubicin's toxic effects on the heart and that CoQ$_{10}$ supplementation might be protective. Animal studies suggest that CoQ$_{10}$ may indeed reduce doxorubicin-associated heart toxicity.[6–10] In a small trial, CoQ$_{10}$ at 50 mg daily given with chemotherapy that included doxorubicin was found to reduce heart complications, compared to participants not taking CoQ$_{10}$.[11]

Please see Appendix D, Safety Issues, for more information.

Vitamin E: Supplementation Possibly Helpful

3 POSITIVE Numerous animal studies and small trials in humans have examined whether vitamin E's antioxidant effects might help prevent the heart toxicity associated with doxorubicin therapy. Many animal studies have found a heart-protective benefit for vitamin E,[12–17] but others have found no apparent benefit.[18–21] Unfortunately, human trials have as yet found little if any heart-protective effect for vitamin E.[22,23,24]

One study found oral vitamin E supplementation helpful for doxorubicin-induced hair loss,[25] but other studies demonstrate no such benefit.[26,27,28]

There is some evidence that the application of dressings containing vitamin E in combination with DMSO (dimethyl sulfoxide) may help prevent skin ulcerations caused by intravenous injection of doxorubicin.[29]

Please see Appendix D, Safety Issues, for more information.

Other Supplements: Supplementation Possibly Helpful

3 POSITIVE Animal studies suggest that the antioxidants selenium,[30,31,32] glutathione,[33,34,35] and vitamin C[36,37] help prevent doxorubicin-related heart damage and increase survival time or delay doxorubicin-related death. Additionally, vitamin C substantially reduced the number of doxorubicin-associated skin ulcerations in animals when injected in combination with the drug.[38]

N-acetyl cysteine, a specially modified form of a dietary amino acid, appears to prevent heart toxicity in mice but not dogs treated with doxorubicin.[39,40] Trials in people have as yet found no benefit.[41,42]

Please see Appendix D, Safety Issues, for more information.

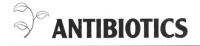

ANTIBIOTICS

Interactions	Rating*
Positive Interactions	
Lactobacillus acidophilus and Other "Friendly Bacteria"	2
Saccharomyces boulardii	2
Vitamin K	3

*Rating Key

1 Significant interaction

2 Possibly significant interaction

3 Interaction of relatively little significance

4 Reported interaction that does not in fact exist or is insignificant

See also **Amoxicillin** (page 12), **Cephalosporins** (page 61), **Ethambutol** (page 81), **Fluoroquinolones** (page 83), **Isoniazid** (page 93), **Nitrofurantoin** (page 113), **Rifampin** (page 157), **Tetracyclines** (page 169), and **Trimethoprim/Sulfamethoxazole** (page 188).

"Antibiotic" is the general term for any drug that kills or hampers the growth of bacteria. Certain interactions apply to most antibiotics in general, and these are discussed here.

There are an enormous number of antibiotics in use today. Some of the drugs in this family include

- amoxicillin (Amoxil, Polymox, PREVPAC, Trimox, Wymox)
- amoxicillin/potassium clavulanate (Augmentin)
- ampicillin (Omnipen, Principen, Totacillin, Marcillin)
- azithromycin (Zithromax)
- bacampicillin (Spectrobid)
- carbenicillin indanyl sodium (Geocillin)
- chloramphenicol (Chloromycetin Kapseals)
- cinoxacin (Cinobac)
- clarithromycin (Biaxin, PREVPAC)
- clindamycin (Cleocin)
- clofazimine (Lamprene)
- cloxacillin sodium (Cloxapen, Tegopen)
- colistin sulfate (Coly-Mycin S, Cortisporin-TC)
- dapsone
- dicloxacillin sodium (Dycill, Dynapen, Pathocil)
- dirithromycin (Dynabac)
- erythromycin (E-Base, Ilosone, EryPed, E.E.S., Ery-Tab, E-Mycin, Eryc, Erythrocin, PCE)
- fosfomycin tromethamine (Monurol)

- kanamycin (Kantrex)
- lincomycin (Lincocin)
- metronidazole (Flagyl, Helidac, Protostat)
- nafcillin sodium (Unipen)
- nalidixic acid (NegGram)
- neomycin (Neo-Tabs, Mycifradin, Neo-fradin)
- novobiocin (Albamycin)
- oxacillin sodium
- paromomycin (Humatin)
- penicillin V (Pen Vee K Beepen-VK, Penicillin VK, Veetids)
- troleandomycin (Tao)
- vancomycin (Vancocin)
- and others

POSITIVE INTERACTIONS

Lactobacillus acidophilus and Other "Friendly Bacteria": Supplementation Probably Helpful

2 POSITIVE A common side effect of antibiotic therapy is diarrhea (about 25 to 30% of people taking antibiotics report this problem). It's primarily caused by the antibiotic's killing of many of the bacteria that normally live in the intestines, allowing other bacteria or fungi to grow in their place. Changes in bacteria can also cause yeast infections. However, if you take "friendly" bacteria (also called **probiotics**; see Appendix D, Safety Issues, for more information) such as *Lactobacillus acidophilus* or *Bifidobacterium longum* at the same time you start antibiotics and continue for some time afterward, you may be able to significantly reduce the risk of these complications.[1,2]

The most well-known probiotic is *Lactobacillus acidophilus*. Others include *L. bulgaricus*, *L. thermophilus*, *L. reuteri*, *S. bulgaricus*, and *B. bifidus*.

Saccharomyces boulardii: Supplementation Possibly Helpful

2 POSITIVE *Saccharomyces boulardii*, a beneficial yeast species related to brewer's yeast, has also been found to prevent antibiotic-induced diarrhea according to most studies,[3–8] but not all of them.[9]

Vitamin K: Supplementation Possibly Helpful

| 3 |
| POSITIVE |

Vitamin K plays a crucial role in blood clotting and also seems to be important for proper bone formation. We get vitamin K from food, and it is also manufactured by bacteria in the intestines.

Antibiotics destroy harmful bacteria as well as "friendly" intestinal bacteria that produce vitamin K. For this reason, it is widely believed that antibiotic use may lead to a vitamin K deficiency. However, this may be a problem only in severely malnourished individuals.[10,11]

Antibiotics in the cephalosporin family may affect vitamin K in a more significant way by interfering with the vitamin after it is absorbed by the body (see **Cephalosporins-Vitamin K;** page 61).

Also see Appendix D, Safety Issues, for more information.

ANTICONVULSANT AGENTS

Negative Interactions	
Ginkgo	3
Glutamine	4
Grapefruit Juice	1
Ipriflavone	2
Kava, Valerian, Passionflower, Hops	2
Nicotinamide	3
St. John's Wort, Dong Quai	3
Vitamin A	3
White Willow	3

Mixed Interactions	
Biotin	3
Folate	2

Positive Interactions	
Calcium	2
Carnitine	2
Vitamin D	2
Vitamin K	2

*Rating Key

1 Significant interaction
2 Possibly significant interaction
3 Interaction of relatively little
   significance
4 Reported interaction that does not
   in fact exist or is insignificant

Anticonvulsant agents are used primarily to prevent seizures in conditions such as epilepsy. Drugs in this category include

- carbamazepine (Atretol, Carbatrol, Epitol, Tegretol, Tegretol XR)
- phenobarbital
- phenytoin (Dilantin) and similar drugs, including ethotoin (Peganone) and mephenytoin (Mesantoin)
- primidone (Mysoline)
- valproic acid (Depakene, Depakote)

NEGATIVE INTERACTIONS

Ginkgo: Possible Harmful Interaction

3 NEGATIVE The herb ginkgo (*Ginkgo biloba*) has been used to treat Alzheimer's disease and ordinary age-related memory loss, among many other uses.

This interaction involves potential contaminants in ginkgo, not ginkgo itself.

A recent study found that a natural nerve toxin present in the seeds of *Ginkgo biloba* made its way into standardized ginkgo extracts prepared from the leaves.[1] This toxin has been associated with convulsions and death in laboratory animals.[2,3,4]

Fortunately, the detected amounts of this toxic substance are considered harmless.[5] However, given the lack of satisfactory standardization of herbal formulations in the United States, it is possible that some batches of product might contain higher contents of the toxin depending on the season of harvest.

In light of these findings, taking a ginkgo product that happened to contain significant levels of the nerve toxin might theoretically prevent an anticonvulsant from working as well as expected.

Glutamine: Possible Harmful Interaction

4 NEGATIVE The amino acid glutamine is converted to glutamate in the body. Glutamate is thought to act as a neurotransmitter (a chemical that enables nerve transmission). Because anticonvulsants work (at least in part) by blocking glutamate pathways in the brain, high dosages of the amino acid glutamine might theoretically diminish an anticonvulsant's effect and increase the risk of seizures.

Grapefruit Juice: Possible Harmful Interaction

1 NEGATIVE Grapefruit juice slows the body's normal breakdown of several drugs, including the anticonvulsant carbamazepine, allowing it to build up to potentially dangerous levels in the blood.[6] A recent study indicates this effect can last for three days or more following the last glass of juice.[7]

Because of this risk, if you take carbamazepine, the safest approach is to avoid grapefruit juice altogether.

Ipriflavone: Possible Harmful Interaction

2 NEGATIVE Ipriflavone, a synthetic isoflavone that slows bone breakdown, is used to treat osteoporosis.

Test tube studies indicate that ipriflavone might increase blood levels of the anticonvulsants carbamazepine and phenytoin when they are taken therapeutically.[8] Ipriflavone was found to inhibit a liver enzyme involved in the body's normal breakdown of these drugs, thus allowing them to build up in the blood. Higher drug levels increase the risk of adverse effects.

Because anticonvulsants are known to contribute to the development of osteoporosis, a concern is that the use of ipriflavone for this drug-induced osteoporosis could result in higher blood levels of the drugs, with potentially serious consequences.

Individuals taking either of these drugs should use ipriflavone only under medical supervision.

Kava, Valerian, Passionflower, Hops: Possible Harmful Interaction

2 NEGATIVE The herb kava (*Piper methysticum*) has a sedative effect and is used for anxiety and insomnia.

Combining kava with anticonvulsants, which possess similar depressant effects, could result in "add-on" or excessive physical depression, sedation, and impairment. In one case report, a 54-year-old man was hospitalized for lethargy and disorientation, side effects attributed to his having taken the combination of kava and the antianxiety agent alprazolam (Xanax) for 3 days.[9]

Other herbs having a sedative effect that might cause problems when combined with anticonvulsants include ashwagandha (*Withania somnifera*), calendula (*Calendula officinalis*), catnip (*Nepeta cataria*), hops (*Humulus lupulus*), lady's slipper (*Cypripedium* species), lemon balm (*Melissa officinalis*), passionflower (*Passiflora incarnata*), sassafras (*Sassafras officinale*), skullcap (*Scutellaria lateriflora*), valerian (*Valeriana officinalis*), and yerba mansa (*Anemopsis californica*).

Because of the potentially serious consequences, you should avoid combining these herbs with anticonvulsants or other drugs that also have sedative or depressant effects, except under medical supervision.

Nicotinamide: Possible Harmful Interaction

3 NEGATIVE Nicotinamide (also called niacinamide) is a compound produced by the body's breakdown of niacin (vitamin B_3). It is a supplemental form that does not possess the flushing side effect or the cholesterol-lowering ability of niacin.

Nicotinamide appears to increase blood levels of carbamazepine and primidone, possibly requiring a reduction in drug dosage to prevent toxic effects.

Carbamazepine blood levels increased in two children with epilepsy after they were given nicotinamide,[10] but the fact that the children were on several anticonvulsant drugs clouds the issue somewhat. Similarly, nicotinamide given to three children on primidone therapy increased blood levels of primidone.[11] It is thought that nicotinamide may interfere with the body's normal breakdown of these anticonvulsant agents, allowing them to build up in the blood.

St. John's Wort, Dong Quai: Possible Harmful Interaction

3 NEGATIVE St. John's wort (*Hypericum perforatum*) is primarily used to treat mild to moderate depression.

The herb dong quai (*Angelica sinensis*) is often recommended for menstrual disorders such as dysmenorrhea, PMS, and irregular menstruation.

The anticonvulsant agents **carbamazepine** (see page 54), **valproic acid** (see page 191), and **phenobarbital** (see page 134) have been reported to cause increased sensitivity to the sun, amplifying the risk of sunburn or skin rash. Because St. John's wort and dong quai may also cause this problem, taking them during treatment with these drugs might add to this risk.

It may be a good idea to wear a sunscreen or protective clothing during sun exposure if you take one of these herbs while using these anticonvulsants. (Since primidone is converted in the body to phenobarbital, the same caution applies with this drug.)

Vitamin A: Possible Harmful Interaction

3 NEGATIVE Although the research on this subject is slim, some evidence suggests that valproic acid may interfere with the body's ability to safely handle vitamin A.[12] For this reason, vitamin A supplements should be taken with caution (if at all) by those on valproic acid. Taking beta carotene, which is converted into vitamin A in the body, may not present a problem.

White Willow: Possible Harmful Interaction

3 NEGATIVE The herb white willow (*Salix alba*), also known as willow bark, is used to treat pain and fever. White willow contains a substance that is converted by the body into a salicylate similar to aspirin.

Higher doses of aspirin may increase phenytoin levels and toxicity during long-term use of both drugs.[13] This raises the concern that white willow might have similar effects on phenytoin, though this has not been proven.

MIXED INTERACTIONS

Biotin: Supplementation Possibly Helpful, but Take at a Different Time of Day

3 MIXED Anticonvulsants may deplete biotin, an essential water-soluble B vitamin, possibly by competing with it for absorption in the intestine. It is not clear, however, whether this effect is great enough to be harmful.

Blood levels of biotin were found to be substantially lower in 404 people with epilepsy on long-term treatment with anticonvulsants compared to 112 untreated people with epilepsy.[14] The effect occurred with phenytoin, carbamazepine, phenobarbital, and primidone. Valproic acid appears to affect biotin to a lesser extent than other anticonvulsants.

A test tube study suggested that anticonvulsants might lower biotin levels by interfering with the way biotin is transported in the intestine.[15]

Biotin supplementation may be beneficial if you are on long-term anticonvulsant therapy. To avoid a potential interaction, take the supplement 2 to 3 hours apart from the drug. It has been suggested that the action of anticonvulsant drugs may be at least partly related to their effect of reducing biotin levels. For this reason, it may be desirable to take enough biotin to prevent a deficiency, but not an excessive amount.

Please see Appendix D, Safety Issues, for more information.

Folate: Supplementation Possibly Helpful

2 MIXED Folate (aka folic acid) is a B vitamin that plays an important role in many vital aspects of health, including preventing neural tube birth defects and possibly reducing the risk of heart disease. Because inadequate intake of folate is widespread, if you are taking any medication that depletes or impairs folate even slightly, you may need supplementation.

Most drugs used for preventing seizures can reduce levels of folate in the body. The low serum folate caused by anticonvulsants can raise homocysteine levels, a condition believed to increase the risk of heart disease.[16]

Adequate folate intake is also necessary to prevent neural tube birth defects such as spina bifida and anencephaly. Because anticonvulsant drugs deplete folate, babies born to women taking anticonvulsants are at increased risk for such birth defects. Anticonvulsants may also play a more direct role in the development of birth defects.[17]

The anticonvulsants carbamazepine, phenobarbital, and primidone appear to lower blood levels of folate by speeding up its normal breakdown by the body and also by decreasing its absorption.[18] Additionally, there is some evidence that primidone (which is converted in the body to phenobarbital) may interfere with folate by competing with it in the body.[19] Valproic acid appears to affect folate by decreasing its absorption.[20]

The interaction between phenytoin and folate is more complex. Phenytoin appears to decrease folate levels by interfering with its absorption in the small intestine[21] as well as by accelerating its normal breakdown by the body.[22,23] On the other hand, high folate levels may speed up the normal breakdown of phenytoin.[24,25] This could mean that taking extra folate might cause an increase in seizures.

It is possible that folate supplementation might also impair the effectiveness of other anticonvulsant drugs.

Therefore, the case for folate supplementation during anticonvulsant therapy is not as simple as it might seem and should be supervised by a physician.

Please see Appendix D, Safety Issues, for more information.

POSITIVE INTERACTIONS

Calcium: Supplementation Probably Helpful, but Take at a Different Time of Day

2 POSITIVE Anticonvulsant drugs may impair calcium absorption and in this way increase the risk of osteoporosis and other bone disorders.

Calcium absorption was compared in 12 people on anticonvulsant therapy (all taking phenytoin and some also taking phenobarbital, primidone, and/or carbamazepine) and 12 people receiving no treatment.[26] Calcium absorption was found to be 27% lower in the treated participants.

An observational study found low calcium blood levels in 48% of 109 people taking anticonvulsants.[27] Other findings in this study suggested that anticonvulsants might also reduce calcium levels by directly interfering with parathyroid hormone, a substance that helps keep calcium levels in proper balance.

A low blood level of calcium can itself trigger seizures, and this might reduce the effectiveness of anticonvulsants.[28]

Calcium supplementation may be beneficial for people taking anticonvulsant drugs. However, some studies indicate that antacids containing calcium carbonate may interfere with the absorption of phenytoin and perhaps other anticonvulsants.[29,30] For this reason, take calcium supplements and anticonvulsant drugs several hours apart if possible.

Please see Appendix D, Safety Issues, for more information.

Carnitine: Supplementation Possibly Helpful

2 POSITIVE Carnitine is an amino acid that has been used for heart conditions, Alzheimer's disease, and intermittent claudication (a possible complication of atherosclerosis in which impaired blood circulation causes severe pain in calf muscles during walking or exercising).

Long-term therapy with anticonvulsant agents, particularly valproic acid, is associated with low levels of carnitine.[31] However, it isn't clear whether the anticonvulsants cause the carnitine deficiency or whether it occurs for other reasons. It has been hypothesized that low carnitine levels may contribute to valproic acid's damaging effects on the liver.[32,33] The risk of this liver damage increases in children younger than 24 months,[34] and carnitine supplementation does seem to be protective.[35] However, in one double-blind crossover study, carnitine supplementation produced no real improvement in "well-being" as assessed by parents of children receiving either valproic acid or carbamazepine.[36]

L-carnitine supplementation may be advisable in certain cases, such as in infants and young children receiving valproic acid (especially those younger than 2 years) who have neurologic disorders and are receiving multiple anticonvulsants.[37]

Please see Appendix D, Safety Issues, for more information.

Vitamin D: Supplementation Possibly Helpful

2 POSITIVE Anticonvulsant drugs may interfere with the activity of vitamin D. As proper handling of calcium by the body depends on vitamin D, this may be another way that these drugs increase the risk of osteoporosis and related bone disorders (see the previous calcium topic).

Anticonvulsants appear to speed up the body's normal breakdown of vitamin D, decreasing the amount of the vitamin in the blood.[38] A survey of 48 people taking both phenytoin and phenobarbital found significantly lower levels of calcium and vitamin D in many of them as compared to 38 untreated individuals.[39] Similar but lesser changes were seen in 13 people taking phenytoin or phenobarbital alone. This effect may be apparent only after several weeks of treatment.

Another study found decreased blood levels of one form of vitamin D but normal levels of another.[40] Because there are two primary forms of vitamin D circulating in the blood, the body might be able to adjust in some cases to keep vitamin D in balance, at least for a time, despite the influence of anticonvulsants.[41]

Adequate sunlight exposure may help overcome the effects of anticonvulsants on vitamin D by stimulating the skin to manufacture the vitamin.[42] Of 450 people on anticonvulsants residing in a Florida facility, none were found to have low blood levels of vitamin D or evidence of bone disease. This suggests that environments providing regular sun exposure may be protective.

Individuals regularly taking anticonvulsants, especially those taking combination therapy and those with limited exposure to sunlight, may benefit from vitamin D supplementation.

Please see Appendix D, Safety Issues, for more information.

Vitamin K: Supplementation Possibly Helpful for Pregnant Women

2
POSITIVE

Phenytoin, carbamazepine, phenobarbital, and primidone speed up the normal breakdown of vitamin K into inactive byproducts, thus depriving the body of active vitamin K. This can lead to bone problems such as osteoporosis. Also, use of these anticonvulsants can lead to a vitamin K deficiency in babies born to mothers taking the drugs, resulting in bleeding disorders or facial bone abnormalities in the newborns.[43,44]

Mothers who take these anticonvulsants may need vitamin K supplementation during pregnancy to prevent these conditions in their newborns.

Please see Appendix D, Safety Issues, for more information.

ANTIDIABETIC AGENTS

Interactions	Rating*
Negative Interactions	
Ipriflavone	3
Potassium Citrate	2
St. John's Wort, Dong Quai	3
Mixed Interactions	
Chromium	2
Ginseng	3
Magnesium	3
Vanadium	3
Vitamin E	3
Other Supplements	3

Positive Interactions	
Calcium	2
Coenzyme Q_{10} (CoQ_{10})	3
Vitamin B_{12}	3

*Rating Key

1   Significant interaction

2   Possibly significant interaction

3   Interaction of relatively little significance

4   Reported interaction that does not in fact exist or is insignificant

Antidiabetic agents include insulin and drugs taken by mouth (oral hypoglycemic drugs) to regulate blood sugar levels. Many of these oral drugs are in the sulfonylurea family.

Insulin is a hormone secreted by the pancreas. People with type 1 diabetes (childhood-onset diabetes) produce little or no insulin at all and require insulin injections. In people with type 2 diabetes (adult-onset diabetes), the most common form of the disease, the pancreas doesn't produce enough insulin or the body is unable to use it properly. Most cases of type 2 diabetes can be managed with oral hypoglycemic drugs, but severe cases may also require insulin injections. Insulin products include Humalog, Humulin, Iletin, Novolin, and Velosulin. Oral hypoglycemic drugs include

- acarbose (Prandase, Precose)
- acetohexamide (Dymelor)
- chlorpropamide (Diabinese)
- glimepiride (Amaryl)
- glipizide (Glucotrol, Glucotrol XL)
- glyburide or glibenclamide (DiaBeta, Glynase, Micronase)
- metformin (Glucophage)
- miglitol (Glyset)
- phenformin
- pioglitazone (Actos)
- repaglinide (Prandin)

- rosiglitazone (Avandia)
- tolazamide (Tolinase)
- tolbutamide (Orinase)
- troglitazone (Rezulin)
- and others

NEGATIVE INTERACTIONS

Ipriflavone: Possible Harmful Interaction

 Ipriflavone, a synthetic isoflavone that slows bone breakdown, is used to treat osteoporosis.

There is some evidence that ipriflavone might increase the effects of oral hypoglycemic drugs by raising their levels in the blood.[1] This could cause your blood sugar levels to fall too low. If you are taking oral hypoglycemic medications, don't take ipriflavone without first consulting your physician.

Potassium Citrate: Possible Harmful Interaction

2 NEGATIVE Potassium citrate and other forms of citrate (e.g., calcium citrate, magnesium citrate) may be used to prevent kidney stones. These agents work by making the urine less acidic.

This effect on the urine may lead to decreased blood levels and therapeutic effects of chlorpropamide and possibly other drugs in the sulfonylurea family.[2] Besides chlorpropamide, drugs in this family include acetohexamide, glipizide, glyburide, tolazamide, and tolbutamide.

For this reason, it may be advisable to avoid these citrate compounds during treatment with sulfonylurea drugs.

St. John's Wort, Dong Quai: Possible Harmful Interaction

3 NEGATIVE St. John's wort (*Hypericum perforatum*) is primarily used to treat mild to moderate depression. The herb dong quai (*Angelica sinensis*) is often recommended for menstrual disorders such as dysmenorrhea, PMS, and irregular menstruation.

Oral hypoglycemic drugs in the sulfonylurea family have been reported to cause increased sensitivity to the sun, amplifying the risk of sunburn or skin rash. Drugs in this family include acetohexamide, chlorpropamide, glipizide, glyburide, tolazamide, and tolbutamide. Because St. John's wort and dong quai may also cause this problem, taking these herbal supplements during treatment with sulfonylurea drugs might add to this risk.

It may be a good idea to wear a sunscreen or protective clothing during sun exposure if you take one of these herbs while using a sulfonylurea medication.

MIXED INTERACTIONS

Chromium: Possible Benefits and Risks

| 2 |
| MIXED |

Supplementation with the trace mineral chromium offers a potential benefit and risk at the same time. It might allow you to cut down on the dose of your insulin or oral hypoglycemic drug, but it also might cause your blood sugar levels to fall too low (hypoglycemia). For this reason, individuals with diabetes should consult with a physician before taking chromium.

Most but not all studies suggest that chromium supplementation can improve blood sugar control in people with diabetes.

A double-blind placebo-controlled trial involving 180 men and women with type 2 diabetes found that blood sugar control improved significantly after 2 months in the group receiving chromium 1,000 mcg and after 4 months in the group receiving chromium 200 mcg.[3] Blood insulin levels decreased significantly in both groups at 2 and 4 months.

A primarily open-label study of 243 individuals with type 1 and type 2 diabetes found that chromium supplementation decreased insulin or oral hypoglycemic medication requirements in a significant percentage of cases.[4]

A double-blind study of 30 pregnant women with gestational diabetes (diabetes brought on by pregnancy) found that supplementation with chromium picolinate significantly improved blood sugar control.[5]

Chromium might also be helpful for diabetes caused by corticosteroid drugs.[6,7]

However, for reasons that aren't clear, some studies have found chromium to have no effect on the body's ability to handle blood sugar.[8,9]

Please see Appendix D, Safety Issues, for more information.

Ginseng: Possible Benefits and Risks

| 3 |
| MIXED |

The herb ginseng is promoted as an adaptogen, a treatment that helps the body adapt to stress and resist illness in general.

Supplementation with ginseng offers a potential benefit and risk at the same time. It might allow you to cut down on the dose of your insulin or oral hypoglycemic drug, but it also might cause your blood sugar levels to fall too low (hypoglycemia). For this reason, individuals with diabetes should consult with a physician before taking ginseng.

In an 8-week double-blind study of 36 people with type 2 diabetes, Asian ginseng (*Panax ginseng*) at 200 mg daily decreased fasting blood sugar levels and improved blood sugar control.[10] Similar effects have been seen with American ginseng (*Panax quinquefolius*).[11]

Please see Appendix D, Safety Issues, for more information.

Magnesium: Possible Benefits and Risks

3 MIXED Magnesium supplementation offers a potential benefit and risk at the same time. It might allow you to cut down on the dose of your insulin or oral hypoglycemic drug, but it also might cause your blood sugar levels to fall too low (hypoglycemia). For this reason, individuals with diabetes should consult with a physician before taking magnesium.

Because diabetes may cause low magnesium levels,[12,13] magnesium supplements are often recommended. However, magnesium supplements might increase the absorption and effect of oral hypoglycemic drugs in the sulfonylurea family such as glyburide.[14,15] Other drugs in this family include acetohexamide, glipizide, glyburide, tolazamide, and tolbutamide. If you take one of these medications, you need to be careful that your blood sugar does not fall too low.

Please see Appendix D, Safety Issues, for more information.

Vanadium: Possible Benefits and Risks

3 MIXED Supplementation with the trace mineral vanadium offers a potential benefit and risk at the same time. It might allow you to cut down on the dose of your insulin or oral hypoglycemic drug, but it also might cause your blood sugar levels to fall too low (hypoglycemia). For this reason, individuals with diabetes should consult with a physician before taking vanadium.

Test tube and animal studies suggest that the trace element vanadium has insulin-like action and beneficial effects on diabetes.[16]

In clinical studies in humans, vanadium reduced daily insulin requirements by 14% in individuals with type 1 diabetes.[17] In those with type 2 diabetes, vanadium increased the body's response to its own insulin.

In a single-blind placebo-controlled trial involving 7 people with type 2 diabetes, vanadyl sulfate (100 mg daily) improved the response to insulin compared to placebo.[18]

Note: Animal studies suggest that vanadium in high doses can accumulate in the body, increasing the risk of toxicity.[19,20]

Please see Appendix D, Safety Issues, for more information.

Vitamin E: Possible Benefits and Risks

3 **MIXED** Vitamin E supplementation offers a potential benefit and risk at the same time. It might allow you to cut down on the dose of your insulin or oral hypoglycemic drug, but it also might cause your blood sugar levels to fall too low (hypoglycemia). For this reason, individuals with diabetes should consult with a physician before taking vitamin E.

One double-blind study involving 15 people with type 2 diabetes suggested that high-dose vitamin E supplementation may reduce oxidative stress and provide additional benefits that improve the body's ability to respond to insulin.[21] Vitamin E was taken at a daily dose of 900 mg for 4 months. Another study in 25 elderly individuals with type 2 diabetes found similar results with 900 mg of vitamin E daily.[22]

Please see Appendix D, Safety Issues, for more information.

Other Supplements: Possible Benefits and Risks

3 **MIXED** Use of the following herbs and supplements might improve blood sugar control and require a reduction in the dose of your antidiabetic agent: aloe (*aloe vera*), bitter melon (*Momordica charantia*), bilberry leaf (*Vaccinium myrtillus*), burdock (*Arctium lappa*), carnitine, *Coccinia indica*, dandelion (*Taraxacum officinale*), fenugreek (*Trigonella foenum-graecum*), garlic (*Allium sativum*), gymnema (*Gymnema sylvestre*), lipoic acid, myrhh onion, pterocarpus (*Pterocarpus marsupium*), and salt bush (*Atriplex halimus*).[23–45]

For this reason, individuals with diabetes should consult with a physician before taking these supplements.

Please see Appendix D, Safety Issues, for more information.

POSITIVE INTERACTIONS

Calcium: Supplementation Possibly Helpful

2 **POSITIVE** The oral hypoglycemic drugs metformin and phenformin are associated with malabsorption of vitamin B_{12}.[46] Of special concern is the finding that this drug-induced B_{12} malabsorption may persist after the drugs are stopped.

A recent study involving 21 people with type 2 diabetes suggests that increased calcium intake may help correct this problem.[47] Low vitamin B_{12} blood levels developed in the 14 participants switched from sulfonylurea drug therapy to metformin. Supplementation with oral calcium carbonate was found to partially reverse this effect, resulting in an average 53%

increase in blood levels of the bioavailable form of B_{12}. Based on findings from earlier studies,[48,49] it is believed that metformin interferes with calcium-dependent intestinal absorption of vitamin B_{12}.

Based on this finding, calcium supplementation may be advisable during therapy with metformin or phenformin, as well as medical monitoring for possible B_{12} deficiency.

Please see Appendix D, Safety Issues, for more information.

Coenzyme Q_{10} (CoQ$_{10}$): Supplementation Possibly Helpful

3 POSITIVE Coenzyme Q_{10} is a vitamin-like substance that plays a fundamental role in the body's energy production.[50,51]

Test tube studies suggest that some oral hypoglycemic drugs interfere with the activity of enzymes containing coenzyme Q_{10}. For this reason, CoQ$_{10}$ supplements might be beneficial, although this has not been proven.

The hypoglycemic drugs, in order of decreasing effect on CoQ$_{10}$ enzymes, were acetohexamide, glyburide, phenformin, and tolazamide. Tolbutamide, glipizide, and chlorpropamide had no effect on these enzymes.[52] There is also some evidence that diabetes itself may impair CoQ$_{10}$ function.

Please see Appendix D, Safety Issues, for more information.

Vitamin B_{12}: Supplementation Possibly Helpful

3 POSITIVE Of 46 randomly selected participants with diabetes taking the oral hypoglycemic drugs metformin or phenformin or both, 30% were found to have malabsorption of vitamin B_{12}.[53] Of special concern is the finding that this drug-induced B_{12} malabsorption may persist after the drugs are stopped.

It would be advisable for your physician to monitor for possible B_{12} deficiency and assess the need for B_{12} supplementation during therapy with metformin or phenformin.

Please see Appendix D, Safety Issues, for more information.

Note: A recent study suggests that increased calcium intake may help correct this problem (see **Calcium** topic above).

ANTIHYPERTENSIVE AGENTS

Interactions	Rating*
Positive Interaction	
Coenzyme Q$_{10}$	3

*Rating Key

1 Significant interaction
2 Possibly significant interaction
3 Interaction of relatively little significance
4 Reported interaction that does not in fact exist or is insignificant

These drugs are used to treat high blood pressure. There is some evidence that the following antihypertensive agents may interact with coenzyme Q$_{10}$:

- clonidine (Catapres, Combipres)
- hydralazine (Apresoline, Hydra-Zide)
- hydrochlorothiazide (Esidrix, HydroDIURIL, Oretic)
- methyldopa (Aldoclor, Aldomet, Aldoril)

POSITIVE INTERACTIONS

Coenzyme Q$_{10}$: Supplementation Possibly Helpful

3 POSITIVE Coenzyme Q$_{10}$ is a vitamin-like substance that plays a fundamental role in the body's energy production.[1,2]

Test tube studies suggest that several drugs used to treat high blood pressure inhibit the action of enzymes that contain coenzyme Q$_{10}$ (CoQ$_{10}$). CoQ$_{10}$ is present naturally in heart muscle and other tissues. It appears to play a fundamental role in producing the energy needed for normal heart function.[3]

This interaction is a concern because antihypertensive medications, in addition to lowering blood pressure, are expected to protect the heart.

Propranolol was the greatest CoQ$_{10}$ enzyme inhibitor of all the drugs tested (see **Beta-Blockers-Coenzyme Q$_{10}$**, page 46). The inhibitory effect of clonidine and hydralazine on CoQ$_{10}$ enzymes was 25% of that found for propranolol.[4] The inhibitory effect of hydrochlorothiazide was slightly less. Methyldopa was found to very weakly inhibit one CoQ$_{10}$ enzyme and to have no significant effect on another. Though the inhibitory action of these drugs falls well below that of propranolol, this effect might be something to keep in mind.

It is possible that CoQ$_{10}$ supplementation might be helpful if you take these blood pressure drugs, particularly if you have a pre-existing CoQ$_{10}$ deficiency. However, there are as yet no proven benefits.

Please see Appendix D, Safety Issues, for more information.

ANTIPSYCHOTIC AGENTS

Interactions	Rating*
Negative Interactions	
Kava	2
Phenylalanine	3
St. John's Wort	2
St. John's Wort, Dong Quai	3
Valerian, Passionflower, Hops	2
Yohimbe	3
Positive Interactions	
Coenzyme Q$_{10}$ (CoQ$_{10}$)	3
Ginkgo	3
Milk Thistle	2
Vitamin E	3

*Rating Key

1 Significant interaction
2 Possibly significant interaction
3 Interaction of relatively little significance
4 Reported interaction that does not in fact exist or is insignificant

Antipsychotic agents are used primarily for the treatment of schizo-phrenia and other forms of psychosis. Phenothiazines are older, traditional antipsychotic drugs that have been in use for decades. The newest family of antipsychotic drugs, called atypical antipsychotics, appears to have fewer side effects than the older drugs.

Phenothiazines include

- acetophenazine (Tindal)
- chlorpromazine (Thorazine)
- fluphenazine (Permitil, Prolixin)
- haloperidol (Haldol, Peridol)
- loxapine (Loxitane)
- mesoridazine (Serentil)
- methotrimeprazine (Nozinan)
- molindone (Moban)
- perphenazine (Etrafon, Triavil, Trilafon)
- pimozide (Orap)
- prochlorperazine (Compazine)
- promazine (Sparine)
- promethazine (Mepergan, Phenergan)
- propiomazine (Largon)
- thiethylperazine (Norzine, Torecan)

- thioridazine (Mellaril)
- thiothixene (Navane)
- trifluoperazine (Stelazine, Suprazine)
- triflupromazine (Vesprin)

Atypical antipsychotics include

- clozapine (Clozaril)
- olanzapine (Zyprexa)
- quetiapine (Seroquel)
- risperidone (Risperdal)

A variety of possible interactions can occur between antipsychotic agents and herbs or supplements. Some of these interactions involve either beneficial or detrimental effects on tardive dyskinesia (TD), a disorder that may occur as a side effect of antipsychotics and other psychotherapeutic drugs. Symptoms of TD include involuntary movements of the tongue, mouth, jaw, eyelid, and face. The condition typically develops after long-term use of these drugs, and in most cases may be permanent.

NEGATIVE INTERACTIONS

Kava: Possible Harmful Interaction

2 NEGATIVE The herb kava has a sedative effect and is used for anxiety and insomnia.

Besides the late-developing complication of tardive dyskinesia, antipsychotic drugs can cause another type of movement disorder: dystonic reactions, which are sudden intense movements of the neck and eyes. There is some evidence that the herb kava (*Piper methysticum*) can increase the risk or severity of this side effect.[1]

Preliminary reports suggest that kava may cause this problem by blocking the effects of dopamine, a neurotransmitter (a chemical that enables nerve transmission). Because antipsychotic drugs also block dopamine, the risk of these movement disorders might be increased even further when kava is combined with antipsychotic agents, although this problem has not yet been reported.

Kava might also work against drugs for Parkinson's disease, which ease symptoms by increasing the effects of dopamine.[2] Again, this has not yet been reported.

Another type of interaction could occur between kava and antipsychotic agents. Because this herb and drug possess similar sedative and depressant effects, combined use could result in "add-on" or excessive physical depression, sedation, and impairment. In one case report, a 54-year-old man was hospitalized for lethargy and disorientation, side effects attributed to his having taken the combination of kava and the antianxiety agent alprazolam (Xanax) for 3 days.[3]

Because of the potentially serious consequences, you should avoid combining kava with antipsychotic agents or other drugs that also have sedative or depressant effects unless advised by your physician.

Phenylalanine: Possible Harmful Interaction

3 NEGATIVE Supplementation with the amino acid phenylalanine might worsen symptoms of tardive dyskinesia (TD) in individuals who already have the condition. It is also possible that long-term phenylalanine use may contribute to the development of TD in individuals whose bodies can't properly handle phenylalanine.

L-phenylalanine is an essential dietary amino acid that is the starting point of the body's synthesis of many neurotransmitters.

A double-blind placebo-controlled trial in 18 males with schizophrenia and TD indicated that ingesting phenylalanine can potentially worsen TD symptoms.[4] Another study found similar results.[5]

It may be best for people taking drugs that are associated with causing TD to avoid taking phenylalanine supplements.

St. John's Wort: Possible Harmful Interaction

2 NEGATIVE The herb St. John's wort (*Hypericum perforatum*) is primarily used to treat mild to moderate depression. While reasonably safe on its own, it can interact with numerous medications.

St. John's wort might reduce blood levels of olanzapine (Zyprexa) and clozapine (Clozaril)[6] by accelerating the body's normal breakdown of these drugs. This could lead to an increase in the severity of psychotic symptoms.

Perhaps even more dangerously, if medication levels have been adjusted for an individual already taking St. John's wort, stopping the herb could then cause these levels to climb into the toxic range.

Based on this information, you should avoid taking St. John's wort with these drugs unless supervised by a physician.

St. John's wort could also increase the risk of sun sensitivity when combined with antipsychotic agents in the phenothiazine family (see **St. John's Wort, Dong Quai** topic).

St. John's Wort, Dong Quai: Possible Harmful Interaction

3 NEGATIVE St. John's wort (*Hypericum perforatum*) is primarily used to treat mild to moderate depression. The herb dong quai (*Angelica sinensis*) is often recommended for menstrual disorders such as dysmenorrhea, PMS, and irregular menstruation.

Phenothiazines can cause increased sensitivity to the sun, amplifying the risk of sunburn or skin rash. Sun sensitivity has also been reported with the atypical antipsychotic risperidone. Because St. John's wort and dong quai may also cause this problem, taking these herbal supplements during antipsychotic therapy might add to this risk.

It may be a good idea to wear a sunscreen or protective clothing during sun exposure if you take one of these herbs while using an antipsychotic drug.

Valerian, Passionflower, Hops: Possible Harmful Interaction

2 NEGATIVE As with kava (see **Kava** topic), other herbs with a sedative effect might cause "add-on" depressant effects when combined with antipsychotic agents. These include valerian (*Valeriana officinalis*), passionflower (*Passiflora incarnata*), and hops (*Humulus lupulus*), as well as ashwagandha (*Withania somnifera*), calendula (*Calendula officinalis*), catnip (*Nepeta cataria*), lady's slipper (*Cypripedium*), lemon balm (*Melissa officinalis*), sassafras (*Sassafras officinale*), skullcap (*Scutellaria lateriflora*), and yerba mansa (*Anemopsis californica*).

Because of the potentially serious consequences, you should avoid combining these herbs with antipsychotic agents or other drugs that also have sedative or depressant effects unless advised by your physician.

Yohimbe: Possible Harmful Interaction

3 NEGATIVE The herb yohimbe (*Pausinystalia yohimbe*) is widely promoted as a treatment for impotence.

Yohimbe is relatively toxic, and can cause problems if used incorrectly. Phenothiazine medications may increase the risk of yohimbe toxicity.[7]

POSITIVE INTERACTIONS

Coenzyme Q$_{10}$ (CoQ$_{10}$): Supplementation Possibly Helpful

3 POSITIVE Coenzyme Q$_{10}$ is a vitamin-like substance that plays a fundamental role in the body's energy production.[8,9]

Antipsychotic drugs in the phenothiazine family have been reported to inhibit the activity of important enzymes containing coenzyme Q$_{10}$.[10]

CoQ$_{10}$ (ubiquinone) is present naturally in heart muscle and other tissues and appears to play a fundamental role in producing the energy needed for normal heart function.[11]

It has been suggested that CoQ$_{10}$ supplementation might help prevent the depressant effects on the heart associated with phenothiazines;[12] however, this has not been proven. A typical supplemental dose of CoQ$_{10}$ is 30 to 100 mg daily.

Please see Appendix D, Safety Issues, for more information.

Ginkgo: Supplementation Possibly Helpful

3 POSITIVE The herb ginkgo (*Ginkgo biloba*) is used to treat Alzheimer's disease and ordinary age-related memory loss, among many other uses.

Preliminary evidence suggests that ginkgo might reduce side effects and increase the efficacy of various antipsychotic medications.[13]

Please see Appendix D, Safety Issues, for more information.

Milk Thistle: Supplementation Possibly Helpful

2 POSITIVE The herbal product silymarin, or milk thistle (*Silybum marianum*), has been used for hepatitis and various other liver-related disorders.

Milk thistle might protect against the liver toxicity sometimes caused by phenothiazine drugs. In a double-blind study involving 60 people receiving antipsychotic therapy, participants were treated with milk thistle (800 mg daily) or placebo.[14] Milk thistle was found to reduce the liver damage associated with antipsychotic agents.

Please see Appendix D, Safety Issues, for more information.

Vitamin E: Supplementation Possibly Helpful

3 POSITIVE The evidence is mixed, but high-dose vitamin E, in some cases, may be helpful in both the treatment and prevention of drug-induced tardive dyskinesia (TD). The basis for using the antioxidant vitamin E in treating TD is the theory that the condition may at least partially result from tissue damage caused by free radicals.

The most recent meta-analysis (data combined from numerous studies) examining treatments for TD found that vitamin E was among the few effective interventions.[15] A meta-analysis of studies looking specifically at vitamin E found that a significant subgroup (28.3%) of individuals showed modest improvement in TD symptoms with vitamin E supplementation.[16]

This analysis covered all such studies published since 1987, including double-blind trials. Vitamin E appeared to be safe and well tolerated. A 1999 review of 18 trials found that 12 of the trials showed positive results for vitamin E in treating TD.[17] People who had TD for less than 5 years appeared to respond better than those with long-standing TD. Another 1999 review of various approaches found vitamin E to be promising both for the treatment and possible prevention of TD.[18]

However, not all studies have found a benefit for vitamin E in TD. A recent randomized, double-blind placebo-controlled trial involving 158 people in 9 treatment centers found vitamin E to have no significant effect on TD.[19] Participants took either vitamin E at 1,600 IU (international units) per day, or placebo, for 1 year. It is possible that differences between the individuals enrolled in this study and those in previous studies may have contributed to this result. Additional factors that may have minimized the potential benefit of vitamin E could have been the increased use of atypical antipsychotic drugs, which appear to carry less risk of TD, or the use of traditional antipsychotics in less-risky lower doses.

Studies have used vitamin E doses of 600 to 1,600 IU per day.[20] For treating TD, a trial of vitamin E, probably for at least 3 months, may be worthwhile.

Please see Appendix D, Safety Issues, for more information.

AZOLE ANTIFUNGAL AGENTS

Interactions	Rating*
Negative Interaction	
Grapefruit Juice	2

*Rating Key

1　Significant interaction

2　Possibly significant interaction

3　Interaction of relatively little significance

4　Reported interaction that does not in fact exist or is insignificant

Azole antifungal agents are used to treat infections caused by fungi such as yeast (e.g., candidiasis), including infections of the hair, nails, mucous membranes, and skin. Drugs in this family include

- fluconazole (Diflucan)
- itraconazole (Sporanox)
- ketoconazole (Nizoral)

NEGATIVE INTERACTIONS

Grapefruit Juice: Possible Harmful Interaction

2 NEGATIVE Grapefruit juice appears to decrease the body's absorption of itraconazole. In a cross-over study, 11 individuals received an oral itraconazole dose of 200 mg with 240 ml of either water or double-strength grapefruit juice immediately after breakfast.[1] Grapefruit juice was associated with a substantial decrease in blood levels of the active drug, which could result in treatment failure.

Grapefruit juice might also produce the opposite effect—increased drug blood levels.[2] Based on how it affects particular enzymes, grapefruit juice could potentially slow the body's normal breakdown of these antifungal drugs. A recent study indicates that, if this effect occurs, it can last for three days or more following the last glass of juice.[3]

However, decreased drug absorption, with lower blood levels, appears to be the predominant effect with itraconazole. Whether this might apply to the other drugs in this family is uncertain.

Based on these findings, if you take one of these drugs, the safest approach is to avoid grapefruit juice altogether.

BENZODIAZEPINES

Interactions	Rating*
Negative Interactions	
Grapefruit Juice	3
Kava, Valerian, Passionflower, Hops	2
Positive Interaction	
Melatonin	3

*Rating Key

1 Significant interaction

2 Possibly significant interaction

3 Interaction of relatively little significance

4 Reported interaction that does not in fact exist or is insignificant

Medications in the benzodiazepine family exert calming and sedative effects and are used to treat anxiety and insomnia. Benzodiazepines are also used as muscle relaxants and anticonvulsants. They work by increasing the effects of the neurotransmitter (a chemical messenger) GABA. Benzodiazepine drugs include

- alprazolam (Xanax)
- chlordiazepoxide hydrochloride (Libritabs, Librium, Limbitrol, Lipoxide, Mitran, Reposans-10, Sereen)
- clonazepam (Klonopin)
- clorazepate dipotassium (Gen-XENE, Tranxene-T, Tranxene-SD)
- diazepam (Diastat, Valium, Valrelease, Vazepam)
- estazolam (ProSom)
- flurazepam hydrochloride (Dalmane, Durapam)
- halazepam (Paxipam)
- lorazepam (Ativan)
- oxazepam (Serax)
- quazepam (Doral)
- temazepam (Razepam, Restoril, Temaz)
- triazolam (Halcion)
- and others

NEGATIVE INTERACTIONS

Grapefruit Juice: Possible Harmful Interaction

3 NEGATIVE Grapefruit juice slows the body's normal breakdown of several drugs, including some benzodiazepines, allowing them to build up to potentially dangerous levels in the blood.[1] A recent study indicates this effect can last for three days or more following the last glass of juice.[2]

Because of this risk, if you take benzodiazepines, the safest approach is to avoid grapefruit juice altogether.

Kava, Valerian, Passionflower, Hops: Possible Harmful Interaction

2 NEGATIVE The herb kava (*Piper methysticum*) has a sedative effect and is used for anxiety and insomnia.

Combining kava with drugs in the benzodiazepine family, which possess similar effects, could result in "add-on" or excessive physical depression, sedation, and impairment. In one case report of a 54-year-old man hospitalized for lethargy and disorientation, these side effects were attributed to his having taken the combination of kava and alprazolam for 3 days.[3]

Experimental studies suggest that kava, similarly to benzodiazepines, exerts its sedative effects at binding sites in the brain called GABA receptors.[4,5,6]

Other herbs with a sedative effect that might cause problems when combined with benzodiazepines include ashwagandha (*Withania somnifera*), calendula (*Calendula officinalis*), catnip (*Nepeta cataria*), hops (*Humulus lupulus*), lady's slipper (*Cypripedium*), lemon balm (*Melissa officinalis*), passionflower (*Passiflora incarnata*), sassafras (*Sassifras officinale*), skullcap (*Scutellaria lateriflora*), valerian (*Valeriana officinalis*), and yerba mansa (*Anemopsis californica*).

Because of the potentially serious consequences, you should avoid combining these herbs with benzodiazepines or other drugs that also have sedative or depressant effects unless advised by your physician.

POSITIVE INTERACTIONS

Melatonin: Supplementation Possibly Helpful

3 POSITIVE Melatonin is a natural hormone that regulates sleep.

Many people who take conventional sleeping pills (most of which are in the benzodiazepine family) find it difficult to quit. The reason is that when you try to stop the medication, you may experience severe insomnia or interrupted sleep. A double-blind placebo-controlled study of 34 individuals who regularly used such medications found that melatonin at a dose of 2 mg nightly (in a controlled-release formulation) could help them discontinue the use of the drugs.[7]

Warning: It can be dangerous to stop using benzodiazepines if you have taken them for a while. Consult your physician before trying melatonin to help handle benzodiazepine withdrawal or before trying to stop benzodiazepine medication under any conditions.

Please see Appendix D, Safety Issues, for more information.

BETA-BLOCKERS

Interactions	Rating*
Negative Interactions	
Calcium	3
Coleus forskohlii	4
Positive Interactions	
Chromium	3
Coenzyme Q_{10} (CoQ_{10})	2

*Rating Key

1 Significant interaction

2 Possibly significant interaction

3 Interaction of relatively little significance

4 Reported interaction that does not in fact exist or is insignificant

Beta-blockers are used to treat high blood pressure as well as a variety of heart conditions. They work by blocking nerve signals that cause the heart to beat faster and the blood pressure to rise. Drugs in this family include

- acebutolol hydrochloride (Sectral)
- alprenolol
- atenolol (Tenoretic, Tenormin)
- betaxolol hydrochloride (Kerlone)
- bisoprolol fumarate (Zebeta)
- carteolol (Cartrol)
- carvedilol (Coreg)
- esmolol hydrochloride (Brevibloc)
- labetalol hydrochloride (Normodyne, Trandate)
- metoprolol (Lopressor, Toprol XL)
- nadolol (Corgard)
- penbutolol (Levatol)
- pindolol (Visken)
- propranolol hydrochloride (Betachron E-R, Inderal, Inderal LA)
- sotalol (Betapace)
- timolol maleate (Blocadren, Timolide)
- and others

NEGATIVE INTERACTIONS

Calcium: Take at a Different Time of Day

3 NEGATIVE It appears that the beta-blocker atenolol may form an unabsorbable complex with calcium in the intestine, leading to reduced blood levels of the drug.[1] This effect might occur with other beta-blockers as well. However, the effect on atenolol levels appears to wear off after a few days. Most likely, under ordinary circumstances, no change in dosage is necessary.

Coleus forskohlii: Possible Harmful Interaction

4 NEGATIVE The herb *Coleus forskohlii* may relax blood vessels, and therefore might have unpredictable effects on blood pressure if combined with beta-blockers.

POSITIVE INTERACTIONS

Chromium: Supplementation Possibly Helpful

3 POSITIVE Although they are helpful for blood pressure control, beta-blockers tend to reduce levels of HDL ("good") cholesterol. This could be counterproductive if your goal in taking beta-blockers is to protect your heart. According to one study, supplementation with the trace mineral chromium can offset this adverse effect.[2]

Please see Appendix D, Safety Issues, for more information.

Coenzyme Q_{10} (CoQ$_{10}$): Supplementation Possibly Helpful

2 POSITIVE Coenzyme Q_{10} is a vitamin-like substance that appears to play a fundamental role in the body's energy production, including that of the heart.[3,4,5]

Test tube studies suggest that beta-blockers inhibit the action of enzymes that contain CoQ$_{10}$.[6] This is potentially worrisome, as the major purpose of blood pressure medications is to protect the heart. Of the beta-blockers tested, propranolol was the greatest CoQ$_{10}$ enzyme inhibitor.[7] Metoprolol's inhibition was only 25% of that for propranolol. Timolol showed no significant inhibition of CoQ$_{10}$ enzymes, which correlates with its low heart-depressant effects.

In addition, beta-blockers can cause depressed heart function and significant fatigue, especially in elderly individuals. This could be partly due to the drugs' effect on CoQ$_{10}$.[8,9]

For these reasons, if you are taking beta-blockers, it is possible that CoQ$_{10}$ supplements would be helpful, particularly if you presently have a CoQ$_{10}$ deficiency. However, there are as yet no proven benefits.

Please see Appendix D, Safety Issues, for more information.

BILE ACID SEQUESTRANTS

Interactions	Rating*
Positive Interactions	
Folate	2
Other Nutrients	3

*Rating Key

1 Significant interaction

2 Possibly significant interaction

3 Interaction of relatively little significance

4 Reported interaction that does not in fact exist or is insignificant

Bile acid sequestrants are taken to reduce cholesterol levels, although drugs in the **statin** (see page 164) family have largely taken their place.

Bile acid sequestrants work by affecting bile acids, substances produced in the liver that help digest dietary fats. Ordinarily, bile acids are reabsorbed and reused. However, bile acid sequestrants interrupt this process by attaching to bile acids in the intestine and carrying them out of the body in the stool. The liver needs cholesterol to make more bile acids, and gets it by removing cholesterol from the blood, thereby lowering cholesterol levels. Medications in the bile acid sequestrant family include

- cholestyramine (Cholybar, Locholest, Prevalite, Questran, Questran Light)
- colestipol (Colestid)
- and others

POSITIVE INTERACTIONS

Folate: Supplementation Probably Helpful

2 POSITIVE Folate (also known as folic acid) is a B vitamin that plays an important role in many vital aspects of health, including preventing neural tube birth defects and possibly reducing the risk of heart disease. Because inadequate intake of folate is widespread, if you are taking any medication that depletes or impairs folate even slightly, you may need supplementation.

Bile acid sequestrants have been reported to impair the absorption of numerous nutrients;[1,2] however, this effect may be important only for folate (see **Other Nutrients**).

In the digestive tract, cholestyramine tends to bind or attach to the folate present in food, thus reducing the amount of the vitamin absorbed into the body. In one study, prolonged treatment with cholestyramine in 18 children resulted in folate deficiency.[3]

Supplementation with folate at 5 mg daily appears to be adequate to prevent folate depletion in individuals taking bile acid sequestrants. However, it may be advisable to check with your doctor before taking folate at this dose.

Please see Appendix D, Safety Issues, for more information.

Other Nutrients: Supplementation Possibly Helpful

3
POSITIVE Bile acid sequestrants have been reported to impair the absorption of numerous other nutrients, including vitamins A, E, K, and B_{12}, as well as iron and calcium.[4,5] However, this effect does not appear to be very significant. In the study mentioned previously, though cholestyramine interfered with the absorption of nutrients other than folate, levels of these nutrients remained in the normal range.[6]

For this reason, you probably don't need to take supplemental doses of these nutrients if you are taking a bile acid sequestrant. On general principles, however, a comprehensive multivitamin-mineral supplement might be good insurance.

Please see Appendix D, Safety Issues, for more information.

BISPHOSPHONATES

Interactions	Rating*
Negative Interaction	
Calcium	3

*Rating Key

1   Significant interaction

2   Possibly significant interaction

3   Interaction of relatively little significance

4   Reported interaction that does not in fact exist or is insignificant

Bisphosphonates are used primarily for the treatment of osteoporosis. They reverse bone loss and help restore bone strength. This family of drugs includes

- alendronate (Fosamax)
- etidronate (Didronel)
- risedronate (Actonel)
- tiludronate (Skelid)

NEGATIVE INTERACTIONS

Calcium: Take at a Different Time of Day

3 NEGATIVE Individuals trying to strengthen their bones by taking bisphosphonates may also benefit by taking the raw material of healthy bones: calcium. However, this may be tricky; although calcium supplements and bisphosphonates are both helpful for treating osteoporosis, some experts suggest that they shouldn't be taken at the same time of day.[1]

While there is no firm evidence for this caution, it might be advisable to take calcium supplements and bisphosphonates at least 2 hours apart. The absorption of bisphosphonates is also diminished by food and probably by other medications. That is why the labeling provided with these drugs instructs that they be taken with plain water at least 30 minutes to 2 hours before the first food of the day.

BROMOCRIPTINE *(Parlodel)*

Interactions	Rating*
Negative Interaction	
Chasteberry	3

*Rating Key

1 Significant interaction

2 Possibly significant interaction

3 Interaction of relatively little significance

4 Reported interaction that does not in fact exist or is insignificant

Bromocriptine is a drug that reduces levels of prolactin, a hormone the body produces during and after pregnancy. Excessive prolactin production may cause a variety of symptoms. Bromocriptine is also used for other purposes, such as treating Parkinson's disease.

NEGATIVE INTERACTION

Chasteberry: Possible Harmful Interaction

3 NEGATIVE The herb chasteberry (*Vitex agnus-castus*) is used for breast discomfort and other PMS symptoms, menstrual cycle irregularities, and female infertility.

Chasteberry appears to exert its effects by reducing levels of prolactin in the body.[1–6] Because bromocriptine also reduces prolactin levels, it's possible that the drug and herb could produce additive effects, which might cause problems. It is therefore best to avoid combining them.

CALCIUM-CHANNEL BLOCKERS

Interactions	Rating*
Negative Interactions	
Calcium	3
Grapefruit Juice	1

*Rating Key

1 Significant interaction

2 Possibly significant interaction

3 Interaction of relatively little significance

4 Reported interaction that does not in fact exist or is insignificant

Calcium-channel blockers are used to treat high blood pressure, angina, irregular heart rhythms, and other heart-related conditions.

The mineral calcium enables nerves to carry impulses and is necessary for muscle contraction. Calcium-channel blockers "block" this process. This effect is used therapeutically to reduce the contraction of the heart and to relax blood vessels, resulting in improved blood flow and oxygen to the heart and reduced blood pressure, among other benefits. Drugs in this family include

- amlodipine (Lotrel, Norvasc)
- bepridil hydrochloride (Vascor)
- diltiazem (Cardizem, Cardizem CD, Cardizem SR, Dilacor XR, Tiamate, Tiazac)
- felodipine (Lexxel, Plendil)
- isradipine (DynaCirc, DynaCirc CR)
- nicardipine hydrochloride (Cardene, Cardene SR)
- nifedipine (Procardia, Procardia XL, Adalat, Adalat CC)
- nimodipine (Nimotop)
- nisoldipine (Sular)
- verapamil (Calan, Calan SR, Covera-HS, Isoptin, Isoptin SR, Tarka, Verelan)
- and others

NEGATIVE INTERACTIONS

Calcium: Possible Harmful Interaction

3 NEGATIVE Since calcium-channel blockers work by blocking calcium, supplementation with this mineral may work against some of their therapeutic effects. Most of the evidence relates to calcium given intravenously (into a vein), but it is possible that oral calcium supplements might produce a similar effect when combined with vitamin D. (Vitamin D increases the absorption and use of calcium by the body.)

Because it antagonizes the action of these drugs, calcium has been given intravenously to counteract the adverse effects caused by an overdose of the calcium-channel blocker verapamil, such as the blood pressure falling too low.[1–4]

There is one case report of oral calcium also interfering with verapamil's actions. An individual whose irregular heart rhythm was successfully treated with verapamil began taking oral supplements of calcium and high-dose calciferol (a form of vitamin D) for osteoporosis.[5] A week later, the irregular heart rhythm reappeared, suggesting that the calcium and vitamin D supplements may have been responsible.

As a precaution, individuals on calcium-channel blockers should not take calcium or vitamin D supplements except under medical supervision.

Grapefruit Juice: Possible Harmful Interaction

1 NEGATIVE Grapefruit juice contains substances that impair the body's normal breakdown of several drugs, including calcium-channel blockers, allowing them to build up to potentially dangerous levels in the blood.[6] A recent study indicates this effect can last for three days or more following the last glass of juice, though the effect declines as time passes and is much greater when drug and juice are taken together.[7]

Because of this risk, if you take calcium-channel blockers, the safest approach is to avoid grapefruit juice altogether.

CARBAMAZEPINE

Trade Names: Atretol, Carbatrol, Epitol, Tegretol, Tegretol XR

Interactions	Rating*
Negative Interactions	
Ginkgo	3
Glutamine	4
Grapefruit Juice	1
Ipriflavone	2
Kava, Valerian, Passionflower, Hops	2
Nicotinamide	3
St. John's Wort, Dong Quai	3
Mixed Interactions	
Biotin	3
Folate	2

Interactions	Rating*
Positive Interactions	
Calcium	2
Carnitine	2
Vitamin D	2
Vitamin K	2

*Rating Key

1 Significant interaction

2 Possibly significant interaction

3 Interaction of relatively little significance

4 Reported interaction that does not in fact exist or is insignificant

Carbamazepine is an anticonvulsant agent used primarily to prevent seizures in conditions such as epilepsy.

Other anticonvulsant agents include **phenobarbital** (see page 134), **phenytoin** (see page 140), **primidone** (see page 146), and **valproic acid** (see page 191). In some cases, combination therapy with two or more anticonvulsant drugs may be used.

NEGATIVE INTERACTIONS

Ginkgo: Possible Harmful Interaction

3 NEGATIVE The herb ginkgo (*Ginkgo biloba*) has been used to treat Alzheimer's disease and ordinary age-related memory loss, among many other conditions.

This interaction involves potential contaminants in ginkgo, not ginkgo itself.

A recent study found that a natural nerve toxin present in the seeds of *Ginkgo biloba* made its way into standardized ginkgo extracts prepared from the leaves.[1] This toxin has been associated with convulsions and death in laboratory animals.[2,3,4]

Fortunately, the detected amounts of this toxic substance are considered harmless.[5] However, given the lack of satisfactory standardization of herbal

formulations in the United States, it is possible that some batches of product might contain higher contents of the toxin depending on the season of harvest.

In light of these findings, taking a ginkgo product that happened to contain significant levels of the nerve toxin might theoretically prevent an anticonvulsant from working as well as expected.

Glutamine: Possible Harmful Interaction

4 NEGATIVE The amino acid glutamine is converted to glutamate in the body. Glutamate is thought to act as a neurotransmitter (chemical that enables nerve transmission). Because anticonvulsants work (at least in part) by blocking glutamate pathways in the brain, high dosages of the amino acid glutamine might theoretically diminish an anticonvulsant's effect and increase the risk of seizures.

Grapefruit Juice: Possible Harmful Interaction

1 NEGATIVE Grapefruit juice slows the body's normal breakdown of several drugs, including the anticonvulsant carbamazepine, allowing it to build up to potentially dangerous levels in the blood.[6] A recent study indicates this effect can last for 3 days or more following the last glass of juice.[7]

Because of this risk, if you use carbamazepine, the safest approach is to avoid grapefruit juice altogether.

Ipriflavone: Possible Harmful Interaction

2 NEGATIVE Ipriflavone, a synthetic isoflavone that slows bone breakdown, is used to treat osteoporosis.

Test tube studies indicate that ipriflavone might increase blood levels of the anticonvulsants carbamazepine and phenytoin when they are taken therapeutically.[8] Ipriflavone was found to inhibit a liver enzyme involved in the body's normal breakdown of these drugs, thus allowing them to build up in the blood. Higher drug levels increase the risk of adverse effects.

Because anticonvulsants are known to contribute to the development of osteoporosis, a concern is that the use of ipriflavone for this drug-induced osteoporosis could result in higher blood levels of the drugs with potentially serious consequences.

Individuals taking either of these drugs should use ipriflavone only under medical supervision.

Kava, Valerian, Passionflower, Hops: Possible Harmful Interaction

2 NEGATIVE The herb kava (*Piper methysticum*) has a sedative effect and is used for anxiety and insomnia.

Combining kava with anticonvulsants, which possess similar depressant effects, could result in "add-on" or excessive physical depression, sedation, and impairment. In one case report, a 54-year-old man was hospitalized for lethargy and disorientation, side effects attributed to his having taken the combination of kava and the antianxiety agent alprazolam (Xanax) for 3 days.[9]

Other herbs having a sedative effect that might cause problems when combined with anticonvulsants include ashwagandha (*Withania somnifera*), calendula (*Calendula officinalis*), catnip (*Nepeta cataria*), hops (*Humulus lupulus*), lady's slipper (*Cypripedium* species), lemon balm (*Melissa officinalis*), passionflower (*Passiflora incarnata*), sassafras (*Sassafras officinale*), skullcap (*Scutellaria lateriflora*), valerian (*Valeriana officinalis*), and yerba mansa (*Anemopsis californica*).

Because of the potentially serious consequences, you should avoid combining these herbs with anticonvulsants or other drugs that also have sedative or depressant effects unless advised by your physician.

Nicotinamide: Possible Harmful Interaction

3 NEGATIVE Nicotinamide (also called niacinamide) is a compound produced by the body's breakdown of niacin (vitamin B_3). It is a supplemental form that does not possess the flushing side effect or the cholesterol-lowering ability of niacin.

Nicotinamide appears to increase blood levels of carbamazepine and primidone, possibly requiring a reduction in drug dosage to prevent toxic effects.

Carbamazepine blood levels increased in two children with epilepsy after they were given nicotinamide,[10] but the fact that the children were on several anticonvulsant drugs clouds the issue somewhat. Similarly, nicotinamide given to three children on primidone therapy increased blood levels of primidone.[11] It is thought that nicotinamide may interfere with the body's normal breakdown of these anticonvulsant agents, allowing them to build up in the blood.

St. John's Wort, Dong Quai: Possible Harmful Interaction

3 NEGATIVE St. John's wort (*Hypericum perforatum*) is primarily used to treat mild to moderate depression.

The herb dong quai (*Angelica sinensis*) is often recommended for menstrual disorders such as dysmenorrhea, PMS, and irregular menstruation.

The anticonvulsant agents carbamazepine, phenobarbital, and valproic acid have been reported to cause increased sensitivity to the sun, amplifying the risk of sunburn or skin rash. Because St. John's wort and dong quai may also cause this problem, taking them during treatment with these drugs might add to this risk.

It may be a good idea to wear a sunscreen or protective clothing during sun exposure if you take one of these herbs while using these anticonvulsants.

MIXED INTERACTIONS

Biotin: Supplementation Possibly Helpful, but Take at a Different Time of Day

3 MIXED Anticonvulsants may deplete biotin, an essential water-soluble B vitamin, possibly by competing with it for absorption in the intestine. It is not clear, however, whether this effect is great enough to be harmful.

Blood levels of biotin were found to be substantially lower in 404 people with epilepsy on long-term treatment with anticonvulsants compared to 112 untreated people with epilepsy.[12] The effect occurred with phenytoin, carbamazepine, phenobarbital, and primidone. Valproic acid appears to affect biotin to a lesser extent than other anticonvulsants.

A test tube study suggested that anticonvulsants might lower biotin levels by interfering with the way biotin is transported in the intestine.[13]

Biotin supplementation may be beneficial if you are on long-term anticonvulsant therapy. To avoid a potential interaction, take the supplement 2 to 3 hours apart from the drug. It has been suggested that the action of anticonvulsant drugs may be at least partly related to their effect of reducing biotin levels. For this reason, it may be desirable to take enough biotin to prevent a deficiency, but not an excessive amount.

Please see Appendix D, Safety Issues, for more information.

Folate: Supplementation Possibly Helpful

2 MIXED Folate (also known as folic acid) is a B vitamin that plays an important role in many vital aspects of health, including preventing neural tube birth defects and possibly reducing the risk of heart disease. Because inadequate intake of folate is widespread, if you are taking any medication that depletes or impairs folate even slightly, you may need supplementation.

Carbamazepine appears to lower blood levels of folate by speeding up its normal breakdown by the body and also by decreasing its absorption.[14] Other antiseizure drugs can also reduce levels of folate in the body.[15–20]

The low serum folate caused by anticonvulsants can raise homocysteine levels, a condition believed to increase the risk of heart disease.[21]

Adequate folate intake is also necessary to prevent neural tube birth defects such as spina bifida and anencephaly. Because anticonvulsant drugs deplete folate, babies born to women taking anticonvulsants are at increased risk for such birth defects. Anticonvulsants may also play a more direct role in the development of birth defects.[22]

However, the case for taking extra folate during anticonvulsant therapy is not as simple as it might seem. It is possible that folate supplementation itself might impair the effectiveness of anticonvulsant drugs, and physician supervision is necessary.

Please see Appendix D, Safety Issues, for more information.

POSITIVE INTERACTIONS

Calcium: Supplementation Probably Helpful, but Take at a Different Time of Day

2 POSITIVE Anticonvulsant drugs may impair calcium absorption and in this way increase the risk of osteoporosis and other bone disorders.

Calcium absorption was compared in 12 people on anticonvulsant therapy (all taking phenytoin and some also taking carbamazepine, phenobarbital, and/or primidone) and 12 people who received no treatment.[23] Calcium absorption was found to be 27% lower in the treated participants.

An observational study found low calcium blood levels in 48% of 109 people taking anticonvulsants.[24] Other findings in this study suggested that anticonvulsants might also reduce calcium levels by directly interfering with parathyroid hormone, a substance that helps keep calcium levels in proper balance.

A low blood level of calcium can itself trigger seizures, and this might reduce the effectiveness of anticonvulsants.[25]

Calcium supplementation may be beneficial for people taking anticonvulsant drugs. However, some studies indicate that antacids containing calcium carbonate may interfere with the absorption of phenytoin and perhaps other anticonvulsants.[26,27] For this reason, take calcium supplements and anticonvulsant drugs several hours apart if possible.

Please see Appendix D, Safety Issues, for more information.

Carnitine: Supplementation Possibly Helpful

2 POSITIVE Carnitine is an amino acid that has been used for heart conditions, Alzheimer's disease, and intermittent claudication (a possible complication of atherosclerosis in which impaired blood circulation causes severe pain in calf muscles during walking or exercising).

Long-term therapy with anticonvulsant agents, particularly valproic acid, is associated with low levels of carnitine.[28] However, it isn't clear whether the anticonvulsants cause the carnitine deficiency or whether it occurs for other reasons. It has been hypothesized that low carnitine levels may contribute to valproic acid's damaging effects on the liver.[29,30] The risk of this liver damage increases in children younger than 24 months,[31] and carnitine supplementation does seem to be protective.[32] However, in one double-blind crossover study, carnitine supplementation produced no real improvement in "well-being" as assessed by parents of children receiving either valproic acid or carbamazepine.[33]

L-carnitine supplementation may be advisable in certain cases, such as in infants and young children (especially those younger than 2 years) who have neurologic disorders and are receiving valproic acid and multiple anticonvulsants.[34]

Please see Appendix D, Safety Issues, for more information.

Vitamin D: Supplementation Possibly Helpful

2 POSITIVE Anticonvulsant drugs may interfere with the activity of vitamin D. As proper handling of calcium by the body depends on vitamin D, this may be another way that these drugs increase the risk of osteoporosis and related bone disorders (see the previous Calcium topic).

Anticonvulsants appear to speed up the body's normal breakdown of vitamin D, decreasing the amount of the vitamin in the blood.[35] A survey of 48 people taking both phenytoin and phenobarbital found significantly lower levels of calcium and vitamin D in many of them as compared to 38 untreated individuals.[36] Similar but lesser changes were seen in 13 people taking phenytoin or phenobarbital alone. This effect may be apparent only after several weeks of treatment.

Another study found decreased blood levels of one form of vitamin D but normal levels of another.[37] Because there are two primary forms of vitamin D circulating in the blood, the body might be able to adjust in some cases

Carbamazepine

to keep vitamin D in balance, at least for a time, despite the influence of anticonvulsants.[38]

Adequate sunlight exposure may help overcome the effects of anticonvulsants on vitamin D by stimulating the skin to manufacture the vitamin.[39] Of 450 people on anticonvulsants residing in a Florida facility, none were found to have low blood levels of vitamin D or evidence of bone disease. This suggests that environments providing regular sun exposure may be protective.

Individuals regularly taking anticonvulsants, especially those taking combination therapy and those with limited exposure to sunlight, may benefit from vitamin D supplementation.

Please see Appendix D, Safety Issues, for more information.

Vitamin K: Supplementation Possibly Helpful for Pregnant Women

2 POSITIVE Phenytoin, carbamazepine, phenobarbital, and primidone speed up the normal breakdown of vitamin K into inactive byproducts, thus depriving the body of active vitamin K. This can lead to bone problems such as osteoporosis. Also, use of these anticonvulsants can lead to a vitamin K deficiency in babies born to mothers taking the drugs, resulting in bleeding disorders or facial bone abnormalities in the newborns.[40]

Mothers who take these anticonvulsants may need vitamin K supplementation during pregnancy to prevent these conditions in their newborns.

Please see Appendix D, Safety Issues, for more information.

CEPHALOSPORINS

Interactions	Rating*
Positive Interaction	
Vitamin K	3

*Rating Key

1   Significant interaction

2   Possibly significant interaction

3   Interaction of relatively little significance

4   Reported interaction that does not in fact exist or is insignificant

These **antibiotics** (see page 19) work somewhat similarly to penicillin, but have been chemically modified to exert a broader spectrum of action in killing infection-causing bacteria. Drugs in this family include

- cefaclor (Ceclor, Ceclor CD)
- cefadroxil (Duricef, Ultracel)
- cefdinir (Omnicef)
- cefixime (Suprax)
- cefpodoxime proxetil (Vantin)
- cefprozil (Cefzil)
- ceftibuten (Cedax)
- cefuroxime (Axetil, Ceftin, Zinacef)
- cephalexin (Cefanex, Keflex, Keftab, Biocef)
- cephradine (Anspor, Velosef)
- loracarbef (Lorabid)
- and others

POSITIVE INTERACTIONS

Vitamin K: Supplementation Possibly Helpful

3 POSITIVE Vitamin K plays a crucial role in blood clotting and also seems to be important for proper bone formation.

Antibiotics destroy harmful bacteria as well as "friendly" intestinal bacteria that produce vitamin K. For this reason, it is widely believed that antibiotic use may lead to a vitamin K deficiency. However, this may be a problem only in severely malnourished individuals.[1,2]

Cephalosporin antibiotics may affect vitamin K in a more important way: by interfering with the vitamin after it is absorbed by the body. Some studies suggest that only those cephalosporins with a certain chemical structure are likely to interact with vitamin K,[3,4] but others indicate that this may be a general effect associated with all antibiotics in the cephalosporin family.[5,6]

This interaction does not appear to be of real concern in well-nourished individuals. However, people with conditions that prevent them from getting proper amounts of vitamin K may need supplemental doses of the vitamin, and these cases should be evaluated by a physician.

Please see Appendix D, Safety Issues, for more information.

CISPLATIN

Interactions	Rating*
Positive Interactions	
Bismuth Subsalicylate	3
Glutathione	3
Magnesium and Potassium	1
Selenium	2
Vitamin E	2
Other Supplements	3

*Rating Key

1 Significant interaction
2 Possibly significant interaction
3 Interaction of relatively little significance
4 Reported interaction that does not in fact exist or is insignificant

The chemotherapy drug cisplatin (Platinol) is used alone or in combination with other drugs to treat various cancers. Unfortunately, it can cause injury to the kidney and bone marrow. The kidney impairment is thought to be at least in part due to oxidative damage caused by free radicals.

Various antioxidants have been studied to see whether they might protect individuals taking cisplatin from kidney damage and other drug-associated toxicity. Other nutrients may offer benefits as well. However, because of concerns that antioxidants could in some cases interfere with the effectiveness of chemotherapy drugs, individuals on chemotherapy should not use these (or any other) supplements except on physician's advice.

POSITIVE INTERACTIONS

Bismuth Subsalicylate: Supplementation Possibly Helpful

3 POSITIVE A small study in humans found a slightly protective effect against kidney toxicity for people receiving bismuth subsalicylate (e.g., Pepto-Bismol), compared to those not receiving the bismuth formulation.[1]

Glutathione: Supplementation Possibly Helpful

3 POSITIVE Glutathione is a natural antioxidant manufactured in the liver.

Based on the observation that cisplatin appears to deplete kidney stores of glutathione,[2] a possible protective effect of glutathione supplementation on cisplatin toxicity has been investigated. However, human trials testing glutathione's ability to prevent cisplatin-induced kidney toxicity[3,4,5] or hearing damage[6,7] have been a disappointment. One problem may be that glutathione supplements taken orally may not be sufficiently absorbed to be effective.

Magnesium and Potassium: Supplementation Probably Helpful

1 POSITIVE Cisplatin-induced kidney damage leads to the loss of important minerals from the body, including magnesium and potassium.[8] It is thought that low magnesium blood levels may play a role in the development of heart and blood vessel complications,[9,10] and both magnesium and potassium supplementation may be necessary during cisplatin therapy.[11–14]

Because proper balance of these minerals in the blood is critical, supplementation should be supervised by a physician.

Please see Appendix D, Safety Issues, for more information.

Selenium: Supplementation Possibly Helpful

2 POSITIVE The trace mineral selenium helps the body manufacture glutathione, a natural antioxidant manufactured in the liver. Evidence from a human study suggests that selenium supplements may help protect the kidneys and bone marrow against cisplatin toxicity.[15]

Numerous animal studies also suggest that selenium in various forms may diminish cisplatin-induced kidney damage[16–20] and allow the use of a larger antitumor dose of cisplatin.[21]

Please see Appendix D, Safety Issues, for more information.

Vitamin E: Supplementation Possibly Helpful

2 POSITIVE Animal studies suggest that vitamin E, an antioxidant, may protect against cisplatin-induced kidney toxicity.[22,23]

Vitamin E also may alleviate oral mucositis (inflammation of the membranes lining the inside of the mouth), a common complication of chemotherapy. In a double-blind trial, 16 people on cisplatin who had developed drug-induced oral mucositis were treated with either vitamin E oil or placebo oil.[24] The condition improved dramatically within 4 days in those using the vitamin E oil compared to no effect for placebo. Another study found that vitamin E oil substantially reduced the duration of oral mucositis in some individuals but not in others.[25]

Please see Appendix D, Safety Issues, for more information.

Other Supplements: Supplementation Possibly Helpful

3 POSITIVE Based on *in vitro* and animal studies, other supplements that might help protect against kidney damage during cisplatin chemotherapy include silibinin (a substance found in milk thistle, *Silybum marianum*),[26] vitamin C,[27] N-acetyl cysteine,[28] and *Ginkgo biloba* extract (containing the antioxidant superoxide dismutase).[29]

Please see Appendix D, Safety Issues, for more information.

CLONIDINE

Trade Name: Catapres

Interactions	Rating*
Negative Interaction	
Yohimbe	2

*Rating Key

1 Significant interaction
2 Possibly significant interaction
3 Interaction of relatively little significance
4 Reported interaction that does not in fact exist or is insignificant

Clonidine is often used to reduce blood pressure as well as to counter symptoms that occur during withdrawal from alcohol and other addictive substances.

NEGATIVE INTERACTIONS

Yohimbe: Possible Harmful Interaction

2 NEGATIVE The herb yohimbe (source of the drug yohimbine) is promoted as a treatment for impotence.

Though the drug yohimbine has been advocated to decrease blood pressure,[1] it may actually increase blood pressure when taken in doses greater than 5 mg.[2] In particular, yohimbine's effect on blood pressure appears to directly oppose that of clonidine,[3,4] although no problems involving this combination have as yet been reported.[5,6]

As a precaution, you should avoid yohimbe if you take clonidine or other drugs for high blood pressure.

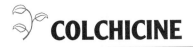

COLCHICINE

Trade Name: ColBENEMID

Interactions	Rating*
Positive Interaction	
Vitamin B$_{12}$	3

*Rating Key

1 Significant interaction

2 Possibly significant interaction

3 Interaction of relatively little significance

4 Reported interaction that does not in fact exist or is insignificant

Although primarily used on a short-term basis for treating attacks of gout, colchicine is increasingly being used as a long-term therapy for gout prevention. This may increase the chance of developing the nutritional deficiency discussed next.

POSITIVE INTERACTIONS

Vitamin B$_{12}$: Supplementation Possibly Helpful

3 POSITIVE Regular use of colchicine may impair the body's absorption of vitamin B$_{12}$. Studies of 20 participants taking oral colchicine found significantly reduced vitamin B$_{12}$ absorption in all but one individual.[1] On a physician's advice, B$_{12}$ supplementation may be beneficial during extended colchicine therapy.

Please see Appendix D, Safety Issues, for more information.

CORTICOSTEROIDS (Glucocorticoids)

Interactions	Rating*
Negative Interaction	
Licorice	1
Mixed Interaction	
Chromium	2
Positive Interactions	
Calcium and Vitamin D	2
DHEA	3
Topical Herbal Treatments	3

*Rating Key

1 Significant interaction
2 Possibly significant interaction
3 Interaction of relatively little significance
4 Reported interaction that does not in fact exist or is insignificant

Corticosteroid drugs (also known as glucocorticoids) act in the body like cortisone, a naturally occurring hormone produced by the adrenal glands. They are strong anti-inflammatory and immunosuppressive medications used in many inflammatory and autoimmune conditions such as arthritis, asthma, inflammatory bowel disease, and systemic lupus erythematosus. Corticosteroids are also prescribed to suppress transplant rejection. Drugs in this family include

- betamethasone (Celestone)
- cortisone acetate (Cortone Acetate)
- dexamethasone (Decadron, Dexameth, Dexone, Hexadrol)
- hydrocortisone (Cortef, Hydrocortone)
- methylprednisolone (Medrol)
- prednisolone (Delta-Cortef, Hydeltrasol, Pediapred, Prelone)
- prednisone (Deltasone, Liquid Pred, Meticorten, Orasone, Panasol-S, Prednicen-M, Sterapred DS)
- triamcinolone (Aristocort, Atolone, Azmacort, Kenacort, Nasacort)
- and others

NEGATIVE INTERACTIONS

Licorice: Possible Harmful Interaction

1 NEGATIVE Licorice root, a member of the pea family, has been used since ancient times as both food and medicine.

Taking licorice (*Glycyrrhiza glabra* or *G. uralensis*) may raise blood levels of corticosteroids and increase their side effects.[1,2,3] In one study, 6 healthy participants were given the synthetic corticosteroid drug prednisolone with or without supplementation with 200 mg of glycyrrhizin, a constituent of licorice.[4] Glycyrrhizin was found to increase blood levels of prednisolone, apparently by interfering with its normal breakdown by the body.

Test tube studies with glycyrrhetinic acid, the major active component of licorice, have found similar effects on the body's natural steroids.[5] Additionally, glycyrrhetinic acid may itself possess a corticosteroid-like effect due to its chemical structure.[6]

For these reasons, licorice ingestion could increase the risk of serious drug side effects and should be avoided. An often unrecognized source of licorice is chewing tobacco.[7]

MIXED INTERACTIONS

Chromium: Possible Benefits and Risks

| 2 |
| MIXED |

A 1999 study demonstrates that supplementation with the trace mineral chromium may help control corticosteroid-induced diabetes.[8] Corticosteroid therapy is known to promote or worsen diabetes, while evidence suggests that chromium supplementation has a positive effect on diabetes.[9,10,11]

In this study, people with diabetes associated with corticosteroid drugs were supplemented with chromium picolinate at a dose of 200 mcg 3 times daily. Elevated blood sugar levels in 47 of 50 participants fell by 40%, despite the fact that their oral antidiabetic drug or insulin dose was reduced by half prior to starting chromium.

This finding illustrates that chromium offers a potential benefit and risk at the same time. Chromium supplementation might allow you to cut down on the dose of your insulin or oral hypoglycemic drug, but it also might cause your blood sugar levels to fall too low (hypoglycemia). For this reason, consult with a physician before taking chromium for any type of diabetes.

Please see Appendix D, Safety Issues, for more information.

POSITIVE INTERACTIONS

Calcium and Vitamin D: Supplementation Probably Helpful

| 2 |
| POSITIVE |

Among the most serious side effects of long-term corticosteroid therapy are reduced bone density and the accelerated development of osteoporosis. This may occur also with inhaled agents. Corticosteroids cause these effects by interfering with the body's absorption of calcium as well as through other mechanisms.

Evidence is coming to light that even low-dose corticosteroid therapy can cause loss of bone mineral density in the lumbar spine. A 2-year, double-blind trial involving 96 people with rheumatoid arthritis found that supplementation with calcium and vitamin D prevented the loss of bone mineral density in the lumbar spine and other areas during low-dose prednisone treatment.[12] Participants were given calcium carbonate (1,000 mg daily) and vitamin D (500 IU daily) together, or placebo.

A recent meta-analysis (data combined from numerous studies) also found significant benefit for calcium and vitamin D supplementation in corticosteroid-treated individuals.[13] The analysis involved a total of 274 individuals taking the supplements for 2 years.

An earlier uncontrolled study of 13 people on prednisone therapy suggests a benefit with calcium supplementation (1,000 mg daily) alone.[14]

However, one double-blind placebo-controlled trial with 62 participants found that supplementation with vitamin D and calcium produced little benefit for people taking prednisone.[15]

There is some evidence that supplementation with calcium and vitamin D may be beneficial for individuals on long-term corticosteroid therapy. Since there may be risks associated with vitamin D treatment, physician monitoring is advisable.

Please see Appendix D, Safety Issues, for more information.

DHEA: Supplementation Possibly Helpful

3 POSITIVE Synthetic supplements of DHEA (dehydroepiandrosterone), a hormone produced by the adrenal glands, are promoted for treating lupus and various other conditions.

There are good theoretical reasons (but little direct evidence) to believe that individuals taking corticosteroids (such as prednisone) might be protected from some drug side effects by taking DHEA at the same time.[16,17]

Please see Appendix D, Safety Issues, for more information.

Topical Herbal Treatments: Possibly Helpful When Applied with Hydrocortisone

3 POSITIVE Aloe (*Aloe vera* or *A. barbadensis*) and licorice are two herbs sometimes used for skin problems. Preliminary evidence suggests that each might help topical corticosteroids such as hydrocortisone work better.[18,19]

In one study, the addition of *Aloe vera* to hydrocortisone appeared to boost hydrocortisone's effects against acute inflammation when the mixture was applied to the skin.[20] Similarly, skin tests in 23 healthy volunteers showed that glycyrrhetinic acid enhanced the effect of hydrocortisone when the two were mixed together and applied to the skin;[21] the findings suggest that glycyrrhetinic acid blocks the skin's normal breakdown of corticosteroids at the site of application.

Please see Appendix D, Safety Issues, for more information.

Cyclosporine

CYCLOSPORINE

Trade Names: Neoral, Sandimmune

Interactions	Rating*
Negative Interactions	
Grapefruit Juice	2
St. John's Wort	2

*Rating Key

1 Significant interaction
2 Possibly significant interaction
3 Interaction of relatively little significance
4 Reported interaction that does not in fact exist or is insignificant

Cyclosporine helps prevent rejection of a transplanted organ by suppressing the immune system.

NEGATIVE INTERACTIONS

Grapefruit Juice: Possible Harmful Interaction

2 NEGATIVE Grapefruit juice slows the body's normal breakdown of several drugs, including cyclosporine, allowing it to build up to potentially excessive levels in the blood.[1] A recent study indicates this effect can last for 3 days or more following the last glass of juice.[2]

If you take cyclosporine, the safest approach is to avoid grapefruit juice altogether.

St. John's Wort: Possible Harmful Interaction

2 NEGATIVE The herb St. John's wort (*Hypericum perforatum*) is primarily used to treat mild to moderate depression.

St. John's wort has the potential to accelerate the body's normal breakdown of certain drugs[3,4] including cyclosporine, resulting in lower blood levels of these drugs.

This interaction appears to have occurred in two people taking cyclosporine, reportedly contributing to heart transplant rejection.[5] These individuals had been doing well after transplantation while taking standard immunosuppressive therapy that included cyclosporine. After starting St. John's wort for depression, however, they began experiencing problems and their blood levels of cyclosporine were found to have dipped below the therapeutic range. After St. John's wort was discontinued, cyclosporine levels returned to normal and no further episodes of rejection occurred.

Numerous cases of transplant rejection episodes involving the heart, kidney, and liver have also been reported in people using the herb.[6]

Based on this evidence, if you are taking cyclosporine, you should not take St. John's wort.

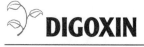

DIGOXIN

Trade Names: Digoxin: Lanoxicaps, Lanoxin
Digitoxin: Crystodigin

Interactions	Rating*
Negative Interactions	
Hawthorn	3
Horsetail	3
Licorice	2
Siberian Ginseng	1
St. John's Wort	1
Positive Interactions	
Calcium	3
Magnesium	3

*Rating Key

1 Significant interaction

2 Possibly significant interaction

3 Interaction of relatively little significance

4 Reported interaction that does not in fact exist or is insignificant

The digitalis drugs digoxin and digitoxin are used for congestive heart failure and other heart conditions. The concerns described below apply equally to both medications.

NEGATIVE INTERACTIONS

Hawthorn: Possible Harmful Interaction

3 NEGATIVE The herb hawthorn is primarily used in the treatment of congestive heart failure.

Because hawthorn (*Crataegus laevigata, C. oxyacantha,* or *C. monogyna*) has effects on the heart somewhat similar to those of digoxin, you shouldn't combine the two treatments except under the supervision of a physician.

Horsetail: Possible Harmful Interaction

3 NEGATIVE One animal study suggests that horsetail (*Equisetum arvense*) can deplete the body of potassium.[1] Because low potassium levels can increase the toxicity of digoxin, it might not be safe to combine horsetail with this drug.

Licorice: Possible Harmful Interaction

2 NEGATIVE Licorice root, a member of the pea family, has been used since ancient times as both food and medicine.

Glycyrrhizic acid, the active ingredient in licorice (*Glycyrrhiza glabra* or *G. uralensis*), promotes potassium loss in the urine,[2,3] and there have been case reports of low blood levels of potassium following long-term or high-dose licorice use.[4,5,6] Low potassium levels can increase the toxicity of digoxin, causing symptoms such as nausea, visual changes, and heart rhythm irregularities.[7,8]

Individuals taking digoxin should avoid licorice. An often-unrecognized source of licorice is chewing tobacco.[9]

However, a special form of licorice known as DGL (deglycyrrhizinated licorice) is a deliberately altered form of the herb that should not affect potassium levels and so should not pose a danger for digoxin users.

Siberian Ginseng: Possible Harmful Interaction

1 NEGATIVE The herb Siberian ginseng (*Eleutherococcus senticosus*) is promoted as an adaptogen, a treatment that helps the body adapt to stress and resist illness in general.

Siberian ginseng appears to interfere with the measurement of digoxin blood levels, but not with the drug itself.

A case report determined that Siberian ginseng caused false high readings for blood levels of digoxin.[10] However, actual digoxin levels were not high, and the person taking ginseng had no adverse symptoms ordinarily associated with high digoxin levels.

Accepting a false measurement as a true value might lead to faulty treatment decisions. For this reason, inform your physician of the possibility of this interaction before combining Siberian ginseng with digoxin.

St. John's Wort: Possible Harmful Interaction

1 NEGATIVE The herb St. John's wort is primarily used to treat mild to moderate depression.

Evidence suggests that St. John's wort (*Hypericum perforatum*) decreases blood levels of digoxin, requiring an increased dosage of the drug to maintain the proper therapeutic effect.[11,12] Conversely, in those who take St. John's wort as well as digoxin, and have found a dose of the drug that maintains normal levels, stopping the herb might cause digoxin levels in the blood to rise dangerously high.

Digoxin

POSITIVE INTERACTIONS

Calcium: Supplementation Possibly Helpful

3 POSITIVE Although the evidence is weak, digoxin may increase the body's loss of calcium, potentially leading to depletion of this mineral.[13] Making sure to get adequate amounts of calcium through either diet or supplements might be advisable; in any case, this is a good idea on general principles.

Please see Appendix D, Safety Issues, for more information.

Magnesium: Supplementation Possibly Helpful, but Take at a Different Time of Day

3 POSITIVE Individuals taking digoxin may have low magnesium levels for several reasons, including the use of other drugs that cause the body to lose magnesium. Low levels of magnesium can increase the toxicity of digoxin, causing symptoms such as nausea, visual changes, and heart rhythm irregularities.[14–17]

For this reason, magnesium supplementation may be beneficial in people taking digoxin. However, evidence suggests that digoxin and magnesium supplements should be taken at least 2 hours apart.[18]

Please see Appendix D, Safety Issues, for more information.

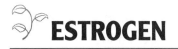

ESTROGEN

Interactions	Rating*
Negative Interactions	
Androstenedione	3
Boron	3
Dong Quai	4
Grapefruit Juice	2
Mixed Interaction	
Ipriflavone	2
Positive Interactions	
Calcium, Vitamin D	1
Magnesium	3

*Rating Key

1 Significant interaction
2 Possibly significant interaction
3 Interaction of relatively little significance
4 Reported interaction that does not in fact exist or is insignificant

Estrogen is used as a component of birth control pills as well as for preventing osteoporosis and heart disease in postmenopausal women.

There are many forms of estrogen. Certain products, such as Ortho Dienestrol Vaginal Cream, contain estrogen in the form of dienestrol.

Medications containing a form of estrogen called estradiol include

- Alora
- Climara
- CombiPatch
- Delestrogen (injectable)
- depGynogen (injectable)
- Depo-Estradiol Cypionate (injectable)
- Depogen (injectable)
- Esclim
- Estrace
- Estraderm
- Estra-L (injectable)
- Estring
- FemPatch
- Gynogen L.A. (injectable)
- Vagifem
- Valergen (injectable)
- Vivelle
- and others

Premarin, Cenestin, Prempro, and Premphase contain another form of the hormone called conjugated estrogens. Additional forms and some of their brand names include

- diethylstilbestrol diphosphate (Stilphostrol)
- estrone (Kestrone-5)
- esterified estrogens (Estratab, Menest)
- estropipate (Ogen, Ortho-Est)
- ethinyl estradiol (Estinyl)
- and others

NEGATIVE INTERACTIONS

Androstenedione: Possible Harmful Interaction

3 NEGATIVE Androstenedione has become popular as a sports supplement, based on the theory that it increases the body's testosterone levels and enhances sports performance. However, the best documented effect of androstenedione is a rise in estrogen levels.[1,2,3]

This finding raises concerns that combining androstenedione with estrogen could increase the risk of estrogen-related side effects.

It would seem best for estrogen users to avoid androstenedione supplementation.

Boron: Possible Harmful Interaction

3 NEGATIVE In some studies, the trace element boron has been found to elevate levels of the body's own estrogen.[4,5] A concern is that combining boron with estrogen therapy might lead to increased estrogen risks and side effects.

For this reason, women on ERT (estrogen replacement therapy) or HRT (hormone replacement therapy, which is estrogen combined with the hormone progestin) should use boron with caution. If supplementation is desired, it might be advisable to do so by means of a diet high in fruits and vegetables, which provides boron safely.

Dong Quai: Interaction Unlikely or Probably Insignificant

4 NEGATIVE The herb dong quai (*Angelica sinensis*) is used for menstrual disorders.

Because dong quai contains beta-sitosterol, a phytoestrogen,[6] there have been concerns that taking the herb with estrogen might add to estrogen-related side effects. However, a 24-week placebo-controlled study of 74 postmenopausal women found no estrogen-like effects or reduction of menopausal symptoms associated with taking dong quai.[7]

Therefore, dong quai seems unlikely to increase estrogen-related side effects.

Grapefruit Juice: Possible Harmful Interaction

2 NEGATIVE Grapefruit juice slows the body's normal breakdown of several drugs, including estrogen, allowing it to build up to potentially excessive levels in the blood.[8] A recent study indicates this effect can last for 3 days or more following the last glass of juice.[9]

If you take estrogen, the safest approach is to avoid grapefruit juice altogether.

MIXED INTERACTIONS

Ipriflavone: Possible Benefits and Risks

 2 MIXED Ipriflavone, a synthetic isoflavone that slows bone breakdown, is used to treat osteoporosis.

When the two are taken together, ipriflavone may increase estrogen's ability to protect bone.[10–14] This may allow you to use a lower dose of estrogen and still receive its beneficial effects.

However, while this combination is probably safe, there is one potential concern: some evidence suggests that when ipriflavone is combined with estrogen, estrogen's effects on the uterus are increased.[15,16] This might mean that risk of uterine cancer would be elevated by the combination.

It should be possible to overcome this risk by taking progesterone along with estrogen, which is standard medical practice in any case. However, this finding does make one wonder whether ipriflavone–estrogen combinations might raise the risk of breast cancer as well, an estrogen side effect that is not easily avoided. At present, there is no available information on this important subject.

Please see Appendix D, Safety Issues, for more information.

POSITIVE INTERACTIONS

Calcium, Vitamin D: Supplementation Probably Helpful

1 POSITIVE People taking estrogen or other drugs for osteoporosis may not realize they still need to take calcium and vitamin D for optimal benefit.[17] The most important nutrient for healthy bones is calcium. Vitamin D is also important because it helps the body absorb and use calcium.

Please see Appendix D, Safety Issues, for more information.

Magnesium: Supplementation Possibly Helpful

3 **POSITIVE** Estrogen enhances the body's use of the mineral magnesium by moving it from the blood into tissues and bone, resulting in lower blood levels of the mineral.[18] A 1991 study in 32 women found a 26% decrease in magnesium levels after 6 months of oral contraceptive (OC) use compared to normal levels before OC use.[19] Similar findings have been observed during estrogen replacement therapy in menopause.[20]

When magnesium levels in the blood fall too low, symptoms may include appetite loss, nausea and vomiting, sleepiness, weakness, muscle spasms, tremors, and personality changes.

Though no problems related to the lower magnesium levels were noted, it is important to maintain proper magnesium levels in the body. For this reason, magnesium supplementation may be advisable in individuals taking OCs who don't get enough magnesium from the diet.

Please see Appendix D, Safety Issues, for more information.

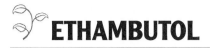

ETHAMBUTOL

Trade Name: Myambutol

Interactions	Rating*
Positive Interaction	
Copper and Zinc	3

*Rating Key

1 Significant interaction

2 Possibly significant interaction

3 Interaction of relatively little significance

4 Reported interaction that does not in fact exist or is insignificant

Ethambutol is often used along with **isoniazid** (see page 93) in the treatment of tuberculosis. These agents work by killing the bacteria that cause the disease.

POSITIVE INTERACTIONS

Copper and Zinc: Supplementation Possibly Helpful

3 POSITIVE Based on animal studies, ethambutol is believed to decrease tissue levels of copper and zinc, supposedly by chelating, or attaching to, these minerals.[1] However, in these studies, the effect was not significant as long as food intake was adequate. To be on the safe side, taking a multivitamin/multimineral tablet containing copper and zinc might be advisable during ethambutol therapy.

Please see Appendix D, Safety Issues, for more information.

ETOPOSIDE

Trade Names: Etopophos, Toposar, VePesid

Interactions	Rating*
Negative Interaction	
St. John's Wort	2

*Rating Key

1 Significant interaction
2 Possibly significant interaction
3 Interaction of relatively little significance
4 Reported interaction that does not in fact exist or is insignificant

Etoposide and related drugs are useful anticancer agents for treatment of breast, prostate, lung, and colon cancers, as well as some types of leukemia.

Drugs related to etoposide are doxorubicin, mitoxantrone, and teniposide.

NEGATIVE INTERACTIONS

St. John's Wort: Possible Harmful Interaction

2 NEGATIVE The herb St. John's wort (*Hypericum perforatum*) is primarily used to treat mild to moderate depression.

Test tube studies have found that hypericin, a constituent of St. John's wort, could reverse the therapeutic effect of etoposide.[1,2] However, the possible influence of hypericin on etoposide's anticancer action in tumor cells in people has not been determined.

As a precaution, individuals taking etoposide or anticancer drugs that work similarly should avoid St. John's wort.

FLUOROQUINOLONES

Interactions	Rating*
Negative Interactions	
Fennel	2
St. John's Wort, Dong Quai	3
Minerals	2

*Rating Key

1 Significant interaction
2 Possibly significant interaction
3 Interaction of relatively little significance
4 Reported interaction that does not in fact exist or is insignificant

Antibiotics in the fluoroquinolone family are used for urinary tract infections as well as other infectious diseases. These drugs exert a broad spectrum of action in killing various infection-causing bacteria (see **Antibiotics,** page 19). Fluoroquinolone antibiotics include

- ciprofloxacin (Cipro)
- enoxacin (Penetrex)
- grepafloxacin (Raxar)
- levofloxacin (Levaquin)
- lomefloxacin (Maxaquin)
- norfloxacin (Noroxin, Chibroxin)
- ofloxacin (Floxin)
- sparfloxacin (Zagam)
- trovafloxacin/alatrofloxacin (Trovan)
- and others

NEGATIVE INTERACTIONS

Fennel: Possible Harmful Interaction

2 NEGATIVE The herb fennel appears to reduce blood levels of ciprofloxacin, possibly impairing its effectiveness.[1] This finding comes from a placebo-controlled study in rats. Fennel might be expected to interfere similarly with other fluoroquinolone antibiotics.

Allowing 2 hours between taking ciprofloxacin and fennel should reduce the potential for an interaction, but may not eliminate it. For this reason, it may be advisable to avoid fennel supplementation during therapy with ciprofloxacin or other antibiotics in this family.

St. John's Wort, Dong Quai: Possible Harmful Interaction

3 NEGATIVE St. John's wort (*Hypericum perforatum*) is primarily used to treat mild to moderate depression.

The herb dong quai (*Angelica sinensis*) is often recommended for menstrual disorders such as dysmenorrhea, PMS, and irregular menstruation.

Fluoroquinolone antibiotics have been reported to cause increased sensitivity to the sun, amplifying the risk of sunburn or skin rash. Because St. John's wort and dong quai may also cause this problem, taking these herbal supplements during treatment with fluoroquinolone drugs might add to the risk.

It may be a good idea to wear a sunscreen or protective clothing during sun exposure if you take one of these herbs with a fluoroquinolone antibiotic.

Minerals: Take at a Different Time of Day

2 NEGATIVE The minerals calcium,[2–6] iron,[7–12] and zinc[13,14] may interfere with the absorption of various fluoroquinolone antibiotics. **Antacids** (see page 13) containing aluminum and magnesium may interact similarly.[15–20] This could weaken the effect of the antibiotic against the infection it is supposed to cure.

Among this family of antibiotics, lomefloxacin and ofloxacin may not interact with minerals as much, but this is not certain. To prevent problems, take mineral supplements and milk/dairy products as far apart as possible from fluoroquinolone antibiotics.

H₂ ANTAGONISTS

Interactions	Rating*
Negative Interaction	
Magnesium	3
Positive Interactions	
Folate	3
Vitamin B₁₂	2
Vitamin D	3
Minerals	3

*Rating Key

1 Significant interaction

2 Possibly significant interaction

3 Interaction of relatively little significance

4 Reported interaction that does not in fact exist or is insignificant

Medications in this family sharply decrease stomach acid production. They are widely used for the treatment of peptic ulcers as well as for mild cases of esophageal reflux (heartburn). Drugs in this family include

- cimetidine (Tagamet, Tagamet HB)
- famotidine (Mylanta AR Acid Reducer, Pepcid, Pepcid AC, Pepcid RPD)
- nizatidine (Axid, Axid AR)
- ranitidine hydrochloride (Zantac, Zantac EFFERdose, Zantac GELdose, Zantac 75)
- and others

NEGATIVE INTERACTIONS

Magnesium: Take at a Different Time of Day

3 NEGATIVE Magnesium-containing **antacids** (see page 13) may reduce the absorption of H₂ antagonists.[1] However, the study on which this concern is based tested an antacid containing both magnesium and aluminum. Therefore, we can't be certain that magnesium alone was the interacting substance. This also makes it unclear whether a magnesium supplement might have a similar effect on H₂ antagonists. Furthermore, there's probably little need for concern, because this type of antacid and H₂ antagonist are often prescribed together for their "one-two punch" against stomach acid, with no apparent problem.

Nonetheless, if you have a choice, it certainly wouldn't hurt to separate the times you take magnesium-containing products and H₂ antagonists.

POSITIVE INTERACTIONS

Folate: Supplementation Possibly Helpful

3 POSITIVE Folate (also known as folic acid) is a B vitamin that plays an important role in many vital aspects of health, including preventing neural tube birth defects and possibly reducing the risk of heart disease. Because inadequate intake of folate is widespread, if you are taking any medication that depletes or impairs folate even slightly, you may need supplementation.

Conditions for folate absorption are best in the slightly acidic part of the intestine nearest to the stomach. There is some evidence that H_2 antagonists, by reducing stomach acid, may interfere with the absorption of folate.[2] This effect appears to be relatively minor. However, because folate is commonly deficient in the diet anyway, folate supplementation in nutritional doses may be worthwhile, especially if you take H_2 antagonists regularly.

Please see Appendix D, Safety Issues, for more information.

Vitamin B₁₂: Supplementation Probably Helpful

2 POSITIVE Vitamin B_{12} in foods is attached to proteins, and adequate stomach acid is required to release it from this bound form. The vitamin is then picked up by a protective stomach substance called intrinsic factor and absorbed from the intestine. H_2 antagonists, by reducing stomach acid, can interfere with the absorption of vitamin B_{12}.

One study found that cimetidine given 4 times daily (1,000 mg total) reduced the absorption of dietary vitamin B_{12} in participants with and without peptic ulcers.[3] Other studies have found similar results with cimetidine[4] as well as ranitidine.[5]

However, supplemental oral vitamin B_{12} can still be absorbed, presumably because it does not have to be split apart from proteins.[6] Therefore, if you take H_2 antagonists, it may be advisable to take vitamin B_{12} supplementation in nutritional doses to make up for malabsorption of the vitamin from foods.

Another way to get around this interaction is to take one nightly dose of the H_2 antagonist. Acid levels may rise enough during the following day to allow greater absorption of B_{12} from food.

Please see Appendix D, Safety Issues, for more information.

Vitamin D: Supplementation Possibly Helpful

3 **POSITIVE** Cimetidine may interfere with the handling of vitamin D by the body.[7,8,9] However, this effect may not be significant enough to matter unless you are not getting enough vitamin D in the first place.

Please see Appendix D, Safety Issues, for more information.

Minerals: Supplementation Possibly Helpful

3 **POSITIVE** By reducing stomach acid levels, H₂ antagonists may interfere with the absorption of iron and zinc and possibly other minerals that are absorbed best under acidic conditions.[10,11] If you are on an H₂ antagonist, taking a general multivitamin/multimineral supplement should help.

Please see Appendix D, Safety Issues, for more information.

HEPARIN

Interactions	Rating*
Negative Interactions	
Garlic	1
Ginkgo	1
Phosphatidylserine	3
Policosanol	1
Vitamin C	3
White Willow	2
Other Supplements	3
Positive Interaction	
Vitamin D	1

*Rating Key

1 Significant interaction

2 Possibly significant interaction

3 Interaction of relatively little significance

4 Reported interaction that does not in fact exist or is insignificant

Heparin is a very strong blood-thinning drug that is delivered by injection. If you receive heparin, make sure you check with your doctor before taking any type of supplement.

NEGATIVE INTERACTIONS

Garlic: Possible Harmful Interaction

1 NEGATIVE The herb garlic (*Allium sativum*) is taken to lower cholesterol, among many other proposed uses.

Because garlic has a blood-thinning effect itself, it might be dangerous to combine garlic with heparin.[1,2]

Two cases have been reported in which the combination of garlic and the blood-thinner warfarin doubled the time it took for blood to clot.[3] Though warfarin thins the blood in a different way than heparin, there are concerns that garlic might interact similarly with heparin.

Ginkgo: Possible Harmful Interaction

1 NEGATIVE The herb ginkgo (*Ginkgo biloba*) has been used to treat Alzheimer's disease and ordinary age-related memory loss, among many other conditions.

Ginkgo thins the blood by reducing the ability of blood-clotting cells called platelets to stick together.[4,5] Because case reports have implicated use of *Ginkgo biloba* in the development of serious bleeding abnormalities,[6,7] combining ginkgo with heparin might be expected to intensify the danger.

Phosphatidylserine: Possible Harmful Interaction

3 NEGATIVE The supplement phosphatidylserine is promoted to treat Alzheimer's disease and ordinary age-related memory loss.

A test tube study suggests that phosphatidylserine might amplify heparin's blood-thinning effects.[8] If this effect were to occur inside the body, it could increase the risk of abnormal bleeding. If you receive heparin, make sure you check with your doctor before taking phosphatidylserine.

Policosanol: Possible Harmful Interaction

1 NEGATIVE Policosanol, derived from sugar cane, has been taken for hyperlipidemia and intermittent claudication.

Human trials suggest that policosanol makes blood platelets more slippery, an action that could potentiate the blood-thinning effects of heparin, possibly causing a risk of abnormal bleeding episodes.[9] A 30-day double-blind placebo-controlled trial of 27 individuals with high cholesterol levels found that policosanol at 10 mg daily markedly reduced the ability of blood platelets to clump together.[10] Another double-blind placebo-controlled study of 37 healthy volunteers found evidence that the blood-thinning effect of policosanol increased as the dose was increased—the larger the policosanol dose, the greater the effect.[11] Yet another double-blind placebo-controlled study of 43 healthy volunteers compared the effects of policosanol (20 mg daily), the blood-thinner aspirin (100 mg daily), and policosanol and aspirin combined at these same doses.[12] The results again showed that policosanol substantially reduced the ability of blood platelets to stick together, and that the combined therapy exhibited additive effects.

Based on these findings, you should not combine heparin and policosanol except under medical supervision.

Vitamin C: Possible Harmful Interaction

3 NEGATIVE Test tube studies suggest that high amounts of vitamin C may reduce the blood-thinning effect of heparin.[13] However, it is not clear whether the interaction is significant enough to make a practical difference.

White Willow: Possible Harmful Interaction

2 NEGATIVE The herb white willow (*Salix alba*), also known as willow bark, is used to treat pain and fever. White willow contains a substance that is converted by the body into a salicylate similar to aspirin.

Since combining aspirin with heparin increases the risk of abnormal bleeding, it would be advisable not to combine white willow with heparin.

Heparin

Other Supplements: Possible Harmful Interaction

3 NEGATIVE Based on their known effects or constituents, the following herbs and supplements might not be safe to combine with heparin, though this has not been proven: bromelain (in the fruit and stem of pineapple, *Ananas comosus*), papaya (*Carica papaya*), chamomile (*Matricaria recutita*), *Coleus forskohlii*, Danshen (*Salvia miltorrhiza*), devil's claw (*Harpogophytum procumbens*), dong quai (*Angelica sinensis*), feverfew (*Tanacetum parthenium*), ginger (*Zingiber officinale*), horse chestnut (*Aesculus hippocastanum*), red clover (*Trifolium pratense*), reishi (*Ganoderma lucidum*), aortic glycosaminoglycans (GAGs), fish oil, OPCs (oligomeric proanthocyanidins), and vitamin E.

POSITIVE INTERACTIONS

Vitamin D: Supplementation Possibly Helpful

1 POSITIVE High doses or long-term use of heparin may interfere with the proper handling of vitamin D by the body;[14] because vitamin D is needed for calcium absorption and utilization, this may in turn lead to bone loss and osteoporosis. Additionally, heparin may directly interfere with bone formation.[15]

This interaction is of special concern during pregnancy, when there is a greater calcium demand and diminished levels of a hormone that pushes calcium into bones. In fact, there have been several reports of fractured and collapsed vertebrae in pregnant women on heparin therapy.[16,17]

Supplementary calcium and vitamin D may help prevent heparin-induced osteoporosis. It might also be advisable to have your bone density checked during long-term heparin therapy.

Please see Appendix D, Safety Issues, for more information.

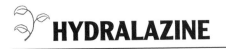

HYDRALAZINE

Trade Names: Apresoline, Hydra-Zide

Interactions	Rating*
Negative Interaction	
Coleus forskohlii	4
Positive Interaction	
Vitamin B$_6$	1

*Rating Key

1 Significant interaction

2 Possibly significant interaction

3 Interaction of relatively little significance

4 Reported interaction that does not in fact exist or is insignificant

Hydralazine relaxes and widens blood vessels and is used to treat high blood pressure. (See also **Antihypertensive Agents**, page 36.)

NEGATIVE INTERACTIONS

Coleus forskohlii: Possible Harmful Interaction

4 NEGATIVE The herb *Coleus forskohlii* relaxes blood vessels and might have unpredictable effects if combined with hydralazine.

POSITIVE INTERACTIONS

Vitamin B$_6$: Supplementation Probably Helpful

1 POSITIVE Hydralazine is known to interfere with vitamin B$_6$. The drug is a structural cousin of **isoniazid** (see page 93) and, like it, can attach to and disable the active form of vitamin B$_6$ (see Vitamin B$_6$ in the full article **Isoniazid** for more information). Taking extra vitamin B$_6$ is considered advisable when taking hydralazine.

Please see Appendix D, Safety Issues, for more information.

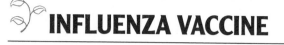 INFLUENZA VACCINE

Trade Names: Fluogen, Fluvirin, Fluzone

Interactions	Rating*
Positive Interaction	
Asian Ginseng	3

*Rating Key

1 Significant interaction
2 Possibly significant interaction
3 Interaction of relatively little significance
4 Reported interaction that does not in fact exist or is insignificant

The influenza vaccine, though not perfect, significantly decreases the risk of getting caught up in the annual flu epidemic. It may also lead to less severe symptoms if influenza does develop.

POSITIVE INTERACTIONS

Asian Ginseng: Supplementation Probably Helpful

3 **POSITIVE** The herb Asian ginseng (*Panax ginseng*) is promoted as an adaptogen, a treatment that helps the body adapt to stress and resist illness.

There is evidence that ginseng may work synergistically with the influenza vaccine.

A double-blind study of 227 individuals found that Asian ginseng might help the vaccine work more effectively, increasing antibody production and decreasing the frequency of colds and flus.[1] The dose used in the study was 100 mg of Asian ginseng taken twice daily for 1 month prior and 2 months after the vaccine was administered.

Please see Appendix D, Safety Issues, for more information.

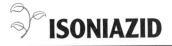

ISONIAZID

Trade Names: Nydrazid, Rifamate, Rifater

Interactions	Rating*
Positive Interactions	
Niacin (Vitamin B$_3$)	2
Vitamin B$_6$	1
Vitamin D	3

*Rating Key

1 Significant interaction

2 Possibly significant interaction

3 Interaction of relatively little significance

4 Reported interaction that does not in fact exist or is insignificant

Isoniazid, a drug used in the treatment of tuberculosis, works by killing the bacteria that cause the disease. Isoniazid can interfere with the body's handling of numerous nutrients. Because this **antibiotic** (see also page 19) is commonly taken for a very long period of time, deficiencies can mount up over the course of treatment, impairing overall health.

POSITIVE INTERACTIONS

Niacin (Vitamin B$_3$): Supplementation Possibly Helpful

| 2 |
| POSITIVE |

Isoniazid appears to interfere with the body's ability to manufacture niacin, apparently by blocking the action of vitamin B$_6$.[1–4] Vitamin B$_6$ is needed to convert the amino acid L-tryptophan to niacin, so disabling B$_6$ can produce either a subtle or an all-out niacin deficiency (known as pellagra).

Niacin supplementation may help prevent the development of pellagra during isoniazid therapy. Though the most effective preventive dosage of niacin has not been determined, supplementation at standard nutritional doses should help.

Please see Appendix D, Safety Issues, for more information.

Vitamin B$_6$: Supplementation Probably Helpful

| 1 |
| POSITIVE |

Individuals who take isoniazid may develop nerve problems such as tingling or numbness in the arms, hands, legs, and feet. The cause appears to be isoniazid's interference with the action of vitamin B$_6$.[5] The drug attaches to and disables the active form of the vitamin.[6,7]

Supplementation with vitamin B$_6$ at 6 to 50 mg daily may prevent these complications. Once nerve symptoms develop, a much higher B$_6$ dose may be required, along with discontinuing the drug.[8] However, in the absence of definite signs of nerve injury, it is important not to exceed the recommended dose of vitamin B_6, because excessive B_6 intake may interfere with isoniazid's antituberculosis activity.[9] Physician supervision is therefore recommended before you take any amount of vitamin B_6 while on isoniazid.

Please see Appendix D, Safety Issues, for more information.

Vitamin D: Supplementation Possibly Helpful

3 POSITIVE Isoniazid may interfere with the conversion of vitamin D to its active forms, resulting in lower blood levels of calcium[10,11] and possible impairment of bone development. In most cases, however, the body seems to be able to adjust in ways that keep these nutrients in proper balance.[12] Still, supplementation with vitamin D at standard nutritional doses might be worthwhile during isoniazid therapy, especially for individuals with increased calcium requirements (such as children and pregnant women, those whose diets are deficient in vitamin D, or individuals who get little sun exposure).[13,14]

Please see Appendix D, Safety Issues, for more information.

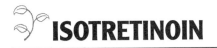

ISOTRETINOIN

Trade Name: Accutane

Interactions	Rating*
Negative Interactions	
St. John's Wort, Dong Quai	3
Vitamin A	1

*Rating Key

1 Significant interaction
2 Possibly significant interaction
3 Interaction of relatively little significance
4 Reported interaction that does not in fact exist or is insignificant

Isotretinoin, chemically related to vitamin A, is used for the treatment of acne and other skin conditions.

NEGATIVE INTERACTIONS

St. John's Wort, Dong Quai: Possible Harmful Interaction

3 NEGATIVE St. John's wort (*Hypericum perforatum*) is primarily used to treat mild to moderate depression.

The herb dong quai (*Angelica sinensis*) is often recommended for menstrual disorders such as dysmenorrhea, PMS, and irregular menstruation.

Isotretinoin has been reported to cause increased sensitivity to the sun, amplifying the risk of sunburn or skin rash. Because St. John's wort and dong quai may also cause this problem, taking these herbal supplements during isotretinoin therapy might add to this risk.

It may be a good idea to wear a sunscreen or protective clothing during sun exposure if you take one of these herbs while using isotretinoin.

Vitamin A: Possible Harmful Interaction

1 NEGATIVE Do not combine vitamin A supplements and isotretinoin. Based on their structural similarities, they might increase each other's toxicity.

ITRACONAZOLE

Trade Name: Sporanox

Interactions	Rating*
Negative Interactions	
Grapefruit Juice	2

*Rating Key

1 Significant interaction
2 Possibly significant interaction
3 Interaction of relatively little significance
4 Reported interaction that does not in fact exist or is insignificant

Itraconazole is an antifungal agent used to treat infections caused by fungi such as yeast (e.g., candidiasis), including infections of the hair, nails, mucous membranes, and skin.

NEGATIVE INTERACTIONS

Grapefruit Juice: Possible Harmful Interaction

2 NEGATIVE Grapefruit juice appears to decrease the body's absorption of itraconazole. In a crossover study, 11 individuals received an oral itraconazole dose of 200 mg with 240 ml of either water or double-strength grapefruit juice immediately after breakfast.[1] Grapefruit juice was associated with a substantial decrease in blood levels of the active drug, which might result in treatment failure.

Additionally, grapefruit juice could potentially interact with itraconazole in a way that could produce the opposite effect—increased blood levels of the drug.[2] Evidence suggests that, if this interaction occurs, it can last for 3 days or more following the last glass of juice.[3] However, decreased drug absorption, with lower blood levels, appears to be the predominant effect.

For these reasons, if you take itraconazole, the safest approach is to avoid grapefruit juice altogether.

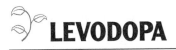

LEVODOPA

Trade Names: Dopar, Larodopa

Interactions	Rating*
Negative Interactions	
5-HTP	2
BCAAs	2
Iron	1
Kava	2
Vitamin B$_6$	1
Mixed Interaction	
S-Adenosylmethionine (SAMe)	3

*Rating Key

1 Significant interaction

2 Possibly significant interaction

3 Interaction of relatively little significance

4 Reported interaction that does not in fact exist or is insignificant

Levodopa, either by itself or in combination with carbidopa (Sinemet), is used in treating Parkinson's disease. This disease is associated with a deficit of dopamine, a neurotransmitter (a chemical messenger in the brain). Levodopa is converted to dopamine in the brain. (See also **Levodopa/Carbidopa**, page 100.)

NEGATIVE INTERACTIONS

5-HTP: Possible Harmful Interaction

2 NEGATIVE The body uses the natural substance 5-hydroxytryptophan (5-HTP) to manufacture serotonin, and supplemental forms of 5-HTP have been used for treating depression and migraine headaches. Since it is converted by the body to serotonin, 5-HTP might have antidepressant properties. For this reason, some people with Parkinson's-related depression have tried it.

However, the combination of 5-HTP and carbidopa might cause a scleroderma-like condition, in which the skin becomes hard and tight.[1,2,3] Because of the risk of this side effect, if you take the combination of levodopa and carbidopa for Parkinson's disease, avoid supplemental 5-HTP.

BCAAs: Possible Harmful Interaction

2 NEGATIVE Branched chain amino acids (BCAAs) in supplement form have been used to improve appetite in cancer patients and to slow the progression of amyotrophic lateral sclerosis (ALS, or Lou Gehrig's disease).

Dietary protein can decrease the effectiveness of levodopa in Parkinson's disease.[4] Because it is the amino acids in proteins that affect levodopa, BCAAs might cause the same problem. Therefore, if you take levodopa for Parkinson's, it may be advisable to avoid BCAAs and other amino acid supplements.

Iron: Take at a Different Time of Day

1 NEGATIVE Iron appears to interfere with the absorption of both levodopa and carbidopa by binding to them. Studies have found that blood levels of levodopa and carbidopa are reduced 30 to 51% and 75%, respectively, by iron supplementation, resulting in a worsening of symptoms of Parkinson's disease.[5] Based on this finding, you should separate the times you take iron and these drugs by as long as possible.

Kava: Possible Harmful Interaction

2 NEGATIVE The herb kava (*Piper methysticum*) has a sedative effect and is used for anxiety and insomnia.

A few case reports suggest that kava might interfere with the action of dopamine in the body.[6] This could at least partially neutralize the therapeutic effects of levodopa. In one individual, parkinsonism symptoms got worse following supplementation with kava extract (150 mg twice daily for 10 days).[7]

Based on these reports, it may be advisable to avoid combining kava with levodopa.

Vitamin B$_6$: Possible Harmful Interaction

1 NEGATIVE Vitamin B$_6$ (pyridoxine) in higher doses can reduce the therapeutic effects of levodopa in Parkinson's disease.

The daily standard nutritional intake for vitamin B$_6$ in adults is 2 mg for men and 1.6 mg for women. In higher doses of 5 to 25 mg and above, the vitamin is known to interfere with levodopa's therapeutic effects. It does this by speeding up the body's normal breakdown of levodopa in the general circulation, leaving less available for conversion to dopamine in the brain.[8] Because this effect appears to occur only with higher pyridoxine doses, you probably don't need to be concerned about an interaction with the amount of vitamin B$_6$ you get in your diet.[9]

Fortunately, most individuals with Parkinson's disease use a combination of levodopa and the drug carbidopa rather than levodopa alone. Carbidopa neutralizes the effect of vitamin B$_6$ on levodopa, making the interaction with B$_6$ unlikely in practice.

MIXED INTERACTIONS

S-Adenosylmethionine (SAMe): Possible Benefits and Risks

3
MIXED

S-Adenosylmethionine is a naturally occurring compound derived from the amino acid methionine and the energy molecule adenosine triphosphate (ATP). SAMe is widely used as a supplement for treatment of osteoarthritis and depression.

Preliminary evidence suggests that levodopa might deplete levels of SAMe in the body.[10,11] This suggests (but definitely does not prove) that individuals taking levodopa might benefit from SAMe supplements.

One short-term (30-day) double-blind study suggests that such combination treatment is safe and might help depression related to Parkinson's disease.[12] However, there are also concerns that SAMe could cause levodopa to be less effective over time.[13]

The bottom line: If you are taking levodopa, consult your physician about whether you should take SAMe as well.

Please see Appendix D, Safety Issues, for more information.

LEVODOPA/CARBIDOPA

Trade Name: Sinemet

Interactions	Rating*
Negative Interactions	
5-HTP	2
BCAAs	2
Iron	1
Kava	2
Mixed Interaction	
S-Adenosylmethionine (SAMe)	3

*Rating Key

1 Significant interaction
2 Possibly significant interaction
3 Interaction of relatively little significance
4 Reported interaction that does not in fact exist or is insignificant

Carbidopa in combination with levodopa is used in treating Parkinson's disease. This disease is associated with a deficit of dopamine, a neurotransmitter (a chemical messenger in the brain). By preventing the breakdown of levodopa in the general circulation, carbidopa enables more levodopa to enter the brain, where it is converted into dopamine. (See also **Levodopa** page 97.)

NEGATIVE INTERACTIONS

5-HTP: Possible Harmful Interaction

2 NEGATIVE The body uses the natural substance 5-hydroxytryptophan (5-HTP) to manufacture serotonin, and supplemental forms of 5-HTP have been used for treating depression and migraine headaches. Since it is converted by the body to serotonin, 5-HTP might have antidepressant properties. For this reason, some people with Parkinson's-related depression have tried it.

However, the combination of 5-HTP and carbidopa might cause a scleroderma-like condition, in which the skin becomes hard and tight.[1,2,3] Because of the risk of this side effect, if you take levodopa/carbidopa for Parkinson's disease, avoid supplemental 5-HTP.

BCAAs: Possible Harmful Interaction

2 NEGATIVE Branched chain amino acids (BCAAs) in supplement form have been used to improve appetite in cancer patients and to slow the progression of amyotrophic lateral sclerosis (ALS, or Lou Gehrig's disease).

Dietary protein can decrease the effectiveness of levodopa in Parkinson's disease.[4] Because it is the amino acids in proteins that affect levodopa, BCAAs might cause the same problem. Therefore, if you take levodopa/carbidopa for Parkinson's, it may be advisable to avoid BCAAs and other amino acid supplements.

Iron: Take at a Different Time of Day

1 NEGATIVE Iron appears to interfere with the absorption of both levodopa and carbidopa by binding to them. Studies have found that blood levels of levodopa and carbidopa are reduced 30 to 51% and 75%, respectively, by iron supplementation, resulting in a worsening of symptoms of Parkinson's disease.[5] Based on this finding, you should separate the times you take iron and these drugs by as long as possible.

Kava: Possible Harmful Interaction

2 NEGATIVE The herb kava (*Piper methysticum*) has a sedative effect and is used for anxiety and insomnia.

A few case reports suggest that kava might interfere with the action of dopamine in the body.[6] This could at least partially neutralize the therapeutic effects of levodopa. In one individual, parkinsonism symptoms got worse following supplementation with kava extract (150 mg twice daily for 10 days).[7]

Based on these reports, it may be advisable to avoid kava during levodopa/carbidopa therapy.

MIXED INTERACTIONS

S-adenosylmethionine (SAMe): Possible Benefits and Risks

3 MIXED S-adenosylmethionine is a naturally occurring compound derived from the amino acid methionine and the energy molecule adenosine triphosphate (ATP). SAMe is widely used as a supplement for treatment of osteoarthritis and depression.

Preliminary evidence suggests that levodopa might deplete levels of SAMe in the body.[8,9] This suggests (but definitely does not prove) that individuals taking levodopa/carbidopa might benefit from SAMe supplements.

One short-term (30-day) double-blind study suggests that such combination treatment is safe and might help depression related to Parkinson's disease.[10] However, there are also concerns that SAMe could cause levodopa to be less effective over time.[11]

The bottom line: If you are taking levodopa/carbidopa, consult your physician about whether you should take SAMe as well.

Please see Appendix D, Safety Issues, for more information.

LOOP DIURETICS

Interactions	Rating*
Negative Interactions	
Licorice	2
St. John's Wort, Dong Quai	3
Positive Interactions	
Magnesium	2
Potassium	1
Vitamin B$_1$ (Thiamin)	2

*Rating Key

1 Significant interaction

2 Possibly significant interaction

3 Interaction of relatively little significance

4 Reported interaction that does not in fact exist or is insignificant

These powerful diuretics reduce fluid accumulation in the body by causing the kidneys to channel more fluid into the urine. This makes them useful for treating high blood pressure and edema (excessive fluid in body tissues). Drugs in this family include

- bumetanide (Bumex)
- ethacrynic acid (Edecrin)
- furosemide (Lasix)
- torsemide (Demadex)
- and others

NEGATIVE INTERACTIONS

Licorice: Possible Harmful Interaction

2 NEGATIVE Licorice root, a member of the pea family, has been used since ancient times as both food and medicine.

Glycyrrhizic acid, the active ingredient in licorice (*Glycyrrhiza glabra* or *G. uralensis*), promotes potassium loss in the urine,[1,2] and there have been case reports of low blood levels of potassium following long-term or high-dose licorice use.[3,4,5] Because loop diuretics also cause potassium loss, individuals taking these drugs should avoid licorice supplementation. An often-unrecognized source of licorice is chewing tobacco.[6]

A special type of licorice known as DGL (deglycyrrhizinated licorice) is a deliberately altered form of the herb that should not affect potassium levels and so should not pose a danger for loop diuretic users.

St. John's Wort, Dong Quai: Possible Harmful Interaction

3 NEGATIVE St. John's wort (*Hypericum perforatum*) is primarily used to treat mild to moderate depression.

The herb dong quai (*Angelica sinensis*) is often recommended for menstrual disorders such as dysmenorrhea, PMS, and irregular menstruation.

Loop diuretics have been reported to cause increased sensitivity to the sun, amplifying the risk of sunburn or skin rash. Because St. John's wort and dong quai may also cause this problem, taking these herbal supplements during treatment with loop diuretics might add to this risk.

It may be a good idea to wear a sunscreen or protective clothing during sun exposure if you take one of these herbs while using a loop diuretic.

POSITIVE INTERACTIONS

Magnesium: Supplementation Probably Helpful

2 POSITIVE Loop diuretics can wash magnesium out of the body in the urine.[7,8,9] In some cases, this may lead to magnesium deficiency. Additionally, untreated magnesium depletion can make it more difficult to correct potassium depletion.[10]

Because magnesium deficiency is common anyway, magnesium supplementation at standard nutritional doses might make sense, especially if you must stay on diuretic therapy for a long time. Adding a type of diuretic that helps counteract magnesium loss is another option.

Please see Appendix D, Safety Issues, for more information.

Potassium: Supplementation Probably Helpful

1 POSITIVE As with magnesium, loop diuretics wash potassium out of the body in the urine. This may cause potassium blood levels to fall too low and produce symptoms such as muscle cramps or weakness. Heart rhythm irregularities may also occur, especially in those taking the heart drug **digoxin** (see page 74).

The classic treatment is to consume high-potassium foods such as bananas and orange juice. Potassium levels can also be raised by potassium supplements and salt substitutes containing potassium. Adding a type of diuretic that helps counteract potassium loss is another option.

Please see Appendix D, Safety Issues, for more information.

Vitamin B₁ (Thiamin): Supplementation Probably Helpful

2
POSITIVE One study suggests that the loop diuretic furosemide may deplete vitamin B$_1$, apparently by washing it out of the body in the urine.[11] Vitamin B$_1$ deficiency was found in 21 of the 23 participants with congestive heart failure taking furosemide, compared to only 2 of the 16 healthy control participants. Another study indicates that malnourishment caused by the congestive heart failure itself may also be a factor in this deficiency.[12]

In any case, there is evidence that supplementation with vitamin B$_1$ may improve heart function in individuals with congestive heart failure who are taking loop diuretics.[13,14]

Please see Appendix D, Safety Issues, for more information.

MAO INHIBITORS

Interactions	Rating*
Negative Interactions	
Asian Ginseng	2
Ephedra	1
Green Tea	2
SAMe, 5-HTP	2
Scotch Broom	1
St. John's Wort	2
Positive Interaction	
Vitamin B$_6$ (Pyridoxine)	2

*Rating Key

1 Significant interaction
2 Possibly significant interaction
3 Interaction of relatively little significance
4 Reported interaction that does not in fact exist or is insignificant

MAO inhibitors (monoamine oxidase inhibitors) were the first antidepressant drugs developed. They increase levels of neurotransmitters (chemicals that enable nerve transmission) by interfering with their normal breakdown in the body.

MAO inhibitors can be dangerous if combined with certain foods, drugs, or supplements. For instance, if you're on MAO inhibitor therapy and ingest tyramine, a substance naturally present in some cheeses, beer, fermented soy products, and other foods, your blood pressure can soar out of control. Drugs in this family include

- furazolidone (Furoxone)
- isocarboxazid (Marplan)
- phenelzine sulfate (Nardil)
- tranylcypromine sulfate (Parnate)
- and others

NEGATIVE INTERACTIONS

Asian Ginseng: Possible Harmful Interaction

2 NEGATIVE The herb Asian ginseng (*Panax ginseng*) is promoted as an adaptogen, a treatment that helps the body adapt to stress and resist illness in general.

According to two case reports, the combination of Asian ginseng and the MAO inhibitor phenelzine caused headache, insomnia, trembling, and other symptoms.[1,2] It is uncertain whether these effects might be related to the ginsenosides present in Asian ginseng[3,4] or to caffeine contamination that can occur with any ginseng product.[5]

In any case, it would be prudent to avoid ginseng–MAO inhibitor combinations until more is known about them.

Ephedra: Harmful Interaction

1
NEGATIVE The herb ephedra (*Ephedra sinica*, *E. intermedia*, or *E. equisetina*) contains ephedrine,[6] a compound that can elevate blood pressure directly and also indirectly by promoting the release of body chemicals that raise blood pressure. The herb is widely promoted as a stimulant and weight-loss aid.

MAO inhibitors prevent the normal breakdown of the stimulant chemicals released in response to ephedra, allowing them to build up unchecked.[7] For this reason, taking an MAO inhibitor along with ephedra could result in serious problems, including possible hypertensive crisis, an emergency condition in which the blood pressure shoots dangerously high.

You can protect yourself by not taking ephedra if you are using an MAO inhibitor. Ephedra is sometimes listed as ma huang or other names on product labels.

Green Tea: Possible Harmful Interaction

2
NEGATIVE Green tea (*Camellia sinensis*) contains strong antioxidant substances that may have cancer-preventive effects.

Because it contains caffeine, green tea should not be combined with MAO inhibitors. Caffeine is a stimulant that may promote the release of body chemicals that elevate blood pressure, thus adding to the effects of MAO inhibitors.

It is best not to mix green tea (or other caffeine sources, including black tea) with MAO inhibitors.

SAMe, 5-HTP: Possible Harmful Interaction

2
NEGATIVE SAMe (s-adenosylmethionine) is a naturally occurring compound derived from the amino acid methionine and the energy molecule adenosine triphosphate (ATP).

The natural substance 5-HTP (5-hydroxytryptophan) is converted by the body to serotonin.

Both SAMe and 5-HTP are sometimes used for depression. However, there may be a risk of serotonin syndrome when combining either of these supplements with MAO inhibitors.

Serotonin is a neurotransmitter involved in depression, and most antidepressants affect serotonin levels.

Serotonin syndrome, a toxic reaction requiring immediate medical attention, is associated with too much serotonin. Symptoms may include anxiety, restlessness, confusion, weakness, tremor, muscle twitching or spasm, high fever, profuse sweating, and rapid heartbeat.

One report describes a case of apparent serotonin syndrome in an individual taking SAMe with clomipramine, a **tricyclic antidepressant** (see page 184) that increases serotonin activity.[8]

Because MAO inhibitors are known to increase the activity of serotonin, the same thing might happen if SAMe were taken with these drugs.

Since 5-HTP is converted to serotonin in the body, it could potentially contribute to serotonin syndrome as well.

Scotch Broom: Harmful Interaction

1 NEGATIVE The herb scotch broom (*Sarothamnus scoparius*) contains tyramine, a substance that can raise blood pressure.[9] As mentioned previously, tyramine is a substance found naturally in some foods. It is normally harmless, because an enzyme called MAO is at work constantly breaking it down to inactive byproducts. However, MAO inhibitors block the action of this protective enzyme, permitting tyramine levels to rise and blood pressure to escalate uncontrolled.

Avoid taking scotch broom with an MAO inhibitor.

St. John's Wort: Possible Harmful Interaction

2 NEGATIVE The herb St. John's wort (*Hypericum perforatum*) is primarily used to treat mild to moderate depression.

Test tube and animal studies suggest that St. John's wort may elevate serotonin levels in the brain.

Symptoms of excess serotonin (serotonin syndrome) have been reported in individuals combining St. John's wort with **SSRI antidepressants** (see page 158) and other serotonin-enhancing drugs.[10,11]

Serotonin syndrome is a serious condition requiring immediate medical attention. Symptoms may include anxiety, restlessness, confusion, weakness, tremor, muscle twitching or spasm, high fever, profuse sweating, and rapid heartbeat.

Because serotonin syndrome is a known risk of combining SSRI antidepressants with MAO inhibitors, it also may be likely to occur with the St. John's wort–MAO inhibitor combination. For this reason, you should avoid St. John's wort if you take an MAO inhibitor.

POSITIVE INTERACTIONS

Vitamin B$_6$ (Pyridoxine): Supplementation Probably Helpful

2
POSITIVE The MAO inhibitors phenelzine and isocarboxazid are structurally similar to the antituberculosis drug **isoniazid** (see page 93), and may likewise attach to and disable the active form of vitamin B$_6$ (see Vitamin B$_6$ in the full chapter on **Isoniazid**). In fact, a nerve disorder related to vitamin B$_6$ deficiency has been reported in an individual taking phenelzine.[12] Vitamin B$_6$ supplementation, in at least nutritional doses, may be good insurance if you are on MAO inhibitor therapy.

Please see Appendix D, Safety Issues, for more information.

METHOTREXATE

Trade Names: Folex PFS, Immunex, Rheumatrex

Interactions	Rating*
Negative Interactions	
Potassium Citrate	3
St. John's Wort, Dong Quai	3
White Willow	2
Positive Interaction	
Folate	1

*Rating Key

1 Significant interaction
2 Possibly significant interaction
3 Interaction of relatively little significance
4 Reported interaction that does not in fact exist or is insignificant

Methotrexate is used in cancer chemotherapy as well as for treating inflammatory diseases such as rheumatoid arthritis and psoriasis.

NEGATIVE INTERACTIONS

Potassium Citrate: Possible Harmful Interaction

3 NEGATIVE Potassium citrate and other forms of citrate (e.g., calcium citrate, magnesium citrate) may be used to prevent kidney stones. These agents work by making the urine less acidic.

This effect on the urine may lead to decreased blood levels and therapeutic effects of methotrexate.[1]

It may be advisable to avoid these citrate compounds during methotrexate therapy except under medical supervision.

St. John's Wort, Dong Quai: Possible Harmful Interaction

3 NEGATIVE St. John's wort (*Hypericum perforatum*) is primarily used to treat mild to moderate depression.

The herb dong quai (*Angelica sinensis*) is often recommended for menstrual disorders such as dysmenorrhea, PMS, and irregular menstruation.

Methotrexate has been reported to cause increased sensitivity to the sun, amplifying the risk of sunburn or skin rash. Because St. John's wort and dong quai may also cause this problem, taking these herbal supplements during methotrexate therapy might add to this risk.

It may be a good idea to wear a sunscreen or protective clothing during sun exposure if you take one of these herbs while using methotrexate.

Methotrexate

White Willow: Possible Harmful Interaction

2 NEGATIVE The herb white willow (*Salix alba*), also known as willow bark, is used to treat pain and fever. White willow contains a substance that is converted by the body into a salicylate similar to aspirin.

Case reports suggest that salicylates can increase methotrexate blood levels and toxicity.[2] For this reason, you should avoid combining white willow with methotrexate.

POSITIVE INTERACTIONS

Folate: Supplementation Possibly Helpful

1 POSITIVE Folate (also known as folic acid) is a B vitamin that plays an important role in many vital aspects of health, including preventing neural tube birth defects and possibly reducing the risk of heart disease. Because inadequate intake of folate is widespread, if you are taking any medication that depletes or impairs folate even slightly, you may need supplementation.

Methotrexate is called a "folate antagonist" because it prevents the body from converting folate to its active form. In fact, this inactivation of folate plays a role in methotrexate's therapeutic effects. This leads to an interesting catch-22: methotrexate use can lead to folate deficiency, but taking extra folate might prevent methotrexate from working properly.

However, evidence suggests that individuals who take methotrexate for rheumatoid arthritis, juvenile rheumatoid arthritis, or psoriasis can use folate supplements to good effect.[3,4,5] Not only does the methotrexate continue to work properly, but its usual side effects may decrease also.

In a double-blind study of individuals taking methotrexate for rheumatoid arthritis and supplemented with various doses of oral folate, methotrexate-related side effects were similar to those in people taking placebo.[6] Moreover, methotrexate's benefits were not blunted by folate. In another study, folate (5 mg daily) eliminated the gastrointestinal side effects associated with oral methotrexate therapy for psoriasis, also without interfering with the drug's therapeutic benefits.[7]

Therefore, folate supplementation may be advisable in individuals taking methotrexate for psoriasis, rheumatoid arthritis, or juvenile rheumatoid arthritis.[8]

Note: This does not necessarily mean that it is safe to take folate supplements if you are using methotrexate for some other condition, such as cancer. We just don't know yet.

Please see Appendix D, Safety Issues, for more information.

METHYLDOPA *(Aldoclor, Aldomet)*

Interactions	Rating*
Negative Interactions	
Iron	1
St. John's Wort, Dong Quai	3

*Rating Key

1 Significant interaction

2 Possibly significant interaction

3 Interaction of relatively little significance

4 Reported interaction that does not in fact exist or is insignificant

Methyldopa is a medication that is sometimes used to control high blood pressure, though it is not a first-line treatment due to various health risks associated with its use. (See also **Antihypertensive Agents**, page 36.)

NEGATIVE INTERACTIONS

Iron: Take at a Different Time of Day

1 NEGATIVE Forms of iron include ferrous fumarate, ferrous gluconate, ferrous sulfate, and iron polysaccharide.

Ferrous sulfate and ferrous gluconate have been found to substantially decrease the absorption of methyldopa and interfere with blood pressure control.

In a trial with 12 participants, absorption of methyldopa was reduced by 73% with ferrous sulfate (325 mg) and by 61% with ferrous gluconate (600 mg).[1] Blood pressure increased in four of five individuals (substantially in three) given ferrous sulfate for 2 weeks. When the iron supplement was stopped, blood pressure declined. Giving an iron supplement even 2 hours before the drug resulted in a 42% fall in methyldopa absorption.[2]

For these reasons, it would be advisable to separate doses of iron and methyldopa by as long as possible.

St. John's Wort, Dong Quai: Possible Harmful Interaction

3 NEGATIVE St. John's wort (*Hypericum perforatum*) is primarily used to treat mild to moderate depression.

The herb dong quai (*Angelica sinensis*) is often recommended for menstrual disorders such as dysmenorrhea, PMS, and irregular menstruation.

Methyldopa has been reported to cause increased sensitivity to the sun, amplifying the risk of sunburn or skin rash. Because St. John's wort and dong quai may also cause this problem, taking these herbal supplements during methyldopa therapy might add to this risk.

It may be a good idea to wear a sunscreen or protective clothing during sun exposure if you take one of these herbs while using methyldopa.

NITROFURANTOIN

Trade Names: Furadantin, Furalan, Furatoin, Macrobid, Macrodantin

Interactions	Rating*
Negative Interaction	
Magnesium	3

*Rating Key

1 Significant interaction

2 Possibly significant interaction

3 Interaction of relatively little significance

4 Reported interaction that does not in fact exist or is insignificant

Nitrofurantoin is sometimes taken on an ongoing basis to prevent bladder infections. In lower doses, the drug retards growth of infection-causing bacteria; in higher doses, it kills bacteria. (See also **Antibiotics**, page 19.)

NEGATIVE INTERACTIONS

Magnesium: Take at a Different Time of Day

3 NEGATIVE Magnesium trisilicate appears to decrease the absorption of nitrofurantoin.[1] In one study, a magnesium-aluminum antacid reduced blood levels of nitrofurantoin by about 25% in 10 volunteers.[2] Whether this effect has practical importance has not been determined, but it is possible that the therapeutic effect of nitrofurantoin might be lessened by magnesium.

For this reason, either avoid this combination or separate doses of magnesium supplements and nitrofurantoin by as long as possible.

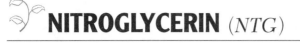

NITROGLYCERIN (NTG)

Trade Names: Deponit, Nitro-Bid, Nitro-Dur, Nitrostat, Nitrol

Interactions	Rating*
Mixed Interaction	
N-Acetyl Cysteine (NAC)	3
Positive Interaction	
Vitamin C	3

*Rating Key

1　Significant interaction
2　Possibly significant interaction
3　Interaction of relatively little significance
4　Reported interaction that does not in fact exist or is insignificant

Nitroglycerin (NTG) is one of the most commonly used treatments for quick relief of anginal pain. Related drugs include isosorbide dinitrate and isosorbide mononitrate.

MIXED INTERACTIONS

N-Acetyl Cysteine (NAC): Possible Benefits and Risks

3 MIXED N-acetyl cysteine (NAC) is a specially modified form of the dietary amino acid cysteine that has various proposed uses.

Nitrates such as nitroglycerin lose some of their effectiveness over time. According to some studies,[1,2] but not all,[3,4] the supplement N-acetyl cysteine might help these drugs work better. However, there's a catch: the combination of NAC and nitroglycerin appears to cause severe headaches.[5,6]

Taking NAC with nitroglycerin may be beneficial in some cases. However, unpleasant side effects probably limit the use of this combination.

Please see Appendix D, Safety Issues, for more information.

POSITIVE INTERACTIONS

Vitamin C: Supplementation Possibly Helpful

3 POSITIVE The body develops a kind of tolerance for nitroglycerin over time. There is some evidence that vitamin C might counteract this tolerance and help nitroglycerin remain effective, possibly due to the antioxidant action of the vitamin.[7,8]

A placebo-controlled study involving nine participants found that 1,000 mg of vitamin C given 3 times daily kept the nitrate drug working up to par during long-term therapy.[9] A double-blind study with 48 participants found similar results for 2,000 mg of vitamin C given 3 times daily during nitroglycerin therapy.[10]

Supplemental vitamin C may be worth trying in people taking continuous nitrate therapy to see if it can help prevent nitrate tolerance.

Please see Appendix D, Safety Issues, for more information.

NITROUS OXIDE

Interactions	Rating*
Positive Interaction	
Vitamin B$_{12}$, Folate	1

*Rating Key

1 Significant interaction

2 Possibly significant interaction

3 Interaction of relatively little significance

4 Reported interaction that does not in fact exist or is insignificant

Nitrous oxide gas is used primarily as a local anesthetic in dentistry as well as in certain phases of cardiac bypass surgery.

POSITIVE INTERACTIONS

Vitamin B$_{12}$, Folate: Supplementation Possibly Helpful

1 POSITIVE Abundant evidence suggests that nitrous oxide inactivates vitamin B$_{12}$,[1,2,3] and this may possibly lead to B$_{12}$ deficiency. The inactivated B$_{12}$ is rapidly replaced,[4] so short-term exposure of healthy individuals to nitrous oxide appears to cause no significant problems. However, long-term exposure can produce anemia and neurologic complications.

Individuals with existing vitamin B$_{12}$ deficiency are especially at risk[5] because their bodies cannot replace B$_{12}$, and seriously ill people have another strike against them.[6] If the deficiency is not identified and managed, the resulting neurologic damage may not be correctable and could be fatal.[7]

The effect on vitamin B$_{12}$ also may lead to folate deficiency in seriously ill people and make matters even worse.[8,9,10]

Professionals regularly exposed to nitrous oxide, such as dentists and dental hygienists, may be at risk as well.

Vitamin B$_{12}$ deficiency should be identified and treated before exposure to nitrous oxide anesthesia. In seriously ill individuals, supplementation with both vitamin B$_{12}$ and folate (or folinic acid, a derivative of folic acid) should be considered.

Please see Appendix D, Safety Issues, for more information.

NONSTEROIDAL ANTI-INFLAMMATORY DRUGS (*NSAIDs*)

Interactions	Rating*
Negative Interactions	
Arginine	3
Feverfew	2
Garlic	2
Ginkgo	2
Policosanol	2
Potassium Citrate	2
St. John's Wort, Dong Quai	3
Vitamin E	2
White Willow	3
Herbs and Supplements	3

Interactions	Rating*
Positive Interactions	
Cayenne	3
Colostrum	3
Folate	2
Licorice	3
Vitamin C	3

*Rating Key

1 Significant interaction

2 Possibly significant interaction

3 Interaction of relatively little significance

4 Reported interaction that does not in fact exist or is insignificant

NSAIDs are used to treat pain, fever, and inflammation. Traditional NSAIDs block COX-1 and COX-2 enzymes that the body uses to manufacture substances called prostaglandins. Since COX-1 prostaglandins are stomach-protective, blocking this enzyme is associated with gastrointestinal toxicity, a known side effect of these drugs. Newer NSAIDs (called COX-2 inhibitors) block primarily COX-2 prostaglandins associated with pain, fever, and inflammation, and are thought to be less risky to the stomach. Drugs in this family include

- aspirin, alternatively called acetylsalicylic acid or ASA (Adprin-B, Anacin, Arthritis Foundation Aspirin, Ascriptin, Aspergum, Asprimox, Bayer, BC, Bufferin, Buffex, Cama, Cope, Easprin, Ecotrin, Empirin, Equagesic, Fiorinal, Fiortal, Halfprin, Heartline, Genprin, Lanorinal, Magnaprin, Measurin, Micrainin, Momentum, Norwich, St. Joseph, ZORprin)
- bromfenac sodium (Duract)
- celecoxib (Celebrex)
- choline salicylate (Arthropan)
- choline salicylate/magnesium salicylate (Tricosal, Trilisate)
- diclofenac potassium (Cataflam, Voltaren Rapide)
- diclofenac sodium (Arthrotec, Voltaren, Voltaren SR, Voltaren-XR)
- diclofenac sodium/misoprostol (Arthrotec)
- diflunisal (Dolobid)

- etodolac (Lodine, Lodine XL)
- fenoprofen calcium (Nalfon)
- flurbiprofen (Ansaid)
- ibuprofen (Advil, Arthritis Foundation Ibuprofen, Bayer Select Ibuprofen, Dynafed IB, Genpril, Haltran, IBU, Ibuprin, Ibuprohm, Menadol, Midol IB, Motrin, Nuprin, Saleto)
- indomethacin (Indochron E-R, Indocin, Indocin SR, Indometacin, Indomethacin SR, Novomethacin)
- ketoprofen (Actron, Orudis, Orudis KT, Oruvail)
- ketorolac tromethamine (Toradol)
- magnesium salicylate (Doan's, Magan, Mobidin, Backache Maximum Strength Relief, Bayer Select Maximum Strength Backache, Momentum Muscular Backache Formula, Nuprin Backache, Mobigesic, Magsal)
- meclofenamate sodium (Mecolfen, Meclomen)
- mefenamic acid (Ponstan, Ponstel)
- nabumetone (Relafen)
- naproxen (EC-Naprosyn, Napron X, Naprosyn)
- naproxen sodium (Aleve, Anaprox, Anaprox DS, Naprelan)
- oxaprozin (Daypro)
- piroxicam (Feldene)
- rofecoxib (Vioxx)
- salsalate or salicylic acid (Amigesic, Argesic-SA, Arthra-G, Disalcid, Marthritic, Mono-Gesic, Salflex, Salgesic, Salsitab)
- sodium salicylate (Pabalate)
- sodium thiosalicylate (Rexolate)
- sulfasalazine (Azulfidine EN-tabs, Salazopyrin, SAS-500)
- sulindac (Clinoril)
- tolmetin sodium (Tolectin, Tolectin DS)
- and others

NEGATIVE INTERACTIONS

Arginine: Possible Harmful Interaction

3 NEGATIVE Arginine is an amino acid found in many foods, including dairy products, meat, poultry, and fish. Supplemental arginine has been proposed as a treatment for various conditions, including heart problems.

Arginine has been found to stimulate the body's production of gastrin, a hormone that increases stomach acid.[1] Because excessive acid can irritate the stomach, there are concerns that arginine could be harmful for individuals taking drugs that are also hard on the stomach (such as NSAIDs).

It may be best not to mix arginine with NSAIDs unless approved by your doctor.

Feverfew: Possible Harmful Interaction

2 NEGATIVE The herb feverfew (*Tanacetum parthenium*) is primarily used for the prevention and treatment of migraine headaches.

NSAIDs are also used for migraines, so there is a chance that some individuals might use both the herb and drug at once, a combination that may present risks.

The biggest concern with NSAIDs is that they can cause stomach ulcers, which may progress to bleeding or perforation without pain or other warning symptoms. This stomach damage is due to drug interference with the body's protective prostaglandins. Newer NSAIDs called COX-2 inhibitors may be less likely to produce this side effect.

Feverfew also affects prostaglandins.[2,3,4] Thus, combining it with an NSAID might increase the risk of stomach problems.

Garlic, Ginkgo: Possible Harmful Interaction

2 NEGATIVE The herb garlic (*Allium sativum*) is taken to lower cholesterol, among many other proposed uses.

One of the possible side effects of garlic is an increased tendency to bleed.[5,6] Therefore, you should not combine garlic and aspirin or other NSAIDs except under medical supervision.

The herb ginkgo is used to treat Alzheimer's disease and ordinary age-related memory loss, among many other uses.

One case report suggests that the combination of ginkgo and aspirin might increase the chance of bleeding problems.[7]

You probably should not take ginkgo while using NSAIDs except under medical supervision.

Policosanol: Possible Harmful Interaction

 Policosanol, derived from sugar cane, has been taken for hyperlipidemia and intermittent claudication.

Human trials suggest that policosanol makes blood platelets more slippery, an action that could potentiate the blood-thinning effects of aspirin and other drugs in this family, possibly causing a risk of abnormal bleeding episodes.[8] A 30-day double-blind placebo-controlled trial of 27 individuals with high cholesterol levels found that policosanol at 10 mg daily markedly reduced the ability of blood platelets to clump together.[9] Another double-blind placebo-controlled study of 37 healthy volunteers found evidence that the blood-thinning effect of policosanol increased as the dose was increased—the larger the policosanol dose, the greater the effect.[10] Yet another double-blind placebo-controlled study of 43 healthy volunteers compared the effects of policosanol (20 mg daily), aspirin (100 mg daily), and policosanol and aspirin combined at these same doses.[11] The results again showed that policosanol substantially reduced the ability of blood platelets to stick together, and that the combined therapy exhibited additive effects.

Based on these findings, it would be advisable to avoid combining aspirin or other NSAIDs with policosanol except under medical supervision.

Potassium Citrate: Possible Harmful Interaction

2 NEGATIVE Potassium citrate and other forms of citrate (e.g., calcium citrate, magnesium citrate) may be used to prevent kidney stones. These agents work by making the urine less acidic.

This effect on the urine may lead to decreased blood levels and therapeutic effects of several drugs, including aspirin and other salicylates (choline salicylate, magnesium salicylate, salsalate, sodium salicylate, sodium thiosalicylate).[12]

It may be advisable to avoid these citrate compounds during therapy with aspirin or salicylates except under medical supervision.

St. John's Wort, Dong Quai: Possible Harmful Interaction

3 NEGATIVE St. John's wort (*Hypericum perforatum*) is primarily used to treat mild to moderate depression.

The herb dong quai (*Angelica sinensis*) is often recommended for menstrual disorders such as dysmenorrhea, PMS, and irregular menstruation.

Certain NSAIDs, including most notably piroxicam, can cause increased sensitivity to the sun, amplifying the risk of sunburn or skin rash. Because St. John's wort and dong quai may also cause this problem, taking these herbal supplements during NSAID therapy might add to this risk.

It may be a good idea to wear a sunscreen or protective clothing during sun exposure if you take one of these herbs while using an NSAID.

Vitamin E: Possible Harmful Interaction

2 NEGATIVE Vitamin E appears to add to aspirin's blood-thinning effects. One study suggests that the combination of aspirin and even relatively small amounts of vitamin E (50 mg daily) may lead to a significantly increased risk of bleeding.[13] In another study of 28,519 men, vitamin E supplementation at a low dose of about 50 IU (international units) daily was associated with an increase in fatal hemorrhagic strokes, the kind of stroke caused by bleeding within the brain.[14] However, there was a reduced risk of the more common ischemic stroke, caused by obstruction of a blood vessel in the brain, and the two effects were found to essentially cancel each other out.

The bottom line: Seek medical advice before combining vitamin E and aspirin.

White Willow: Possible Harmful Interaction

3 NEGATIVE The herb white willow (*Salix alba*), also known as willow bark, is used to treat pain and fever.

White willow contains a substance that is converted by the body into a salicylate similar to aspirin. It is therefore possible that taking NSAIDs and white willow could lead to increased risk of side effects, just as would occur if you combined NSAIDs with aspirin.

Herbs and Supplements: Possible Harmful Interaction

3 NEGATIVE Based on their known effects or constituents, the herbs dong quai (*Angelica sinensis*), garlic (*Allium sativum*), ginger (*Zingiber officinale*), horse chestnut (*Aesculus hippocastanum*), and red clover (*Trifolium pratense*), and the substances aortic glycosaminoglycans (GAGs), fish oil, and OPCs (oligomeric proanthocyanidins) might conceivably present an increased risk of bleeding if combined with aspirin.

POSITIVE INTERACTIONS

Cayenne: Supplementation Possibly Helpful

3 POSITIVE Cayenne (*Capsicum annuum* or *C. frutescens*) and other hot peppers used in chili and various dishes contain as their "hot" ingredient capsaicin, a substance that is thought to be stomach-protective.

For years, people have believed that spicy foods were a cause of stomach ulcers. However, preliminary evidence suggests that cayenne peppers might actually help protect the stomach against ulcers caused by aspirin and possibly other NSAIDs.[15,16,17]

In a study involving 18 healthy human volunteers, one group received chili powder, water, and aspirin; the control group received only water and aspirin.[18] Chili powder was found to significantly protect the stomach against damage from aspirin, a known stomach irritant. It was suggested that this protective effect might result from capsaicin-induced stimulation of blood flow in the lining of the stomach.

Further support for this theory comes from a study in rats which found that capsaicin protected the stomach against damage caused by aspirin, ethanol (drinking alcohol), and acid.[19] Increasing the dose of capsaicin brought even greater benefit, as did increasing the time between giving capsaicin and the other agents. An earlier study in rats found that capsaicin exerted similar protection against aspirin damage.[20]

Some researchers have used this data to advocate chili or capsaicin as treatment for peptic ulcer disease,[21] but check with your doctor before trying to self-treat this serious condition.

Please see Appendix D, Safety Issues, for more information.

Colostrum: Supplementation Possibly Helpful

3 POSITIVE Colostrum is the fluid that new mothers' breasts produce during the first day or two after birth. It gives newborns a rich mixture of antibodies and growth factors that help them get a good start.

According to one study involving rats, taking colostrum from cows (bovine colostrum) as a supplement might help protect against the ulcers caused by NSAIDs.[22]

Please see Appendix D, Safety Issues, for more information.

Folate: Supplementation Possibly Helpful

2 POSITIVE Folate (also known as folic acid) is a B vitamin that plays an important role in many vital aspects of health, including preventing neural tube birth defects and possibly reducing the risk of heart disease. Because inadequate intake of folate is widespread, if you are taking any medication that depletes or impairs folate even slightly, you may need supplementation.

There is some evidence that NSAIDs might produce this effect. In test tube studies, many NSAIDs have been found to interfere with folate activity.[23,24,25] In addition, a study of 25 people with arthritis receiving the drug sulfasalazine found evidence of folate deficiency.[26] In another report, a woman taking 650 mg of aspirin every 4 hours for 3 days experienced a significant fall in blood levels of folate.[27]

Based on this preliminary evidence, folate supplementation may be warranted if you are taking drugs in the NSAID family.

Please see Appendix D, Safety Issues, for more information.

Licorice: Supplementation Possibly Helpful

3 POSITIVE Licorice root (*Glycyrrhiza glabra* or *G. uralensis*), a member of the pea family, has been used since ancient times as both food and medicine.

Preliminary evidence suggests that a specific form of licorice called DGL (deglycyrrhizinated licorice) might help protect the stomach against damage caused by the use of aspirin and possibly other NSAIDs. (DGL is a modified version of licorice that is safer to use.)

In a double-blind study of 9 healthy human volunteers, participants were given aspirin alone (325 mg) or aspirin (325 mg) plus DGL (175 mg).[28] Stomach damage (as measured by blood loss) was found to be about 20% less when DGL was given with aspirin. As part of the same study, DGL was also found to reduce stomach damage caused by aspirin in rats, though the benefit was small. It is possible that larger doses of DGL might provide greater protection.

Please see Appendix D, Safety Issues, for more information.

Vitamin C: Supplementation Possibly Helpful

3 POSITIVE Test tube studies suggest that aspirin promotes the loss of vitamin C through the urine,[29,30] which could lead to tissue depletion of the vitamin. In addition, low vitamin C levels have been noted in individuals with rheumatoid arthritis, and this has been attributed to aspirin therapy taken for this condition.[31]

If you take aspirin regularly, vitamin C supplementation may be advisable.

Please see Appendix D, Safety Issues, for more information.

ORAL CONTRACEPTIVES (OCs, Birth Control Pills)

Interactions	Rating*
Negative Interactions	
Androstenedione	3
Copper	3
Licorice	2
Milk Thistle	3
St. John's Wort	2
St. John's Wort, Dong Quai	3
Positive Interactions	
Folate	4
Magnesium	3
Soy	4
Vitamin B$_2$ (Riboflavin)	3

Interactions	Rating*
Positive Interactions *(cont.)*	
Vitamin B$_6$	4
Vitamin B$_{12}$	4
Vitamin C	3
Zinc	3

*Rating Key

1 Significant interaction
2 Possibly significant interaction
3 Interaction of relatively little significance
4 Reported interaction that does not in fact exist or is insignificant

Oral contraceptives (OCs), or birth control pills, are some of the most effective contraceptive drugs. They work by suppressing ovulation (discharge of the egg from the ovary).

NEGATIVE INTERACTIONS

Androstenedione: Possible Harmful Interaction

3 NEGATIVE Androstenedione has become popular as a sports supplement, based on the theory that it increases the body's testosterone levels and enhances sports performance. However, the best-documented effect of androstenedione is a rise in estrogen levels.[1,2,3]

This finding raises concerns that combining androstenedione with OCs could increase the risk of estrogen-related side effects.

It would seem best for OC users to avoid androstenedione supplementation.

Copper: Possible Harmful Interaction

3 NEGATIVE Oral contraceptives appear to increase blood levels of the trace mineral copper.[4,5] The latest OCs may elevate copper levels to a greater extent, possibly due to the newer progestins used in them.[6]

Elevated levels of copper might not be good for you. Epidemiologic studies suggest that high copper levels in the blood are associated with increased risk of heart disease.[7,8] However, such studies do not prove that copper is a direct cause of increased heart disease risk; other unidentified factors may play a role.

Nonetheless, it may not be a good idea to take copper supplements while using OCs.

Licorice: Possible Harmful Interaction

2 NEGATIVE Licorice root (*Glycyrrhiza glabra* or *G. uralensis*), a member of the pea family, has been used since ancient times as both food and medicine.

Licorice ingestion may worsen certain side effects associated with OCs. Glycyrrhizic acid, the active ingredient in licorice, produces side effects similar to those experienced by some women taking OCs, including fluid retention, high blood pressure, and low blood levels of potassium.[9–12] The compounding of side effects has been reported to occur in two women taking this combination.[13]

Because these adverse effects can have serious health consequences, women taking OCs should consult with a physician before taking licorice. Licorice flavored candies should not be a problem, but chewing tobacco may contain substantial amounts of the herb.

Milk Thistle: Possible Harmful Interaction

3 NEGATIVE The herb milk thistle (*Silybum marianum*) is used to treat various liver diseases.

One report has noted that an ingredient of milk thistle, silibinin, can inhibit a bacterial enzyme called beta-glucuronidase. This enzyme helps OCs work.[14] Taking milk thistle could therefore reduce the effectiveness of OCs.

OC users might wish to avoid milk thistle supplements.

St. John's Wort: Possible Harmful Interaction

2 NEGATIVE The herb St. John's wort (*Hypericum perforatum*) is primarily used to treat mild to moderate depression.

Case reports and the known actions of St. John's wort suggest that this herb may interfere with the effectiveness of OCs.[15]

St. John's wort has been reported to cause breakthrough bleeding in women taking OCs, a sign of diminished pill effect and a warning of potential contraceptive failure.

The herb appears to speed up the body's normal breakdown of the estrogen component in many OC pills. This tends to lower the amount of working estrogen in the blood, and is comparable to taking a weakened pill.

For this reason, OC users should probably avoid St. John's wort supplements until more is known.

St. John's Wort, Dong Quai: Possible Harmful Interaction

3 NEGATIVE St. John's wort (*Hypericum perforatum*) is primarily used to treat mild to moderate depression.

The herb dong quai (*Angelica sinensis*) is often recommended for menstrual disorders such as dysmenorrhea, PMS, and irregular menstruation.

OCs have been reported to cause increased sensitivity to the sun, amplifying the risk of sunburn or skin rash. Because St. John's wort and dong quai may also cause this problem, taking these herbal supplements while taking OCs might add to this risk.

It may be a good idea to wear a sunscreen or protective clothing during sun exposure if you take one of these herbs while using OCs.

POSITIVE INTERACTIONS

Folate: Interaction Unlikely or Probably Insignificant

4 POSITIVE Folate (also known as folic acid) is a B vitamin that plays an important role in many vital aspects of health, including preventing neural tube birth defects and possibly reducing the risk of heart disease. Because inadequate intake of folate is widespread, if you are taking any medication that depletes or impairs folate even slightly, you may need supplementation.

Oral contraceptives have been reported to lower folate levels in the body in most, but not all studies. However, this effect does not appear to be strong enough to cause a folate deficiency under ordinary circumstances.

A 1991 controlled study following 29 women taking OCs over 4 cycles found no effect on folate levels,[16] suggesting that folate supplementation is not routinely required for women taking OCs. A 1993 study found decreased blood levels of folate after folate supplementation in OC users compared to controls, but no evidence of folate deficiency.[17] Similar results were reported in an observational study of 229 adolescent females taking

OCs.[18] Studies involving high-estrogen OCs also have found no evidence of folate deficiency.[19]

Only OC users with increased folate needs because of specific medical conditions may need folate supplementation. However, as folate deficiency is common anyway, supplementation of this vitamin in standard nutritional doses may be a good idea on general principle.

Please see Appendix D, Safety Issues, for more information.

Magnesium: Supplementation Possibly Helpful

3 POSITIVE Estrogen enhances the body's use of the mineral magnesium by moving it from the blood into tissues and bone, resulting in lower blood levels of magnesium.[20] A 1991 study in 32 women found a 26% decrease in magnesium levels after 6 months of OC use compared to normal levels before OC use.[21]

When magnesium levels in the blood fall too low, symptoms may include appetite loss, nausea and vomiting, sleepiness, weakness, muscle spasms, tremors, and personality changes.

Though no problems related to the lower magnesium levels were noted in the study, it is important to maintain proper magnesium levels in the body. For this reason, magnesium supplementation may be advisable for individuals taking OCs who don't get enough magnesium from their diets.

Please see Appendix D, Safety Issues, for more information.

Soy: Interaction Unlikely or Probably Insignificant

4 POSITIVE Soy protein is present in many food items, including soybeans, soymilk, and tofu. Estrogen-like chemicals called phytoestrogens are present in the isoflavone constituents of soy.

Concerns have been expressed by some experts that soy or soy isoflavones might interfere with the action of OCs. However, one study of 40 women suggests that such concerns are groundless.[22] More studies are needed to confirm this finding.

Please see Appendix D, Safety Issues, for more information.

Vitamin B$_2$ (Riboflavin): Supplementation Possibly Helpful

3 POSITIVE Numerous studies indicate that OC use may deplete vitamin B$_2$ in the body to some extent, especially in those taking OCs for a long period of time.[23,24,25] Under ordinary circumstances, however, OC use appears unlikely to produce any real problems related to lack of vitamin B$_2$.

Though OC use is generally unlikely to deplete vitamin B_2 significantly, supplementation in standard nutritional doses may be advisable on general principle.

Please see Appendix D, Safety Issues, for more information.

Vitamin B_6: Interaction Unlikely or Probably Insignificant

4 POSITIVE Although it has sometimes been reported that OCs may adversely affect vitamin B_6 status, more recent studies do not appear to bear this out. In a placebo-controlled study involving 115 women taking OCs, no significant effects on the body's vitamin B_6 supplies were found.[26] Similarly, a placebo-controlled study of 14 young women found that 6 cycles of triphasic low-dose OC use did not alter vitamin B_6 levels in either blood or tissue in most of the women consuming an adequate diet.[27] Another 6-month study in 55 women taking various brands of low-dose OCs also found no negative effects on vitamin B_6.[28]

Though OCs appear not to affect vitamin B_6 status under ordinary circumstances, B_6 deficiency is relatively common.[29] For this reason, vitamin B_6 supplementation in standard nutritional doses may be appropriate on general principles.

Please see Appendix D, Safety Issues, for more information.

Vitamin B_{12}: Interaction Unlikely or Probably Insignificant

4 POSITIVE An observational study of 229 adolescent females taking OCs found decreased vitamin B_{12} levels in their blood.[30] In a placebo-controlled study, OC use decreased blood levels of vitamin B_{12}, but did not significantly change the overall amount of B_{12} in the body.[31] Other evidence indicates that the low vitamin B_{12} levels associated with OC use may be "false low readings" caused by the particular way B_{12} is carried in the blood. For this reason, a vitamin B_{12} deficiency would not be expected to occur as a result of OC use.[32]

Under ordinary circumstances, vitamin B_{12} supplementation may not be necessary in OC users.

Please see Appendix D, Safety Issues, for more information.

Vitamin C: Supplementation Possibly Helpful

3 POSITIVE Oral contraceptives appear to depress blood levels of vitamin C. In a 1972 study, researchers controlled vitamin C intake in 6 young women over 2 menstrual cycles; 4 participants took OCs and 2 served as controls.[33] Compared to the controls, those taking OCs had lower blood levels of vitamin C. Reduced vitamin C levels in OC users have also been reported in numerous other studies.[34–37]

It should be noted that these studies were performed in the days of high-estrogen OCs. It isn't clear whether today's low-estrogen OCs would produce similar effects.

Nonetheless, vitamin C supplementation might be advisable for OC users on general principles.

Please see Appendix D, Safety Issues, for more information.

Zinc: Supplementation Possibly Helpful

3 POSITIVE Although there is disagreement, most studies have found that OCs (at least OCs of the high-estrogen type used at the time the studies were performed) may reduce blood levels of the trace mineral zinc.[38]

Though the importance of this effect is unclear, marginal zinc deficiency is relatively common.[39–45] For this reason, zinc supplementation at standard nutritional levels might be beneficial in women taking OCs.

Please see Appendix D, Safety Issues, for more information.

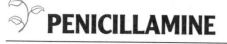

PENICILLAMINE

Trade Names: Cuprimine, Depen

Interactions	Rating*
Negative Interactions	
Copper	1
Iron	1
Magnesium	2
Positive Interaction	
Vitamin B₆ (Pyridoxine)	3

*Rating Key

1 Significant interaction

2 Possibly significant interaction

3 Interaction of relatively little significance

4 Reported interaction that does not in fact exist or is insignificant

The drug penicillamine is primarily used to treat Wilson's disease (an inherited disorder affecting copper metabolism, causing cirrhosis and brain and eye problems) and rheumatoid arthritis.

NEGATIVE INTERACTIONS

Copper: Possible Harmful Interaction

1 NEGATIVE Wilson's disease is a defect in the body's handling of the trace mineral copper, which results in abnormal deposits of copper in organs including the brain, liver, kidneys, and eyes. Penicillamine is used to capture copper from these tissues and ferry it out of the body through the urine.

Individuals with Wilson's disease should therefore avoid taking supplements containing copper.

Iron: Take at a Different Time of Day

1 NEGATIVE Iron may interfere with the absorption of penicillamine. It is thought that penicillamine attaches to iron, thus reducing the absorption of the drug. This effect would be expected to reduce iron absorption as well.

In a crossover study of six healthy men, a single dose of penicillamine (500 mg) was given alone or after a dose of ferrous sulfate (300 mg), an iron supplement.[1] Blood levels of penicillamine in the men receiving iron were only 35% of the penicillamine levels in those taking the drug alone.

To avoid this problem if you are using penicillamine, take the drug at least 2 hours apart from iron preparations. Forms of iron include ferrous fumarate, ferrous gluconate, ferrous sulfate, and iron polysaccharide.

Magnesium: Take at a Different Time of Day

2 NEGATIVE Magnesium may reduce the absorption of penicillamine. As with iron, it is thought that the drug binds with magnesium, reducing the absorption of each.

In a crossover study of six healthy men, a single dose of penicillamine (500 mg) was given either alone or after a 30-ml dose of magnesium-containing **antacid** (see page 13).[2] Blood levels of penicillamine in the men receiving the antacid were only 66% of the penicillamine levels in those taking the drug alone. However, the antacid in this study contained both magnesium and aluminum, and no attempt was made to distinguish effects between the two.

To avoid this potential problem if you are using penicillamine, take the drug at least 2 hours apart from magnesium preparations.

POSITIVE INTERACTIONS

Vitamin B$_6$ (Pyridoxine): Supplementation Possibly Helpful

3 POSITIVE Indirect evidence suggests that penicillamine therapy could deplete vitamin B$_6$, possibly leading to a B$_6$ deficiency.[3] In this test tube study, blood samples drawn from individuals taking penicillamine for rheumatoid arthritis were compared to those of control participants not taking the drug. Despite this finding, no symptoms of B$_6$ deficiency were observed.

Penicillamine's effect on vitamin B$_6$ may be important only in individuals with poor nutritional status. However, as this vitamin is commonly deficient in the diet,[4,5,6] B$_6$ supplementation in standard nutritional doses may be advisable on general principles.

Please see Appendix D, Safety Issues, for more information.

PENTOXIFYLLINE

Trade Name: Trental

Interactions	Rating*
Negative Interactions	
Garlic	2
Ginkgo	2
Policosanol	2
White Willow	3
Herbs and Supplements	3

*Rating Key

1 Significant interaction
2 Possibly significant interaction
3 Interaction of relatively little significance
4 Reported interaction that does not in fact exist or is insignificant

Pentoxifylline, a drug that makes the blood less "sticky," is used to increase blood circulation in conditions such as intermittent claudication (a possible complication of atherosclerosis in which impaired blood circulation causes severe pain in calf muscles during walking or exercising).

NEGATIVE INTERACTIONS

Garlic, Ginkgo: Possible Harmful Interaction

2 NEGATIVE The herb garlic (*Allium sativum*) is taken to lower cholesterol, among many other proposed uses.

One of the possible side effects of garlic is an increased tendency to bleed.[1,2] Therefore, you should not combine garlic and pentoxifylline except under medical supervision.

The herb ginkgo (*Ginkgo biloba*) has been used to treat Alzheimer's disease and ordinary age-related memory loss, among many other uses.

Ginkgo appears to reduce the ability of platelets (blood-clotting cells) to stick together.[3] Several case reports suggest that this blood-thinning effect of ginkgo may be associated with an increased risk of serious abnormal bleeding episodes in individuals taking the herb.[4,5,6]

Because of these risks, you should not combine ginkgo and pentoxifylline without physician supervision.

Policosanol: Possible Harmful Interaction

 Policosanol is a blood thinner and might add to the blood-thinning effects of pentoxifylline; therefore, you should not combine the two except under medical supervision.

White Willow: Possible Harmful Interaction

3 NEGATIVE The herb white willow (*Salix alba*), also known as willow bark, is used to treat pain and fever. White willow contains a substance that is converted by the body into a salicylate similar to the blood-thinner aspirin. For this reason, white willow might add to the effects of pentoxifylline, possibly thinning the blood too much.

It may be advisable to avoid white willow while taking pentoxifylline except under medical supervision.

Herbs and Supplements: Possible Harmful Interaction

3 NEGATIVE Herbs and supplements that impair the blood's ability to coagulate (clot) might add to the effects of pentoxifylline, possibly increasing the risk of excessive bleeding. This includes most prominently vitamin E.

Numerous other substances could conceivably present this risk, including aortic glycosaminoglycans (GAGs), bromelain (from the fruit and stem of pineapple, *Ananas comosus*), chamomile (*Matricaria recutita*), *Coleus forskohlii*, danshen (*Salvia miltorrhiza*), dong quai (*Angelica sinensis*), feverfew (*Tanacetum parthenium*), fish oil, ginger (*Zingiber officinale*), horse chestnut (*Aesculus hippocastanum*), OPCs (oligomeric proanthocyanidins), papaya (*Carica papaya*), and red clover (*Trifolium pratense*).

PHENOBARBITAL

Interactions	Rating*
Negative Interactions	
Ginkgo	3
Glutamine	4
Kava, Valerian, Passionflower, Hops	2
Nicotinamide	3
St. John's Wort, Dong Quai	3
Mixed Interactions	
Biotin	3
Folate	2

Interactions	Rating*
Positive Interactions	
Calcium	2
Carnitine	2
Vitamin D	2
Vitamin K	2

*Rating Key

1 Significant interaction

2 Possibly significant interaction

3 Interaction of relatively little significance

4 Reported interaction that does not in fact exist or is insignificant

Phenobarbital is a barbiturate with anticonvulsant action that may be used to prevent seizures in conditions such as epilepsy.

Other anticonvulsant agents include **carbamazepine** (see page 54), **phenytoin** (see page 140), **primidone** (see page 146), and **valproic acid** (see page 191). In some cases, combination therapy with two or more anticonvulsant drugs may be used.

NEGATIVE INTERACTIONS

Ginkgo: Possible Harmful Interaction

3 NEGATIVE The herb ginkgo (*Ginkgo biloba*) has been used to treat Alzheimer's disease and ordinary age-related memory loss, among many other conditions.

This interaction involves potential contaminants in ginkgo, not ginkgo itself.

A recent study found that a natural nerve toxin present in the seeds of *Ginkgo biloba* made its way into standardized ginkgo extracts prepared from the leaves.[1] This toxin has been associated with convulsions and death in laboratory animals.[2,3,4]

Fortunately, the detected amounts of this toxic substance are considered harmless.[5] However, given the lack of satisfactory standardization of herbal formulations in the United States, it is possible that some batches of product might contain higher contents of the toxin depending on the season of harvest.

In light of these findings, taking a ginkgo product that happened to contain significant levels of the nerve toxin might theoretically prevent an anticonvulsant from working as well as expected.

Glutamine: Possible Harmful Interaction

4 NEGATIVE The amino acid glutamine is converted to glutamate in the body. Glutamate is thought to act as a neurotransmitter (a chemical that enables nerve transmission). Because anticonvulsants work (at least in part) by blocking glutamate pathways in the brain, high dosages of the amino acid glutamine might theoretically diminish an anticonvulsant's effect and increase the risk of seizures.

Kava, Valerian, Passionflower, Hops: Possible Harmful Interaction

2 NEGATIVE The herb kava (*Piper methysticum*) has a sedative effect and is used for anxiety and insomnia.

Combining kava with anticonvulsants, which possess similar depressant effects, could result in "add-on" or excessive physical depression, sedation, and impairment. In one case report, a 54-year-old man was hospitalized for lethargy and disorientation, side effects attributed to his having taken the combination of kava and the antianxiety agent alprazolam (Xanax) for 3 days.[6]

Other herbs having a sedative effect that might cause problems when combined with anticonvulsants include ashwagandha (*Withania somnifera*), calendula (*Calendula officinalis*), catnip (*Nepeta cataria*), hops (*Humulus lupulus*), lady's slipper (*Cypripedium* species), lemon balm (*Melissa officinalis*), passionflower (*Passiflora incarnata*), sassafras (*Sassafras officinale*), skullcap (*Scutellaria lateriflora*), valerian (*Valeriana officinalis*), and yerba mansa (*Anemopsis californica*).

Because of the potentially serious consequences, you should avoid combining these herbs with anticonvulsants or other drugs that also have sedative or depressant effects, unless advised by your physician.

Nicotinamide: Possible Harmful Interaction

3 NEGATIVE Nicotinamide (also called niacinamide) is a compound produced by the body's breakdown of niacin (vitamin B_3). It is a supplemental form that does not possess the flushing side effect or the cholesterol-lowering ability of niacin.

Nicotinamide appears to increase blood levels of carbamazepine and primidone (which is converted in the body to phenobarbital), possibly requiring a reduction in drug dosage to prevent toxic effects.

Carbamazepine blood levels increased in two children with epilepsy after they were given nicotinamide,[7] but the fact that the children were on several anticonvulsant drugs clouds the issue somewhat. Similarly, nicotinamide given to three children on primidone therapy increased blood levels of primidone.[8] It is thought that nicotinamide may interfere with the body's normal breakdown of these anticonvulsant agents, allowing them to build up in the blood.

St. John's Wort, Dong Quai: Possible Harmful Interaction

3 NEGATIVE St. John's wort (*Hypericum perforatum*) is primarily used to treat mild to moderate depression.

The herb dong quai (*Angelica sinensis*) is often recommended for menstrual disorders such as dysmenorrhea, PMS, and irregular menstruation.

The anticonvulsant agents phenobarbital, valproic acid and carbamazepine have been reported to cause increased sensitivity to the sun, amplifying the risk of sunburn or skin rash. Because St. John's wort and dong quai may also cause this problem, taking them during treatment with these drugs might add to this risk.

It may be a good idea to wear a sunscreen or protective clothing during sun exposure if you take one of these herbs while using these anticonvulsants.

MIXED INTERACTIONS

Biotin: Supplementation Possibly Helpful, but Take at a Different Time of Day

3 MIXED Anticonvulsants may deplete biotin, an essential water-soluble B vitamin, possibly by competing with it for absorption in the intestine. It is not clear, however, whether this effect is great enough to be harmful.

Blood levels of biotin were found to be substantially lower in 404 people with epilepsy on long-term treatment with anticonvulsants compared to 112 untreated people with epilepsy.[9] The effect occurred with phenytoin, carbamazepine, phenobarbital, and primidone. Valproic acid appears to affect biotin to a lesser extent than other anticonvulsants.

A test tube study suggested that anticonvulsants might lower biotin levels by interfering with the way biotin is transported in the intestine.[10]

Biotin supplementation may be beneficial if you are on long-term anticonvulsant therapy. To avoid a potential interaction, take the supplement 2 to 3 hours apart from the drug. It has been suggested that the action of anticonvulsant drugs may be at least partly related to their effect of reducing biotin levels. For this reason, it may be desirable to take enough biotin to prevent a deficiency, but not an excessive amount.

Please see Appendix D, Safety Issues, for more information.

Folate: Supplementation Possibly Helpful

2 MIXED Folate (also known as folic acid) is a B vitamin that plays an important role in many vital aspects of health, including preventing neural tube birth defects and possibly reducing the risk of heart disease. Because inadequate intake of folate is widespread, if you are taking any medication that depletes or impairs folate even slightly, you may need supplementation.

Phenobarbital appears to lower blood levels of folate by speeding up its normal breakdown by the body and also by decreasing its absorption.[11] Other antiseizure drugs can also reduce levels of folate in the body.[12–17]

The low serum folate caused by anticonvulsants can raise homocysteine levels, a condition believed to increase the risk of heart disease.[18]

Adequate folate intake is also necessary to prevent neural tube birth defects such as spina bifida and anencephaly. Because anticonvulsant drugs deplete folate, babies born to women taking anticonvulsants are at increased risk for such birth defects. Anticonvulsants may also play a more direct role in the development of birth defects.[19]

However, the case for taking extra folate during anticonvulsant therapy is not as simple as it might seem. It is possible that folate supplementation might itself impair the effectiveness of anticonvulsant drugs, and physician supervision is necessary.

Please see Appendix D, Safety Issues, for more information.

POSITIVE INTERACTIONS

Calcium: Supplementation Probably Helpful, but Take at a Different Time of Day

 **2 POSITIVE** Anticonvulsant drugs may impair calcium absorption and in this way increase the risk of osteoporosis and other bone disorders.

Calcium absorption was compared in 12 people on anticonvulsant therapy (all taking phenytoin and some also taking phenobarbital, primidone, and/or carbamazepine) and 12 people receiving no treatment.[20] Calcium absorption was found to be 27% lower in the treated participants.

An observational study found low calcium blood levels in 48% of 109 people taking anticonvulsants.[21] Other findings in this study suggested that anticonvulsants might also reduce calcium levels by directly interfering with parathyroid hormone, a substance that helps keep calcium levels in proper balance.

A low blood level of calcium can itself trigger seizures, and this might reduce the effectiveness of anticonvulsants.[22]

Calcium supplementation may be beneficial for people taking anticonvulsant drugs. However, some studies indicate that antacids containing calcium carbonate may interfere with the absorption of phenytoin and perhaps other anticonvulsants.[23,24] For this reason, take calcium supplements and anticonvulsant drugs several hours apart if possible.

Please see Appendix D, Safety Issues, for more information.

Carnitine: Supplementation Possibly Helpful

2 POSITIVE Carnitine is an amino acid that has been used for heart conditions, Alzheimer's disease, and intermittent claudication (a possible complication of atherosclerosis in which impaired blood circulation causes severe pain in calf muscles during walking or exercising).

Long-term therapy with anticonvulsant agents, particularly valproic acid, is associated with low levels of carnitine.[25] However, it isn't clear whether the anticonvulsants cause the carnitine deficiency or whether it occurs for other reasons. It has been hypothesized that low carnitine levels may contribute to valproic acid's damaging effects on the liver.[26,27] The risk of this liver damage increases in children younger than 24 months,[28] and carnitine supplementation does seem to be protective.[29] However, in one double-blind crossover study, carnitine supplementation produced no real improvement in "well-being" as assessed by parents of children receiving either valproic acid or carbamazepine.[30]

L-carnitine supplementation may be advisable in certain cases, such as in infants and young children (especially those younger than 2 years) who have neurologic disorders and are receiving valproic acid and multiple anticonvulsants.[31]

Please see Appendix D, Safety Issues, for more information.

Vitamin D: Supplementation Possibly Helpful

2 POSITIVE Anticonvulsant drugs may interfere with the activity of vitamin D. As proper handling of calcium by the body depends on vitamin D, this may be another way that these drugs increase the risk of osteoporosis and related bone disorders (see the previous calcium topic).

Anticonvulsants appear to speed up the body's normal breakdown of vitamin D, decreasing the amount of the vitamin in the blood.[32] A survey of 48 people taking both phenobarbital and phenytoin found significantly lower levels of calcium and vitamin D in many of them as compared to 38 untreated individuals.[33] Similar but lesser changes were seen in 13 people taking phenobarbital or phenytoin alone. This effect may be apparent only after several weeks of treatment.

Another study found decreased blood levels of one form of vitamin D but normal levels of another.[34] Because there are two primary forms of vitamin D circulating in the blood, the body might be able to adjust in some cases to keep vitamin D in balance, at least for a time, despite the influence of anticonvulsants.[35]

Adequate sunlight exposure may help overcome the effects of anticonvulsants on vitamin D by stimulating the skin to manufacture the vitamin.[36] Of 450 people on anticonvulsants residing in a Florida facility, none were found to have low blood levels of vitamin D or evidence of bone disease. This suggests that environments providing regular sun exposure may be protective.

Individuals regularly taking anticonvulsants, especially those taking combination therapy and those with limited exposure to sunlight, may benefit from vitamin D supplementation.

Please see Appendix D, Safety Issues, for more information.

Vitamin K: Supplementation Possibly Helpful for Pregnant Women

2 POSITIVE Phenobarbital, primidone, phenytoin, and carbamazepine speed up the normal breakdown of vitamin K into inactive byproducts, thus depriving the body of active vitamin K. This can lead to bone problems such as osteoporosis. Also, use of these anticonvulsants can lead to a vitamin K deficiency in babies born to mothers taking the drugs, resulting in bleeding disorders or facial bone abnormalities in the newborns.[37,38]

Mothers who take these anticonvulsants may need vitamin K supplementation during pregnancy to prevent these conditions in their newborns.

Please see Appendix D, Safety Issues, for more information.

PHENYTOIN

Trade Name: Dilantin

Interactions	Rating*
Negative Interactions	
Ginkgo	3
Glutamine	4
Ipriflavone	2
Kava, Valerian, Passionflower, Hops	2
White Willow	3
Mixed Interactions	
Biotin	3
Folate	2

Interactions	Rating*
Positive Interactions	
Calcium	2
Carnitine	2
Vitamin D	2
Vitamin K	2

*Rating Key

1 Significant interaction

2 Possibly significant interaction

3 Interaction of relatively little significance

4 Reported interaction that does not in fact exist or is insignificant

Phenytoin is an anticonvulsant agent used primarily to prevent seizures in conditions such as epilepsy. Drugs similar to phenytoin are ethotoin (Peganone) and mephenytoin (Mesantoin).

Other anticonvulsant agents include **carbamazepine** (see page 54), **phenobarbital** (see page 134), **primidone** (see page 146), and **valproic acid** (see page 191). In some cases, combination therapy with two or more anticonvulsant drugs may be used.

NEGATIVE INTERACTIONS

Ginkgo: Possible Harmful Interaction

3 NEGATIVE The herb ginkgo (*Ginkgo biloba*) has been used to treat Alzheimer's disease and ordinary age-related memory loss, among many other conditions.

This interaction involves potential contaminants in ginkgo, not ginkgo itself.

A recent study found that a natural nerve toxin present in the seeds of *Ginkgo biloba* made its way into standardized ginkgo extracts prepared from the leaves.[1] This toxin has been associated with convulsions and death in laboratory animals.[2,3,4]

Fortunately, the detected amounts of this toxic substance are considered harmless.[5] However, given the lack of satisfactory standardization of herbal

formulations in the United States, it is possible that some batches of product might contain higher contents of the toxin depending on the season of harvest.

In light of these findings, taking a ginkgo product that happened to contain significant levels of the nerve toxin might theoretically prevent an anticonvulsant from working as well as expected.

Glutamine: Possible Harmful Interaction

4 NEGATIVE The amino acid glutamine is converted to glutamate in the body. Glutamate is thought to act as a neurotransmitter (a chemical that enables nerve transmission). Because anticonvulsants work (at least in part) by blocking glutamate pathways in the brain, high dosages of the amino acid glutamine might theoretically diminish an anticonvulsant's effect and increase the risk of seizures.

Ipriflavone: Possible Harmful Interaction

2 NEGATIVE Ipriflavone, a synthetic isoflavone that slows bone breakdown, is used to treat osteoporosis.

Test tube studies indicate that ipriflavone might increase blood levels of the anticonvulsants phenytoin and carbamazepine when they are taken therapeutically.[6] Ipriflavone was found to inhibit a liver enzyme involved in the body's normal breakdown of these drugs, thus allowing them to build up in the blood. Higher drug levels increase the risk of adverse effects.

Because anticonvulsants are known to contribute to the development of osteoporosis, a concern is that the use of ipriflavone for this drug-induced osteoporosis could result in higher blood levels of the drugs, with potentially serious consequences.

Individuals taking either of these drugs should use ipriflavone only under medical supervision.

Kava, Valerian, Passionflower, Hops: Possible Harmful Interaction

2 NEGATIVE The herb kava (*Piper methysticum*) has a sedative effect and is used for anxiety and insomnia.

Combining kava with anticonvulsants, which possess similar depressant effects, could result in "add-on" or excessive physical depression, sedation, and impairment. In one case report, a 54-year-old man was hospitalized for lethargy and disorientation, side effects attributed to his having taken the combination of kava and the antianxiety agent alprazolam (Xanax) for 3 days.[7]

Other herbs having a sedative effect that might cause problems when combined with anticonvulsants include ashwagandha (*Withania somnifera*), calendula (*Calendula officinalis*), catnip (*Nepeta cataria*), hops (*Humulus lupulus*), lady's slipper (*Cypripedium* species), lemon balm (*Melissa officinalis*), passionflower (*Passiflora incarnata*), sassafras (*Sassafras officinale*), skullcap (*Scutellaria lateriflora*), valerian (*Valeriana officinalis*), and yerba mansa (*Anemopsis californica*).

Because of the potentially serious consequences, you should avoid combining these herbs with anticonvulsants or other drugs that also have sedative or depressant effects, unless advised by your physician.

White Willow: Possible Harmful Interaction

3 NEGATIVE The herb white willow (*Salix alba*), also known as willow bark, is used to treat pain and fever. White willow contains a substance that is converted by the body into a salicylate similar to aspirin.

Higher doses of aspirin may increase phenytoin levels and toxicity during long-term use of both drugs.[8] This raises the concern that white willow might have similar effects on phenytoin, though this has not been proven.

MIXED INTERACTIONS

Biotin: Supplementation Possibly Helpful, but Take at a Different Time of Day

3 MIXED Anticonvulsants may deplete biotin, an essential water-soluble B vitamin, possibly by competing with it for absorption in the intestine. It is not clear, however, whether this effect is great enough to be harmful.

Blood levels of biotin were found to be substantially lower in 404 people with epilepsy on long-term treatment with anticonvulsants compared to 112 untreated people with epilepsy.[9] The effect occurred with phenytoin, carbamazepine, phenobarbital, and primidone. Valproic acid appears to affect biotin to a lesser extent than other anticonvulsants.

A test tube study suggested that anticonvulsants might lower biotin levels by interfering with the way biotin is transported in the intestine.[10]

Biotin supplementation may be beneficial if you are on long-term anticonvulsant therapy. To avoid a potential interaction, take the supplement 2 to 3 hours apart from the drug. It has been suggested that the action of anticonvulsant drugs may be at least partly related to their effect of reducing biotin levels. For this reason, it may be desirable to take enough biotin to prevent a deficiency, but not an excessive amount.

Please see Appendix D, Safety Issues, for more information.

Folate: Supplementation Possibly Helpful

2 MIXED Folate (also known as folic acid) is a B vitamin that plays an important role in many vital aspects of health, including preventing neural tube birth defects and possibly reducing the risk of heart disease. Because inadequate intake of folate is widespread, if you are taking any medication that depletes or impairs folate even slightly, you may need supplementation.

Most drugs used for preventing seizures can reduce levels of folate in the body.[11–16]

The low serum folate caused by anticonvulsants can raise homocysteine levels, a condition believed to increase the risk of heart disease.[17]

Adequate folate intake is also necessary to prevent neural tube birth defects such as spina bifida and anencephaly. Because anticonvulsant drugs deplete folate, babies born to women taking anticonvulsants are at increased risk for such birth defects. Anticonvulsants may also play a more direct role in the development of birth defects.[18]

The interaction between phenytoin and folate is fairly complex. Phenytoin appears to decrease folate levels by interfering with its absorption in the small intestine[19] as well as by accelerating its normal breakdown by the body.[20,21] On the other hand, high folate levels may speed up the normal breakdown of phenytoin.[22,23] This could mean that taking extra folate might cause an increase in seizures.

For this reason, folate supplementation during phenytoin therapy should be supervised by a physician.

Please see Appendix D, Safety Issues, for more information.

POSITIVE INTERACTIONS

Calcium: Supplementation Probably Helpful, but Take at a Different Time of Day

2 POSITIVE Anticonvulsant drugs may impair calcium absorption and in this way increase the risk of osteoporosis and other bone disorders.

Calcium absorption was compared in 12 people on anticonvulsant therapy (all taking phenytoin and some also taking phenobarbital, primidone, and/or carbamazepine) and 12 people receiving no treatment.[24] Calcium absorption was found to be 27% lower in the treated participants.

An observational study found low calcium blood levels in 48% of 109 people taking anticonvulsants.[25] Other findings in this study suggested that anticonvulsants might also reduce calcium levels by directly interfering with parathyroid hormone, a substance that helps keep calcium levels in proper balance.

A low blood level of calcium can itself trigger seizures, and this might reduce the effectiveness of anticonvulsants.[26]

Calcium supplementation may be beneficial for people taking anticonvulsant drugs. However, some studies indicate that antacids containing calcium carbonate may interfere with the absorption of phenytoin and perhaps other anticonvulsants.[27,28] For this reason, take calcium supplements and anticonvulsant drugs several hours apart if possible.

Please see Appendix D, Safety Issues, for more information.

Carnitine: Supplementation Possibly Helpful

2 POSITIVE Carnitine is an amino acid that has been used for heart conditions, Alzheimer's disease, and intermittent claudication (a possible complication of atherosclerosis in which impaired blood circulation causes severe pain in calf muscles during walking or exercising).

Long-term therapy with anticonvulsant agents, particularly valproic acid, is associated with low levels of carnitine.[29] However, it isn't clear whether the anticonvulsants cause the carnitine deficiency or whether it occurs for other reasons. It has been hypothesized that low carnitine levels may contribute to valproic acid's damaging effects on the liver.[30,31] The risk of this liver damage increases in children younger than 24 months,[32] and carnitine supplementation does seem to be protective.[33] However, in one double-blind crossover study, carnitine supplementation produced no real improvement in "well-being" as assessed by parents of children receiving either valproic acid or carbamazepine.[34]

L-carnitine supplementation may be advisable in certain cases, such as in infants and young children (especially those younger than 2 years) who have neurologic disorders and are receiving valproic acid and multiple anticonvulsants.[35]

Please see Appendix D, Safety Issues, for more information.

Vitamin D: Supplementation Possibly Helpful

2 POSITIVE Anticonvulsant drugs may interfere with the activity of vitamin D. As proper handling of calcium by the body depends on vitamin D, this may be another way that these drugs increase the risk of osteoporosis and related bone disorders (see the previous calcium topic).

Anticonvulsants appear to speed up the body's normal breakdown of vitamin D, decreasing the amount of the vitamin in the blood.[36] A survey of 48 people taking both phenytoin and phenobarbital found significantly lower levels of calcium and vitamin D in many of them as compared to 38 untreated individuals.[37] Similar but lesser changes were seen in 13 people taking phenytoin or phenobarbital alone. This effect may be apparent only after several weeks of treatment.

Another study found decreased blood levels of one form of vitamin D but normal levels of another.[38] Because there are two primary forms of vitamin D circulating in the blood, the body might be able to adjust in some cases to keep vitamin D in balance, at least for a time, despite the influence of anticonvulsants.[39]

Adequate sunlight exposure may help overcome the effects of anticonvulsants on vitamin D by stimulating the skin to manufacture the vitamin.[40] Of 450 people on anticonvulsants residing in a Florida facility, none were found to have low blood levels of vitamin D or evidence of bone disease. This suggests that environments providing regular sun exposure may be protective.

Individuals regularly taking anticonvulsants, especially those taking combination therapy and those with limited exposure to sunlight, may benefit from vitamin D supplementation.

Please see Appendix D, Safety Issues, for more information.

Vitamin K: Supplementation Possibly Helpful for Pregnant Women

2 POSITIVE Phenytoin, carbamazepine, phenobarbital, and primidone speed up the normal breakdown of vitamin K into inactive byproducts, thus depriving the body of active vitamin K. This can lead to bone problems such as osteoporosis. Also, use of these anticonvulsants can lead to a vitamin K deficiency in babies born to mothers taking the drugs, resulting in bleeding disorders or facial bone abnormalities in the newborns.[41,42]

Mothers who take these anticonvulsants may need vitamin K supplementation during pregnancy to prevent these conditions in their newborns.

Please see Appendix D, Safety Issues, for more information.

PRIMIDONE

Trade Name: Mysoline

Interactions	Rating*
Negative Interactions	
Ginkgo	3
Glutamine	4
Kava, Valerian, Passionflower, Hops	2
Nicotinamide	3
St. John's Wort, Dong Quai	3
Mixed Interactions	
Biotin	3
Folate	2

Interactions	Rating*
Positive Interactions	
Calcium	2
Carnitine	2
Vitamin D	2
Vitamin K	2

*Rating Key

1　Significant interaction

2　Possibly significant interaction

3　Interaction of relatively little significance

4　Reported interaction that does not in fact exist or is insignificant

Primidone is an anticonvulsant agent used primarily to prevent seizures in conditions such as epilepsy.

Other anticonvulsant agents include **carbamazepine** (see page 54), **phenobarbital** (see page 134), **phenytoin** (see page 140), and **valproic acid** (see page 191). Primidone is converted in the body to phenobarbital. In some cases, combination therapy with two or more anticonvulsant drugs may be used.

NEGATIVE INTERACTIONS

Ginkgo: Possible Harmful Interaction

3 NEGATIVE The herb ginkgo (*Ginkgo biloba*) has been used to treat Alzheimer's disease and ordinary age-related memory loss, among many other uses.

This interaction involves potential contaminants in ginkgo, not ginkgo itself.

A recent study found that a natural nerve toxin present in the seeds of *Ginkgo biloba* made its way into standardized ginkgo extracts prepared from the leaves.[1] This toxin has been associated with convulsions and death in laboratory animals.[2,3,4]

Fortunately, the detected amounts of this toxic substance are considered harmless.[5] However, given the lack of satisfactory standardization of herbal

formulations in the United States, it is possible that some batches of product might contain higher contents of the toxin depending on the season of harvest.

In light of these findings, taking a ginkgo product that happened to contain significant levels of the nerve toxin might theoretically prevent an anticonvulsant from working as well as expected.

Glutamine: Possible Harmful Interaction

4 **NEGATIVE** The amino acid glutamine is converted to glutamate in the body. Glutamate is thought to act as a neurotransmitter (chemical that enables nerve transmission). Because anticonvulsants work (at least in part) by blocking glutamate pathways in the brain, high dosages of the amino acid glutamine might theoretically diminish an anticonvulsant's effect and increase the risk of seizures.

Kava, Valerian, Passionflower, Hops: Possible Harmful Interaction

2 **NEGATIVE** The herb kava (*Piper methysticum*) has a sedative effect and is used for anxiety and insomnia.

Combining kava with anticonvulsants, which possess similar depressant effects, could result in "add-on" or excessive physical depression, sedation, and impairment. In one case report, a 54-year-old man was hospitalized for lethargy and disorientation, side effects attributed to his having taken the combination of kava and the antianxiety agent alprazolam (Xanax) for 3 days.[6]

Other herbs having a sedative effect that might cause problems when combined with anticonvulsants include ashwagandha (*Withania somnifera*), calendula (*Calendula officinalis*), catnip (*Nepeta cataria*), hops (*Humulus lupulus*), lady's slipper (*Cypripedium* species), lemon balm (*Melissa officinalis*), passionflower (*Passiflora incarnata*), sassafras (*Sassafras officinale*), skullcap (*Scutellaria lateriflora*), valerian (*Valeriana officinalis*), and yerba mansa (*Anemopsis californica*).

Because of the potentially serious consequences, you should avoid combining these herbs with anticonvulsants or other drugs that also have sedative or depressant effects, unless advised by your physician.

Nicotinamide: Possible Harmful Interaction

3 **NEGATIVE** Nicotinamide (also called niacinamide) is a compound produced by the body's breakdown of niacin (vitamin B_3). It is a supplemental form that does not possess the flushing side effect or the cholesterol-lowering ability of niacin.

Nicotinamide appears to increase blood levels of primidone and carbamazepine, possibly requiring a reduction in drug dosage to prevent toxic effects.

Carbamazepine blood levels increased in two children with epilepsy after they were given nicotinamide,[7] but the fact that the children were on several anticonvulsant drugs clouds the issue somewhat. Similarly, nicotinamide given to three children on primidone therapy increased blood levels of primidone.[8] It is thought that nicotinamide may interfere with the body's normal breakdown of these anticonvulsant agents, allowing them to build up in the blood.

St. John's Wort, Dong Quai: Possible Harmful Interaction

3 NEGATIVE St. John's wort (*Hypericum perforatum*) is primarily used to treat mild to moderate depression.

The herb dong quai (*Angelica sinensis*) is often recommended for menstrual disorders such as dysmenorrhea, PMS, and irregular menstruation.

The anticonvulsant agents valproic acid, carbamazepine, and phenobarbital have been reported to cause increased sensitivity to the sun, amplifying the risk of sunburn or skin rash. (Primidone is converted in the body to phenobarbital.) Because St. John's wort and dong quai may also cause this problem, taking them during treatment with these drugs might add to this risk.

It may be a good idea to wear a sunscreen or protective clothing during sun exposure if you take one of these herbs while using these anticonvulsants.

MIXED INTERACTIONS

Biotin: Supplementation Possibly Helpful, but Take at a Different Time of Day

3 MIXED Anticonvulsants may deplete biotin, an essential water-soluble B vitamin, possibly by competing with it for absorption in the intestine. It is not clear, however, whether this effect is great enough to be harmful.

Blood levels of biotin were found to be substantially lower in 404 people with epilepsy on long-term treatment with anticonvulsants compared to 112 untreated people with epilepsy.[9] The effect occurred with phenytoin, carbamazepine, phenobarbital, and primidone. Valproic acid appears to affect biotin to a lesser extent than other anticonvulsants.

A test tube study suggested that anticonvulsants might lower biotin levels by interfering with the way biotin is transported in the intestine.[10]

Biotin supplementation may be beneficial if you are on long-term anticonvulsant therapy. To avoid a potential interaction, take the supplement 2 to 3 hours apart from the drug. It has been suggested that the action of anticonvulsant drugs may be at least partly related to their effect of reducing biotin levels. For this reason, it may be desirable to take enough biotin to prevent a deficiency, but not an excessive amount.

Please see Appendix D, Safety Issues, for more information.

Folate: Supplementation Possibly Helpful

| 2 |
| MIXED |

Folate (aka folic acid) is a B vitamin that plays an important role in many vital aspects of health, including preventing neural tube birth defects and possibly reducing the risk of heart disease. Because inadequate intake of folate is widespread, if you are taking any medication that depletes or impairs folate even slightly, you may need supplementation.

Primidone appears to lower blood levels of folate by speeding up its normal breakdown by the body and also by decreasing its absorption.[11] Other antiseizure drugs can also reduce levels of folate in the body.[12–16] The low serum folate caused by anticonvulsants can raise homocysteine levels, a condition believed to increase the risk of heart disease.[17]

Adequate folate intake is also necessary to prevent neural tube birth defects such as spina bifida and anencephaly. Because anticonvulsant drugs deplete folate, babies born to women taking anticonvulsants are at increased risk for such birth defects. Anticonvulsants may also play a more direct role in the development of birth defects.[18]

However, the case for taking extra folate during anticonvulsant therapy is not as simple as it might seem. It is possible that folate supplementation might itself impair the effectiveness of anticonvulsant drugs, and physician supervision is necessary.

Please see Appendix D, Safety Issues, for more information.

POSITIVE INTERACTIONS

Calcium: Supplementation Probably Helpful, but Take at a Different Time of Day

| 2 |
| POSITIVE |

Anticonvulsant drugs may impair calcium absorption and in this way increase the risk of osteoporosis and other bone disorders.

Calcium absorption was compared in 12 people on anticonvulsant therapy (all taking phenytoin and some also taking primidone, phenobarbital, and/or carbamazepine) and 12 people receiving no treatment.[19] Calcium absorption was found to be 27% lower in the treated participants.

An observational study found low calcium blood levels in 48% of 109 people taking anticonvulsants.[20] Other findings in this study suggested that anticonvulsants might also reduce calcium levels by directly interfering with parathyroid hormone, a substance that helps keep calcium levels in proper balance.

A low blood level of calcium can itself trigger seizures, and this might reduce the effectiveness of anticonvulsants.[21]

Calcium supplementation may be beneficial for people taking anticonvulsant drugs. However, some studies indicate that antacids containing calcium carbonate may interfere with the absorption of phenytoin and perhaps other anticonvulsants.[22,23] For this reason, take calcium supplements and anticonvulsant drugs several hours apart if possible.

Please see Appendix D, Safety Issues, for more information.

Carnitine: Supplementation Possibly Helpful

2 POSITIVE Carnitine is an amino acid that has been used for heart conditions, Alzheimer's disease, and intermittent claudication (a possible complication of atherosclerosis in which impaired blood circulation causes severe pain in calf muscles during walking or exercising).

Long-term therapy with anticonvulsant agents, particularly valproic acid, is associated with low levels of carnitine.[24] However, it isn't clear whether the anticonvulsants cause the carnitine deficiency or whether it occurs for other reasons. It has been hypothesized that low carnitine levels may contribute to valproic acid's damaging effects on the liver.[25,26] The risk of this liver damage increases in children younger than 24 months,[27] and carnitine supplementation does seem to be protective.[28] However, in one double-blind crossover study, carnitine supplementation produced no real improvement in "well-being" as assessed by parents of children receiving either valproic acid or carbamazepine.[29]

L-carnitine supplementation may be advisable in certain cases, such as in infants and young children (especially those younger than 2 years) who have neurologic disorders and are receiving valproic acid and multiple anticonvulsants.[30]

Please see Appendix D, Safety Issues, for more information.

Vitamin D: Supplementation Possibly Helpful

2 POSITIVE Anticonvulsant drugs may interfere with the activity of vitamin D. As proper handling of calcium by the body depends on vitamin D, this may be another way that these drugs increase the risk of osteoporosis and related bone disorders (see the previous Calcium topic).

Anticonvulsants appear to speed up the body's normal breakdown of vitamin D, decreasing the amount of the vitamin in the blood.[31] A survey of 48 people taking both phenytoin and phenobarbital (primidone is converted in the body to phenobarbital) found significantly lower levels of calcium and vitamin D in many of them as compared to 38 untreated individuals.[32] Similar but lesser changes were seen in 13 people taking phenytoin or phenobarbital alone. This effect may be apparent only after several weeks of treatment.

Another study found decreased blood levels of one form of vitamin D but normal levels of another.[33] Because there are two primary forms of vitamin D circulating in the blood, the body might be able to adjust in some cases to keep vitamin D in balance, at least for a time, despite the influence of anticonvulsants.[34]

Adequate sunlight exposure may help overcome the effects of anticonvulsants on vitamin D by stimulating the skin to manufacture the vitamin.[35] Of 450 people on anticonvulsants residing in a Florida facility, none were found to have low blood levels of vitamin D or evidence of bone disease. This suggests that environments providing regular sun exposure may be protective.

Individuals regularly taking anticonvulsants, especially those taking combination therapy and those with limited exposure to sunlight, may benefit from vitamin D supplementation.

Please see Appendix D, Safety Issues, for more information.

Vitamin K: Supplementation Possibly Helpful for Pregnant Women

2 POSITIVE Primidone, phenobarbital, phenytoin, and carbamazepine speed up the normal breakdown of vitamin K into inactive byproducts, thus depriving the body of active vitamin K. This can lead to bone problems such as osteoporosis. Also, use of these anticonvulsants can lead to a vitamin K deficiency in babies born to mothers taking the drugs, resulting in bleeding disorders or facial bone abnormalities in the newborns.[36,37]

Mothers who take these anticonvulsants may need vitamin K supplementation during pregnancy to prevent these conditions in their newborns.

Please see Appendix D, Safety Issues, for more information.

PROTEASE INHIBITORS

Interactions	Rating*
Negative Interactions	
Grapefruit Juice	1
St. John's Wort	1

*Rating Key

1 Significant interaction

2 Possibly significant interaction

3 Interaction of relatively little significance

4 Reported interaction that does not in fact exist or is insignificant

Protease inhibitors are used to manage HIV infection. They work by blocking the activity of HIV protease, an enzyme that enables the virus to generate the proteins it needs to grow. Protease inhibitors include

- amprenavir (Agenerase)
- indinavir (Crixivan)
- nelfinavir (Viracept)
- ritonavir (Norvir)
- saquinavir (Fortovase)
- saquinavir mesylate (Invirase)

Note: Saquinavir mesylate (Invirase) is being phased out in favor of saquinavir (Fortovase).

NEGATIVE INTERACTIONS

Grapefruit Juice: Possible Harmful Interaction

1 NEGATIVE Grapefruit juice impairs the body's normal breakdown of several drugs, allowing them to build up to potentially excessive levels in the blood.[1] Saquinavir mesylate as well as other protease inhibitors may be affected. A recent study indicates this effect can last for 3 days or more following the last glass of juice.[2]

Because this could increase the risk of drug side effects, if you take protease inhibitors, the safest approach is to avoid grapefruit juice altogether.

St. John's Wort: Possible Harmful Interaction

1 NEGATIVE The herb St. John's wort (*Hypericum perforatum*) is primarily used to treat mild to moderate depression.

St. John's wort has the potential to accelerate the body's normal breakdown of certain drugs,[3,4] including protease inhibitors, resulting in lower blood levels of these drugs. In fact, a study in eight healthy volunteers found that the herb decreased blood levels of the protease inhibitor indinavir by an average of 57%.[5] This is a substantial reduction that could lead to failure of the drug to keep the HIV virus in check. Similar effects are expected to occur with other protease inhibitors.

Based on present evidence, the FDA has issued a warning against combining St. John's wort with protease inhibitors.

It is especially important to be aware of this interaction because individuals with a chronic illness such as HIV often become depressed and may choose to self-treat with St. John's wort. Additionally, it was reported in the past that St. John's wort might have anti-HIV effects. However, this hypothesis has been proven incorrect.

The bottom line, based on the current evidence: If you have HIV, don't take St. John's wort!

PROTON PUMP INHIBITORS

Interactions	Rating*
Negative Interactions	
St. John's Wort	2
Positive Interaction	
Folate	3
Vitamin B$_{12}$	2
Minerals	3

*Rating Key

1 Significant interaction
2 Possibly significant interaction
3 Interaction of relatively little significance
4 Reported interaction that does not in fact exist or is insignificant

Proton pump inhibitors are the most powerful medications for reducing stomach acid levels; in fact, they almost completely shut down the stomach's ability to produce acid. (Their science fiction–sounding name comes from the last step of the acid-secreting process, called the "proton pump.") Proton pump inhibitors are used for stomach ulcers as well as for the treatment of moderate to severe esophageal reflux, commonly known as heartburn. Drugs in this family include

- lansoprazole (Prevacid, PREVPAC)
- omeprazole (Prilosec)
- rabeprazole sodium (Aciphex)
- and others

NEGATIVE INTERACTIONS

St. John's Wort: Possible Harmful Interaction

2 NEGATIVE The herb St. John's wort (*Hypericum perforatum*) is primarily used to treat mild to moderate depression.

St. John's wort can increase your sensitivity to the sun, amplifying the risk of sunburn or skin rash. Proton pump inhibitors might increase this risk even more.[1]

It would be advisable for individuals taking this combination to avoid lengthy sun exposure or to protect themselves by wearing protective clothing and using a sunscreen.

POSITIVE INTERACTIONS

Folate: Supplementation Possibly Helpful

3 POSITIVE Folate (also known as folic acid) is a B vitamin that plays an important role in many vital aspects of health, including preventing neural tube birth defects and possibly reducing the risk of heart disease. Because inadequate intake of folate is widespread, if you are taking any medication that depletes or impairs folate even slightly, you may need supplementation.

Conditions for folate absorption are best in the slightly acidic part of the intestine nearest to the stomach. For this reason, medications that reduce acidity, such as proton pump inhibitors, might be expected to interfere with folate absorption.

One study found that **H_2 antagonists** (see page 85), another group of drugs that reduce stomach acidity, may interfere with the absorption of folate,[12] though this effect appears to be relatively minor. Because proton pump inhibitors reduce stomach acid even more than H_2 antagonists, it stands to reason that they may affect folate in a similar or even greater manner.

Because folate is commonly deficient in the diet anyway, folate supplementation in nutritional doses may be worthwhile, especially if you take proton pump inhibitors regularly.

Please see Appendix D, Safety Issues, for more information.

Vitamin B_{12}: Supplementation Probably Helpful

2 POSITIVE If you take proton pump inhibitors, you may need vitamin B_{12} supplementation.

Vitamin B_{12} in foods is attached to proteins, and adequate stomach acid is required to release it from this bound form.[13,14] The vitamin is then picked up by a protective stomach substance called intrinsic factor and absorbed from the intestine. Proton pump inhibitors, by reducing stomach acid, can interfere with the absorption of vitamin B_{12}.

Studies suggest that treatment with proton pump inhibitors might significantly reduce the absorption of vitamin B_{12} from food.[15,16] In one study, after 2 weeks of treatment, vitamin B_{12} absorption decreased by 72% in participants taking 20 mg of omeprazole daily and 88% in those taking 40 mg daily.[17]

However, vitamin B_{12} taken in supplement form can still be absorbed, presumably because it does not have to be split apart from proteins.[18] Therefore, if you take proton pump inhibitors, it may be advisable to take vitamin

B_{12} supplementation in nutritional doses to make up for malabsorption of the vitamin from foods.

Interestingly, there is some evidence that cranberry juice might increase B_{12} absorption in individuals taking proton pump inhibitors,[19] possibly because the juice is somewhat acidic.

Please see Appendix D, Safety Issues, for more information.

Minerals: Supplementation Possibly Helpful

3 **POSITIVE** Like other acid-blocking drugs, proton pump inhibitors may interfere with the absorption of iron and zinc and possibly other minerals that are absorbed best under acidic conditions.[20,21]

Taking a general multivitamin/multimineral supplement should help overcome these mineral absorption problems when using a proton pump inhibitor.

Please see Appendix D, Safety Issues, for more information.

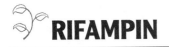

RIFAMPIN

Trade Names: Rifadin, Rifampicin, Rifamate, Rifater

Interactions	*Rating**
Positive Interaction	
Vitamin D	3

*Rating Key

1 Significant interaction

2 Possibly significant interaction

3 Interaction of relatively little significance

4 Reported interaction that does not in fact exist or is insignificant

Rifampin, depending on the dose used, either kills or stops the growth of the bacteria that cause tuberculosis. The drug is often used along with **isoniazid** (see page 93) for the treatment of tuberculosis.

POSITIVE INTERACTIONS

Vitamin D: Supplementation Possibly Helpful

3 POSITIVE Rifampin may interfere with the body's formation of an important form of vitamin D.[1] Since vitamin D is necessary for the proper absorption of calcium, concerns have been raised that rifampin therapy may impair bone development.

However, the body appears to be able to adjust to this effect so that vitamin D deficiency or other problems are unlikely to occur.[2,3] Even so, supplementation with vitamin D at standard nutritional doses might be worthwhile during rifampin therapy. Supplementation may be especially important for individuals with increased calcium requirements, such as children and pregnant women, people whose diets are deficient in vitamin D, or individuals who get little sun exposure.[4]

Please see Appendix D, Safety Issues, for more information.

SELECTIVE SEROTONIN-REUPTAKE INHIBITORS (SSRIs)

Interactions	Rating*
Negative Interactions	
5-HTP (5-Hydroxytryptophan), SAMe (S-Adenosylmethionine)	2
St. John's Wort	2
Positive Interaction	
Ginkgo	2

*Rating Key

1   Significant interaction

2   Possibly significant interaction

3   Interaction of relatively little significance

4   Reported interaction that does not in fact exist or is insignificant

Since the development of Prozac, the first of the selective serotonin-reuptake inhibitors (SSRIs), this family of drugs has been expanding. The SSRIs are used for both severe and mild to moderate depression as well as for a variety of other conditions. These drugs work primarily by increasing the activity of the neurotransmitter (chemical messenger) serotonin in the brain. SSRI antidepressants include

- citalopram (Celexa)
- fluoxetine (Prozac)
- fluvoxamine (Luvox)
- paroxetine (Paxil)
- sertraline (Zoloft)
- and others

Other antidepressants that increase serotonin activity include

- nefazodone (Serzone)
- trazodone (Desyrel)
- venlafaxine (Effexor)

NEGATIVE INTERACTIONS

5-HTP (5-Hydroxytryptophan), SAMe (S-Adenosylmethionine): Possible Harmful Interaction

2 NEGATIVE The body uses the natural substance 5-hydroxytryptophan (5-HTP) to manufacture serotonin, and supplemental forms have been used for treating depression and migraine headaches.

S-Adenosylmethionine (SAMe) is a naturally occurring compound derived from the amino acid methionine and the energy molecule adenosine triphosphate (ATP). SAMe is widely used as a supplement for treating osteoarthritis and depression.

Based on one case report and current thinking about how they work, SAMe and 5-HTP should not be taken with SSRIs, as they might increase the risk of serotonin syndrome.

This syndrome is a toxic reaction brought on by too much serotonin activity. The condition requires immediate medical attention, with symptoms including anxiety, restlessness, confusion, weakness, tremor, muscle twitching or spasm, high fever, profuse sweating, and rapid heartbeat.

The report describes a case of apparent serotonin syndrome in an individual taking SAMe with clomipramine, a **tricyclic antidepressant** (see page 184) that increases serotonin activity.[1]

Although SAMe is not currently known to affect serotonin, it does appear to have antidepressant effects and may in some way increase serotonin activity.

Because SSRIs increase serotonin activity even more than clomipramine, a similar problem might occur if you combine SAMe with an SSRI.

The supplement 5-HTP is used by the body to manufacture serotonin, so it could also increase the risk of serotonin syndrome when combined with an SSRI.

St. John's Wort: Possible Harmful Interaction

2 NEGATIVE The herb St. John's wort (*Hypericum perforatum*) is primarily used to treat mild to moderate depression. One of its actions appears to be increasing the activity of serotonin in the brain.

If you are taking an SSRI medication, do not take the herb St. John's wort at the same time. It is possible that your serotonin levels might be raised too high, causing a dangerous condition called serotonin syndrome[2,3] (please see previous topic).

Several case reports appear to bear this out. Serotonin syndrome was reported in five elderly individuals who began using St. John's wort while taking sertraline (four reports) or nefazodone (one report).[4] One individual had symptoms resembling serotonin syndrome after combining paroxetine (50 mg daily) and St. John's wort (600 mg daily).[5] Another person taking St. John's wort with two other serotonin-enhancing drugs was reported to experience serotonin syndrome.[6]

Furthermore, if you wish to switch from an SSRI to St. John's wort, you may need to wait a few weeks for the SSRI to wash out of your system before it is safe to start taking the herb. The waiting time required depends on which SSRI you are taking. Ask your physician or pharmacist for advice.

POSITIVE INTERACTIONS

Ginkgo: Supplementation Possibly Helpful

2
POSITIVE The herb ginkgo (*Ginkgo biloba*) has been used to treat Alzheimer's disease and ordinary age-related memory loss, among many other uses.

SSRIs can cause many sexual side effects, including inability to achieve orgasm (in women) and impotence (in men). Ginkgo appears to help reverse these problems.

This particular benefit of ginkgo is one of those interesting chance discoveries. An elderly man who was experiencing SSRI-related sexual dysfunction[7] began taking *Ginkgo biloba* for its purported enhancement of memory. After 4 weeks on the herb, he was surprised and pleased to report that his sexual function had improved. When he tried stopping the herb, the problems resurfaced; on restarting it, the prior benefits returned.

This prompted his physician to investigate ginkgo further. Evidence from preliminary studies now suggests that ginkgo can help both men and women with sexual difficulties caused by SSRIs.[8,9]

Though double-blind studies are needed to confirm these findings, the preliminary results are impressive enough to consider a trial of ginkgo if you are experiencing this problem. As there are some potential safety issues with ginkgo, check with your physician first.

Please see Appendix D, Safety Issues, for more information.

SPIRONOLACTONE

Trade name: Aldactone

Interactions	Rating*
Negative Interactions	
Arginine	3
Licorice	1
Magnesium	3
Potassium	1
White Willow	3

*Rating Key

1 Significant interaction

2 Possibly significant interaction

3 Interaction of relatively little significance

4 Reported interaction that does not in fact exist or is insignificant

Spironolactone is a diuretic (an agent that reduces fluid accumulation in the body). It is a member of the potassium-sparing family of diuretics, which were developed to avoid the potassium loss that is common with **loop** (see page 102) and **thiazide diuretics** (see page 174). Potassium-sparing diuretics, though not very powerful by themselves, cause the body to retain potassium and may be used in combination with these other diuretics when needed. Other drugs in this family include **amiloride** (Midamor, Moduretic; see page 7) and **triamterene** (Dyrenium, Maxzide; see page 181).

NEGATIVE INTERACTIONS

Arginine: Possible Harmful Interaction

3 NEGATIVE Arginine is an amino acid found in many foods, including dairy products, meat, poultry, and fish. Supplemental arginine has been proposed as a treatment for various conditions, including heart problems.

Based on experience with arginine given intravenously (into a vein), it is possible that the use of high-dose oral arginine might alter potassium levels in the body, especially in people with severe liver disease.[1] This is a potential concern for individuals who take spironolactone or other potassium-sparing diuretics.

Unless your doctor advises otherwise, it might be best to avoid arginine supplementation if you take spironolactone.

Licorice: Possible Harmful Interaction

1 NEGATIVE Licorice root (*Glycyrrhiza glabra* or *G. uralensis*), a member of the pea family, has been used since ancient times as both food and medicine.

Potassium-sparing diuretics such as spironolactone cause the body to retain potassium and are ordinarily prescribed to take advantage of this effect. Licorice has the opposite effect, causing the body to lose potassium,[2-5] and thus directly counteracts the effect of these drugs. In fact, spironolactone can correct the low potassium levels brought about by excessive licorice ingestion.[6]

Based on these findings, licorice should not be combined with spironolactone except to treat licorice toxicity, which must be supervised by a physician.

Magnesium: Possible Harmful Interaction

3 NEGATIVE Preliminary evidence from animal studies suggests that spironolactone and other potassium-sparing diuretics might cause the body to retain magnesium along with potassium.[7]

Therefore, taking magnesium supplements might conceivably increase the risk of magnesium levels climbing too high and producing toxic effects such as weakness, low blood pressure, and impaired breathing. As a precaution, it may be best to avoid magnesium supplementation while taking spironolactone except under medical supervision.

Potassium: Possible Harmful Interaction

1 NEGATIVE When taking potassium-sparing diuretics such as spironolactone, you generally should not take potassium supplements, since this could raise your potassium levels too high.

Besides potassium supplementation, potassium levels may be raised by high-potassium diets and salt substitutes containing potassium. Symptoms of potassium toxicity include nausea, vomiting, irritability, diarrhea, and changes in heart function.

Treatments that combine thiazide diuretics (which cause potassium loss) and potassium-sparing diuretics can affect potassium levels unpredictably.

If you are taking spironolactone alone or in combination with other diuretics, do not increase your intake of potassium except on the advice of your physician.

White Willow: Possible Harmful Interaction

3 NEGATIVE The herb white willow (*Salix alba*), also known as willow bark, is used to treat pain and fever. White willow contains a substance that is converted by the body into a salicylate similar to aspirin (**NSAIDs**; see page 117).

Because aspirin appears to interfere with the action of spironolactone,[8] there are concerns that white willow might have a similar effect. Based on this observation, it may be advisable to avoid combining white willow with spironolactone.

STATIN DRUGS (*HMG-CoA Reductase Inhibitors*)

Interactions	Rating*
Negative Interactions	
Chaparral, Comfrey, Coltsfoot	2
Grapefruit Juice	1
Niacin (Vitamin B$_3$)	2
Red Yeast Rice	2
Positive Interaction	
Coenzyme Q$_{10}$ (CoQ$_{10}$)	2

*Rating Key

1 Significant interaction

2 Possibly significant interaction

3 Interaction of relatively little significance

4 Reported interaction that does not in fact exist or is insignificant

The statin drugs, also known as HMG-CoA reductase inhibitors, are the most popular and powerful medications for lowering cholesterol. They work by interfering with HMG-CoA reductase, an enzyme necessary for the body's manufacture of cholesterol. Drugs in this family include

- atorvastatin calcium (Lipitor)
- cerivastatin (Baycol)
- fluvastatin (Lescol)
- lovastatin (Mevacor)
- pravastatin (Pravachol)
- simvastatin (Zocor)
- and others

NEGATIVE INTERACTIONS

Chaparral, Comfrey, Coltsfoot: Possible Harmful Interaction

2 NEGATIVE The herb chaparral (*Larrea tridentate* or *L. mexicana*) has been promoted for use in arthritis, cancer, and various other conditions, but there is insufficient evidence supporting its effectiveness. There are, however, concerns about its apparent liver toxicity.

Several cases of chaparral-induced liver damage have been reported, some of them severe enough to require liver transplantation.[1–6]

Based on these reports, combining chaparral with other agents that are hard on the liver, such as statin drugs, may amplify the risk of potential liver problems.[7] Other herbs that are toxic to the liver include comfrey (*Symphytum officinale*) and coltsfoot (*Tussilago farfara*).

Grapefruit Juice: Possible Harmful Interaction

1 NEGATIVE Grapefruit juice impairs the body's normal breakdown of several drugs, including statins, allowing them to build up to potentially excessive levels in the blood.[8] A recent study indicates that this effect can last for 3 days or more following the last glass of juice.[9]

Because this could increase the risk of serious drug side effects, if you take interacting statins, the safest approach is to avoid grapefruit juice altogether. Grapefruit juice may not affect fluvastatin or pravastatin because these drugs are broken down differently than other statins.[10]

Niacin (Vitamin B$_3$): Possible Harmful Interaction

2 NEGATIVE Niacin (nicotinic acid) is vitamin B$_3$. In high doses, niacin is effective in lowering cholesterol levels. Its other form, niacinamide (nicotinamide), does not affect cholesterol.

Combination therapy with statins and niacin is a very effective treatment for certain types of cholesterol disorders. However, there have been concerns that high-dose niacin in combination with statin drugs could increase the risk of drug-induced muscle damage and kidney injury. The good news is that recent studies suggest this risk may be slight, especially in people with normal kidney function.[11,12]

Nonetheless, a doctor's supervision is necessary during treatment with this combination.

Red Yeast Rice: Possible Harmful Interaction

2 NEGATIVE Red yeast rice is an herbal cholesterol-lowering therapy. It contains a mixture of statins; its primary statin ingredient is lovastatin, making it most closely resemble the prescription drug Mevacor.

Based on the similarity of red yeast rice to statin drugs, the two should not be combined without medical supervision.

POSITIVE INTERACTIONS

Coenzyme Q$_{10}$ (CoQ$_{10}$): Supplementation Probably Helpful

2 POSITIVE Coenzyme Q$_{10}$ (CoQ$_{10}$) is a vitamin-like substance that plays a fundamental role in the body's energy production[13,14] and appears to be important for normal heart function.[15]

Statin drugs inhibit the enzyme necessary for the body's synthesis of both cholesterol and CoQ_{10}. Several studies (including two double-blind trials) have found that these drugs reduce CoQ_{10} levels in the body.[16,17,18] Because statin drugs are used to protect the heart by lowering cholesterol levels, their effect of inhibiting CoQ_{10} production might be counterproductive.

Furthermore, statin-induced lowering of tissue CoQ_{10} levels may worsen heart function in people with cardiomyopathy, a disease of the heart muscle.[19] Individuals most vulnerable to this effect appear to be those with low CoQ_{10} levels and impaired heart function to begin with. When the study participants were given oral CoQ_{10} supplementation (100 to 200 mg/day), their CoQ_{10} blood levels increased and their deteriorating heart function improved.

Fortunately, taking CoQ_{10} supplements prevents the lowering of CoQ_{10} levels caused by statin drugs, and does so without interfering with their therapeutic effects.[20]

Based on this evidence, CoQ_{10} supplementation may be advisable when taking statin drugs, especially for individuals with poor heart function.

Please see Appendix D, Safety Issues, for more information.

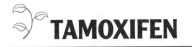
TAMOXIFEN

Interactions	Rating*
Negative Interactions	
Tangeretin	3
Positive Interaction	
Gamma Linolenic Acid (GLA)	2

*Rating Key

1 Significant interaction

2 Possibly significant interaction

3 Interaction of relatively little significance

4 Reported interaction that does not in fact exist or is insignificant

Tamoxifen is an anti-estrogen drug used in treating breast cancer. Estrogen accelerates the growth of some breast cancers, and tamoxifen works by taking its place at estrogen binding sites in breast tissue.

NEGATIVE INTERACTIONS

Tangeretin: Possible Harmful Interaction

3 NEGATIVE In test tube studies, tangeretin, a citrus flavonoid present in tangerines, showed effects similar to tamoxifen in suppressing human breast cancer cells, and combining the two showed additive benefits.[1]

Surprisingly, however, the opposite effect was found when researchers tried to confirm the promising test tube findings in mice that were deliberately injected with human breast cancer cells.[2] Not only did tangeretin fail to stall tumor growth in the mice, it was found to reverse the anti-cancer effects of tamoxifen when the two agents were given together! Whether tangeretin might exert similar effects in humans is not known, but at this point it would certainly seem advisable to avoid excessive intake of tangeretin during tamoxifen therapy.

POSITIVE INTERACTIONS

Gamma Linolenic Acid (GLA): Supplementation Possibly Helpful

2 POSITIVE Gamma Linolenic Acid (GLA) is an omega-6 fatty acid present at high concentrations in borage and evening primrose oils. It has been used for treatment of PMS symptoms and cyclic mastalgia (breast pain that cycles with the menstrual period), as well as numerous other conditions.

In contrast to tangeretin, discussed previously, GLA appears to enhance the benefits of tamoxifen in estrogen-sensitive breast cancer.[3] In one study, 38 persons with breast cancer took 8 capsules of GLA (2.8 g) daily in addition to tamoxifen, while the control group, consisting of 47 persons with breast cancer, took the same dose of tamoxifen alone. After 6 weeks, it was evident that those taking GLA and tamoxifen exhibited a faster treatment response compared to those taking only tamoxifen.

This evidence suggests that high-dose GLA may enhance the beneficial effects of tamoxifen in individuals with breast cancer.

Please see Appendix D, Safety Issues, for more information.

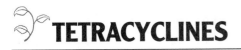

TETRACYCLINES

Interactions	Rating*
Negative Interactions	
Potassium Citrate	2
St. John's Wort, Dong Quai	3
Minerals	2

*Rating Key

1   Significant interaction

2   Possibly significant interaction

3   Interaction of relatively little significance

4   Reported interaction that does not in fact exist or is insignificant

Tetracycline antibiotics are used to treat certain infections such as chlamydia; they are also used for the long-term treatment of acne. Depending on the dose, tetracyclines can either kill or stop the growth of infection-causing bacteria. (See also **Antibiotics**, page 19.) Drugs in this family include

- demeclocycline hydrochloride (Declomycin)
- doxycycline (Bio-Tab, Doryx, Doxy-Caps, Doxychel, Monodox, Novodoxylin, Periostat, Vibramycin, Vibra-Tabs)
- minocycline hydrochloride (Dynacin, Minocin, Vectrin)
- oxytetracycline hydrochloride (Terramycin, Uri-Tet, Urobiotic)
- tetracycline hydrochloride (Achromycin V, Helidac, Panmycin, Robitet, Sumycin, Teline, Tetracap, Tetracyn, Tetralan)
- and others

NEGATIVE INTERACTIONS

Potassium Citrate: Possible Harmful Interaction

2 NEGATIVE Potassium citrate and other forms of citrate (e.g., calcium citrate, magnesium citrate) may be used to prevent kidney stones. These agents work by making the urine less acidic.

This effect on the urine may lead to decreased blood levels and therapeutic effects of several drugs, including tetracycline antibiotics.[1]

It may be advisable to avoid these citrate compounds during treatment with tetracyclines except under medical supervision.

St. John's Wort, Dong Quai: Possible Harmful Interaction

3 NEGATIVE St. John's wort (*Hypericum perforatum*) is primarily used to treat mild to moderate depression.

The herb dong quai (*Angelica sinensis*) is often recommended for menstrual disorders such as dysmenorrhea, PMS, and irregular menstruation.

Tetracycline antibiotics have been reported to cause increased sensitivity to the sun, amplifying the risk of sunburn or skin rash. Because St. John's wort and dong quai may also cause this problem, taking these herbal supplements during tetracycline treatment might add to this risk.

It may be a good idea to wear a sunscreen or protective clothing during sun exposure if you take one of these herbs with a tetracycline antibiotic.

Minerals: Take at a Different Time of Day

2 NEGATIVE Numerous minerals can interfere with the absorption of antibiotics in the tetracycline family, including aluminum (found in many antacids), bismuth (in Pepto-Bismol), calcium, magnesium, iron, and zinc.[2–5] The minerals attach to tetracycline and form compounds that cannot be absorbed—they simply pass through the digestive tract and out of the body. For the same reason, mineral absorption is also impaired.[6]

To prevent absorption problems when using tetracyclines, take them 3 to 4 hours apart from milk and dairy products containing calcium and from supplements containing these other minerals.

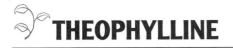

THEOPHYLLINE

Interactions	Rating*
Negative Interactions	
Cayenne	2
Ipriflavone	1
St. John's Wort	2
Positive Interaction	
Vitamin B₆ (Pyridoxine)	2

*Rating Key

1 Significant interaction

2 Possibly significant interaction

3 Interaction of relatively little significance

4 Reported interaction that does not in fact exist or is insignificant

Once among the most common treatments for asthma, theophylline is no longer widely used, having been replaced by drugs that cause fewer side effects. One problem with theophylline is that it has a narrow therapeutic range, which means that toxic symptoms can develop at doses only slightly higher than those necessary to produce benefits; similarly, a dose that is only slightly too low may prove ineffective.

Theophylline is also sometimes used for sleep apnea.

NEGATIVE INTERACTIONS

Cayenne: Possible Harmful Interaction

2 NEGATIVE Cayenne (*Capsicum annuum* or *C. frutescens*) and other hot peppers used in chili and various dishes contain as their "hot" ingredient capsaicin, a substance that is thought to be stomach-protective.

Some evidence suggests that oral cayenne might increase the body's absorption of theophylline,[1] which could lead to an increased risk of theophylline toxicity.

Based on this finding, it may be advisable to avoid ingesting cayenne if you take theophylline.

Ipriflavone: Possible Harmful Interaction

1 NEGATIVE Ipriflavone, a synthetic isoflavone that slows bone breakdown, is used to treat osteoporosis.

Ipriflavone appears to slow the body's normal breakdown of theophylline to inactive forms, allowing the drug to build up in the blood.[2,3] A rise in theophylline blood levels may increase the risk of toxic symptoms such as nervousness and even seizures.

In one individual, blood levels of theophylline increased while ipriflavone was taken, then decreased when ipriflavone was stopped.[4] Although there was no evidence of theophylline toxicity in this particular case, the finding raises an important concern. Some people using theophylline for asthma may also be taking **corticosteroids** (see page 68) for the same condition. In an attempt to prevent corticosteroid-associated osteoporosis, they may decide to take ipriflavone, thus potentially increasing their risk of theophylline toxicity.

If you take theophylline, you should avoid ipriflavone supplementation unless supervised by a physician.

St. John's Wort: Possible Harmful Interaction

2 NEGATIVE The herb St. John's wort (*Hypericum perforatum*) is primarily used to treat mild to moderate depression.

Evidence suggests St. John's wort can lower blood levels of theophylline, making it less effective.[5,6] The herb appears to accelerate the body's normal breakdown of theophylline to inactive forms.

In one case report, a 42-year-old woman was doing well on a certain dose of theophylline until she began taking St. John's wort (standardized to 0.3% hypericin) at 300 mg daily.[7] After she started the herb, the dose of theophylline required to maintain proper blood levels of the drug increased almost three-fold.

When she stopped taking St. John's wort, her theophylline levels climbed dangerously high. This is an example of a "hidden" risk associated with this type of interaction. Because St. John's wort had been holding down drug levels, abruptly stopping the herb was like releasing the brakes, allowing her theophylline levels to surge.

Because of this risk, you should not combine St. John's wort and theophylline except under a physician's supervision.

POSITIVE INTERACTIONS

Vitamin B$_6$ (Pyridoxine): Supplementation Probably Helpful

2 POSITIVE Theophylline appears to impair the normal conversion of vitamin B$_6$ into its active form, pyridoxal 5'-phosphate (PLP).[8] For this reason, long-term theophylline treatment may deplete the body's stores of this vitamin.[9,10] Supplementation may overcome this effect and prevent vitamin B$_6$ deficiency.

In a 6-week placebo-controlled trial, giving vitamin B_6 (pyridoxal HCl) at 15 mg daily in combination with slow-release theophylline kept B_6 levels within the normal range.[11] In a 16-week trial during which theophylline depleted participants' vitamin B_6, giving B_6 (pyridoxine HCl) at 10 mg daily for 1 week raised vitamin levels back to normal.[12]

These findings have led a number of researchers to suspect that some of the many side effects of theophylline could be caused, at least in part, by interference with vitamin B_6 activity. In fact, preliminary evidence suggests that vitamin B_6 supplementation may reduce adverse nervous system effects associated with theophylline, such as hand tremor.[13] This makes sense based on prior evidence indicating an association between B_6 deficiency and the body's release of chemicals that stimulate the central nervous system.[14]

Based on this evidence and the prevalence of vitamin B_6 deficiency in the diet,[15] vitamin B_6 supplementation may be advisable during long-term theophylline therapy.

Please see Appendix D, Safety Issues, for more information.

THIAZIDE DIURETICS

Trade Names: Diucardin, Diuril, Enduron, Exna, Hydrodiuril, Hydromox, Hyrex, Metahydrin, Renee, Saluron

Interactions	Rating*
Negative Interactions	
Calcium	1
Licorice	2
St. John's Wort, Dong Quai	3
Positive Interactions	
Magnesium	2
Potassium	1
Zinc	3

*Rating Key

1 Significant interaction

2 Possibly significant interaction

3 Interaction of relatively little significance

4 Reported interaction that does not in fact exist or is insignificant

Thiazide diuretics reduce fluid accumulation in the body, which makes them useful for treating high blood pressure and edema (excessive fluid in body tissues). They may be used alone or to enhance the effects of other drugs. Thiazide diuretics are often combined with potassium-sparing diuretics (**triamterene**; see page 181) in an attempt to cancel out any effect on potassium.

NEGATIVE INTERACTIONS

Calcium: Possible Harmful Interaction

1 NEGATIVE Instead of causing loss of calcium in the urine as with other minerals, thiazide diuretics promote calcium retention by the body.[1–4] This tends to increase calcium blood levels.

Ordinarily, the body can adjust and this is not likely to cause a problem. However, extra calcium intake from calcium-containing antacids or calcium supplements can drive levels of the mineral too high. Early symptoms of high calcium levels include constipation, appetite loss, nausea and vomiting, and abdominal pain. If high calcium levels are prolonged, kidney stones containing calcium may form and other serious effects might occur.

Vitamin D increases calcium absorption, so taking this vitamin supplement may compound the problem.

If you are using thiazide diuretics, consult with your physician before taking calcium and vitamin D supplements.

Licorice: Possible Harmful Interaction

2 NEGATIVE Licorice root (*Glycyrrhiza glabra* or *G. uralensis*), a member of the pea family, has been used since ancient times as both food and medicine.

Licorice root could enhance the potassium loss caused by thiazides.[5] Glycyrrhizic acid, the active ingredient in licorice, appears to promote potassium loss in the urine,[6,7] and there have been case reports of low blood levels of potassium following licorice use.[8,9,10]

If you are using thiazide diuretics, you should avoid licorice root. An often-unrecognized source of licorice is chewing tobacco.[11] Licorice-flavored candies, however, should not be a problem.

Another option is to use a specific form of licorice known as DGL (deglycyrrhizinated licorice). It is a deliberately altered form of the herb that should not affect potassium levels and therefore should not pose a danger for thiazide diuretic users.

St. John's Wort, Dong Quai: Possible Harmful Interaction

3 NEGATIVE St. John's wort (*Hypericum perforatum*) is primarily used to treat mild to moderate depression.

The herb dong quai (*Angelica sinensis*) is often recommended for menstrual disorders such as dysmenorrhea, PMS, and irregular menstruation.

Thiazide diuretics have been reported to cause increased sensitivity to the sun, amplifying the risk of sunburn or skin rash. Because St. John's wort and dong quai may also cause this problem, taking these herbal supplements during treatment with thiazide diuretics might add to this risk.

It may be a good idea to wear a sunscreen or protective clothing during sun exposure if you take one of these herbs while using a thiazide diuretic.

POSITIVE INTERACTIONS

Magnesium: Supplementation Probably Helpful

 2 POSITIVE Thiazide diuretics can promote loss of magnesium in the urine.[12,13,14] In some cases, this may lead to magnesium deficiency. Additionally, untreated magnesium depletion can make it more difficult to correct potassium depletion.[15]

As magnesium deficiency is common anyway, magnesium supplementation at standard nutritional doses might make sense, especially if you must stay on diuretic therapy for a long time. Adding a type of diuretic that helps counteract magnesium loss is another option.

Please see Appendix D, Safety Issues, for more information.

Potassium: Supplementation Probably Helpful

1 **POSITIVE** As with magnesium, thiazide diuretics wash potassium out of the body in the urine. This may cause potassium blood levels to fall too low and produce symptoms such as muscle cramps or weakness. Heart rhythm irregularities may also occur, especially in individuals also taking the heart drug **digoxin** (see page 74).

The classic treatment is to consume high-potassium foods such as bananas and orange juice. Potassium levels can also be raised by potassium supplements and salt substitutes containing potassium. Adding a type of diuretic that helps counteract potassium loss is another option.

Treatments that combine thiazide diuretics with potassium-sparing diuretics (which cause potassium retention) can affect potassium levels unpredictably. If you are taking such combination treatment, do not increase your intake of potassium except on the advice of your physician.

Please see Appendix D, Safety Issues, for more information.

Zinc: Supplementation Possibly Helpful

3 **POSITIVE** Thiazide diuretics can promote loss of zinc in the urine.[16] Long-term use of these diuretics may result in significant depletion of the mineral, particularly in individuals with conditions that put them at extra risk for zinc depletion, including alcoholism, cirrhosis of the liver, kidney disease, diabetes, gastrointestinal disorders, and pregnancy.[17,18]

As zinc deficiency is relatively common, zinc supplementation in nutritional doses may be advisable, especially if you regularly take thiazide diuretics. Using the smallest effective dose of the drug may be a simple way to help prevent zinc depletion, but you should not make dose changes without your physician's approval. Generally, zinc supplements should also contain copper to prevent zinc-induced copper deficiency.

Please see Appendix D, Safety Issues, for more information.

THYROID HORMONE

Interactions	Rating*
Negative Interactions	
Calcium	2
Iron	1
Soy	2

*Rating Key

1 Significant interaction

2 Possibly significant interaction

3 Interaction of relatively little significance

4 Reported interaction that does not in fact exist or is insignificant

Thyroid hormone supplements are primarily used to treat hypothyroidism, a condition caused by deficient secretion of thyroid hormone by the thyroid gland. Forms of thyroid hormone include

- dextrothyroxine (Choloxin)
- levothyroxine (Levoid, Levothroid, Levoxine, Levoxyl, Synthroid)
- liothyronine (Cytomel, Triostat)
- liotrix (Euthroid, Thyrolar)
- thyroglobulin (Proloid)
- thyroid (Armour Thyroid)

NEGATIVE INTERACTIONS

Calcium: Take at a Different Time of Day

2 NEGATIVE Two case reports suggest that calcium carbonate interferes with the body's absorption of thyroid hormone when both were taken at the same time.[1,2]

A prospective cohort study has validated these case reports.[3] Twenty individuals with hypothyroidism stabilized on long-term levothyroxine therapy were included in the trial. Participants were given calcium carbonate (1200 mg daily of elemental calcium) for 3 months. During the period the calcium supplement was taken, thyroid hormone blood levels declined. But after calcium supplementation was stopped, thyroid levels climbed back up, slightly surpassing the levels measured at the beginning of the study.

It is thought that calcium chelates (combines) with thyroid hormone, thus reducing its absorption.

To prevent this interaction, take thyroid hormone and calcium supplements as far apart as possible.

Iron: Take at a Different Time of Day

1 NEGATIVE Iron salts (including ferrous fumarate, ferrous gluconate, ferrous sulfate, and iron polysaccharide) may impair the effect of the thyroid hormone levothyroxine, probably by forming a complex with it and decreasing its absorption.[4]

To prevent a problem, take iron supplements as far apart as possible from thyroid hormones.

Soy: Possible Harmful Interaction

2 NEGATIVE Soy formula may interfere with the absorption of thyroid medication in infants.[5] In addition, soy may directly interfere with thyroid function.[6,7] The result may be a need to increase the infant's dosage of thyroid medication. However, if you stop giving an infant soy formula, the thyroid dosage may need to be decreased. Of course, all changes relating to thyroid treatment should be managed by a physician.

Based on these findings, individuals with impaired thyroid function should use soy (e.g., soybeans, soy milk, tofu) with caution.

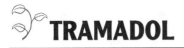 TRAMADOL

Trade Name: Ultram

Interactions	Rating*
Negative Interactions	
St. John's Wort, SAMe (S-Adenosylmethionine), 5-HTP (5-Hydroxytryptophan)	2

*Rating Key

1   Significant interaction

2   Possibly significant interaction

3   Interaction of relatively little significance

4   Reported interaction that does not in fact exist or is insignificant

Tramadol is a unique non-narcotic and non-antiinflammatory analgesic used for the treatment of moderate pain.

NEGATIVE INTERACTIONS

St. John's Wort, SAMe (S-Adenosylmethionine), 5-HTP (5-Hydroxytryptophan): Possible Harmful Interaction

2 NEGATIVE The herb St. John's wort (*Hypericum perforatum*) is primarily used to treat mild to moderate depression.

S-Adenosylmethionine (SAMe) is a naturally occurring compound derived from the amino acid methionine and the energy molecule adenosine triphosphate (ATP). SAMe is widely used as a supplement for treating osteoarthritis and depression.

The body uses the natural substance 5-hydroxytryptophan (5-HTP) to manufacture serotonin, and supplemental forms have been used for treating depression and migraine headaches.

One of the many effects of tramadol is increasing the activity of serotonin, a chemical messenger in the brain. For this reason, tramadol may contribute to the development of serotonin syndrome when combined with other serotonin-enhancing agents such as St. John's wort and 5-HTP. Although SAMe is not currently known to affect serotonin, it does appear to have antidepressant effects and may in some way increase serotonin activity.

Serotonin syndrome, a toxic reaction requiring immediate medical attention, is associated with too much serotonin. Symptoms may include anxiety, restlessness, confusion, weakness, tremor, muscle twitching or spasm, high fever, profuse sweating, and rapid heartbeat.

Two case reports possibly implicate tramadol in serotonin syndrome. One report involved the combination of tramadol and the serotonin-enhancing antidepressant sertraline (Zoloft).[1] Another report involved the use of tramadol in combination with an **MAO inhibitor** (see page 105) and the **tricyclic antidepressant** (see page 184) clomipramine (Anafranil), both of which possess high serotonin activity (see also **SSRIs**, page 158).[2]

Because the herb St. John's Wort[3,4] and the supplement SAMe[5] have also been associated with serotonin syndrome when combined with serotonin-enhancing drugs, mixing these supplements with tramadol might cause similar problems. The supplement 5-HTP (5-Hydroxytryptophan), which is converted in the body to serotonin, could have a similar effect in combination with tramadol.

For these reasons, it would be advisable for individuals taking tramadol to avoid these supplements.

TRIAMTERENE

Trade names: Dyrenium, Maxzide

Interactions	Rating*
Negative Interactions	
Arginine	3
Licorice	1
Magnesium	3
Potassium	1
Positive Interaction	
Folate	3

*Rating Key

1 Significant interaction

2 Possibly significant interaction

3 Interaction of relatively little significance

4 Reported interaction that does not in fact exist or is insignificant

Triamterene is a diuretic (an agent that reduces fluid accumulation in the body). It is a member of the potassium-sparing family of diuretics, which were developed to avoid the potassium loss that is common with **loop** (see page 102) and **thiazide diuretics** (see page 174). Potassium-sparing diuretics, though not very powerful by themselves, cause the body to retain potassium and may be used in combination with these other diuretics when needed. Other drugs in this family include **amiloride** (Midamor, Moduretic; see page 7) and **spironolactone** (Aldactone; see page 161).

NEGATIVE INTERACTIONS

Arginine: Possible Harmful Interaction

3 NEGATIVE Arginine is an amino acid found in many foods, including dairy products, meat, poultry, and fish. Supplemental arginine has been proposed as a treatment for various conditions, including heart problems.

Based on experience with arginine given intravenously (into a vein), it is possible that the use of high-dose oral arginine might alter potassium levels in the body, especially in people with severe liver disease.[1] This is a potential concern for individuals who take triamterene or other potassium-sparing diuretics.

Unless your doctor advises otherwise, it might be best to avoid arginine supplementation if you take triamterene.

Licorice: Possible Harmful Interaction

1 NEGATIVE Licorice root (*Glycyrrhiza glabra* or *G. uralensis*), a member of the pea family, has been used since ancient times as both food and medicine.

Potassium-sparing diuretics such as triamterene cause the body to retain potassium and are ordinarily prescribed to take advantage of this effect. Licorice has the opposite effect, causing the body to lose potassium,[2–5] and thus directly counteracts the effect of these drugs. In fact, the potassium-sparing diuretic spironolactone has been found to correct the low potassium levels brought about by excessive licorice ingestion.[6]

Based on these findings, licorice should not be combined with potassium-sparing diuretics except to treat licorice toxicity, which must be supervised by a physician.

Magnesium: Possible Harmful Interaction

3 NEGATIVE Preliminary evidence from animal studies suggests that triamterene and other potassium-sparing diuretics might cause the body to retain magnesium along with potassium.[7]

Therefore, taking magnesium supplements might conceivably increase the risk of magnesium levels climbing too high and producing toxic effects such as weakness, low blood pressure, and impaired breathing. As a precaution, it may be best to avoid magnesium supplementation while taking triamterene except under medical supervision.

Potassium: Possible Harmful Interaction

1 NEGATIVE When taking potassium-sparing diuretics such as triamterene, you generally should not take potassium supplements, since this could raise your potassium levels too high.

Besides potassium supplementation, potassium levels may be raised by high-potassium diets and salt substitutes containing potassium. Symptoms of potassium toxicity include nausea, vomiting, irritability, diarrhea, and changes in heart function.

Treatments that combine thiazide diuretics (which cause potassium loss) and potassium-sparing diuretics can affect potassium levels unpredictably.

If you are taking triamterene alone or in combination with other diuretics, do not increase your intake of potassium except on the advice of your physician.

POSITIVE INTERACTIONS

Folate: Supplementation Possibly Helpful

| **3** |
| POSITIVE |

Folate (also known as folic acid) is a B vitamin that plays an important role in many vital aspects of health, including preventing neural tube birth defects and possibly reducing the risk of heart disease. Because inadequate intake of folate is widespread, if you are taking any medication that depletes or impairs folate even slightly, you may need supplementation.

Triamterene bears a structural resemblance to folate, and the body might mistakenly use the drug in place of folate in some instances.[8] Because of this, triamterene taken regularly in high doses might cause symptoms related to folate deficiency in individuals with risk factors for folate depletion.

An observational study indicated that triamterene at daily doses of 50 to 150 mg did not cause folate deficiency.[9] In contrast, the use of higher daily doses of triamterene (150 to 600 mg) was associated with a folate-related anemia.[10] Confusing the issue somewhat is that the study participants had liver disease, which could have contributed to this effect.

Typical triamterene doses should not significantly affect folate status in most individuals. However, because of the prevalence of folate deficiency in the general population, folate supplementation at standard nutritional doses may be advisable on general principles.

Please see Appendix D, Safety Issues, for more information.

TRICYCLIC ANTIDEPRESSANTS

Interactions	Rating*
Negative Interactions	
Kava, Valerian, Passionflower, Hops	2
St. John's Wort, Dong Quai	3
St. John's Wort, SAMe (S-Adenosylmethionine), 5-HTP (5-Hydroxytryptophan)	2
Mixed Interaction	
Grapefruit Juice	2
Positive Interaction	
Coenzyme Q_{10} (CoQ_{10})	3

*Rating Key

1 Significant interaction
2 Possibly significant interaction
3 Interaction of relatively little significance
4 Reported interaction that does not in fact exist or is insignificant

For many years, the tricyclics were the most popular antidepressants. Although largely replaced today by the less side-effect prone **SSRI** (see page 158) drugs (such as Prozac), tricyclic antidepressants are still used in certain cases. These drugs appear to work by increasing the activity of various neurotransmitters (chemical messengers) in the brain. Antidepressants in this family include

- amitriptyline hydrochloride (Elavil, Emitrip, Endep, Enovil, Etrafon, Limbitrol, Triavil)
- amoxapine (Asendin)
- clomipramine hydrochloride (Anafranil)
- desipramine hydrochloride (Norpramin, Pertofrane)
- doxepin hydrochloride (Adapin, Sinequan, Zonalon)
- imipramine (Janimine, Tipramine, Tofranil)
- nortriptyline hydrochloride (Aventyl, Pamelor)
- protriptyline hydrochloride (Vivactil)
- trimipramine maleate (Surmontil)
- and others

NEGATIVE INTERACTIONS

Kava, Valerian, Passionflower, Hops: Possible Harmful Interaction

 The herb kava (*Piper methysticum*) has a sedative effect and is used for anxiety and insomnia. Combining kava with tricyclic antidepressants, which possess similar physical depressant effects, could result in "add-on" or excessive physical depression, sedation, and impairment. In one case report of a 54-year-old man hospitalized for lethargy and disorientation, these side effects were attributed to his having taken both kava and the antianxiety agent alprazolam (Xanax) for 3 days.[1]

Other herbs with a sedative effect that might cause problems when combined with tricyclic antidepressants include ashwagandha (*Withania somnifera*), calendula (*Calendula officinalis*), catnip (*Nepeta cataria*), hops (*Humulus lupulus*), lady's slipper (*Cypripedium*), lemon balm (*Melissa officinalis*), passionflower (*Passiflora incarnata*), sassafras (*Sassafras officinale*), skullcap (*Scutellaria lateriflora*), valerian (*Valeriana officinalis*), and yerba mansa (*Anemopsis californica*).

Because of the potentially serious consequences, you should avoid combining these herbs with tricyclic antidepressants or other drugs that have sedative or depressant effects, unless advised by your physician.

St. John's Wort, Dong Quai: Possible Harmful Interaction

 St. John's wort (*Hypericum perforatum*) is primarily used to treat mild to moderate depression.

The herb dong quai (*Angelica sinensis*) is often recommended for menstrual disorders such as dysmenorrhea, PMS, and irregular menstruation.

Tricyclic antidepressants have been reported to cause increased sensitivity to the sun, amplifying the risk of sunburn or skin rash. Because St. John's wort and dong quai may also cause this problem, taking these herbal supplements during treatment with these drugs might add to this risk.

It may be a good idea to wear a sunscreen or protective clothing during sun exposure if you take one of these herbs while using tricyclic antidepressants.

St. John's Wort, SAMe (S-Adenosylmethionine), 5-HTP (5-Hydroxytryptophan): Possible Harmful Interaction

 The herb St. John's wort (*Hypericum perforatum*) is primarily used to treat mild to moderate depression.

S-adenosylmethionine (SAMe) is a naturally occurring compound derived from the amino acid methionine and the energy molecule adenosine triphosphate (ATP). SAMe is widely used as a supplement for treating osteoarthritis and depression.

The body uses the natural substance 5-hydroxytryptophan (5-HTP) to manufacture serotonin, and supplemental forms have been used for treating depression and migraine headaches.

Most tricyclic antidepressants increase, to some degree, the effects of serotonin, a chemical messenger in the brain. For this reason, tricyclics may contribute to the development of serotonin syndrome when combined with other serotonin-enhancing agents such as St. John's wort and 5-HTP. Although SAMe is not currently known to affect serotonin, it does appear to have antidepressant effects and may in some way increase serotonin activity.

Serotonin syndrome, a toxic reaction requiring immediate medical attention, is associated with too much serotonin. Symptoms may include anxiety, restlessness, confusion, weakness, tremor, muscle twitching or spasm, high fever, profuse sweating, and rapid heartbeat.

A report of apparent serotonin syndrome involved an individual taking SAMe while using clomipramine (Anafranil), a tricyclic antidepressant with high serotonin activity.[2]

Several case reports have involved other classes of serotonin-enhancing antidepressants. Serotonin syndrome was reported in five elderly individuals who began using St. John's wort while taking antidepressants—four reports involved sertraline (Zoloft) and one involved nefazodone (Serzone).[3] One individual experienced symptoms resembling serotonin syndrome after combining paroxetine (Paxil) and St. John's wort.[4] Another person taking St. John's wort with two other serotonin-enhancing drugs was reported to experience serotonin syndrome.[5]

The supplement 5-HTP, which is converted in the body to serotonin, could have a similar effect.

Based on this evidence, you should avoid these supplements if you take a tricyclic antidepressant.

MIXED INTERACTIONS

Grapefruit Juice: Possible Benefits and Risks

2 MIXED Grapefruit juice slows the body's normal breakdown of several drugs, including the tricyclic antidepressant clomipramine, resulting in increased blood levels of the drug.[6] A recent study indicates this effect can last for 3 days or more following the last glass of juice.[7] Interestingly, this interaction has been used to improve symptom control in obsessive compulsive disorder (OCD). However, since drug side effects may also be increased, you should not combine grapefruit juice with clomipramine except under a physician's supervision.

POSITIVE INTERACTIONS

Coenzyme Q_{10} (CoQ_{10}): Supplementation Possibly Helpful

3
POSITIVE

Coenzyme Q_{10} is a vitamin-like substance that plays a fundamental role in the body's energy production[8,9] and appears to be important for normal heart function.[10,11]

Preliminary evidence suggests that tricyclic antidepressants might interfere with enzymes containing CoQ_{10}.[12,13] Based on this observation, it has been suggested (but not proven) that CoQ_{10} supplementation might help prevent the heart-related side effects that can occur with the use of tricyclic antidepressants.

Please see Appendix D, Safety Issues, for more information.

TRIMETHOPRIM-SULFAMETHOXAZOLE (TMP-SMZ)

Trade Names: Bactrim, Cotrim, Septra, Sulfatrim

Interactions	Rating*
Negative Interactions	
PABA	2
Potassium	2
St. John's Wort, Dong Quai	3
Positive Interactions	
Folate	1
N-acetyl cysteine (NAC)	4

*Rating Key

1 Significant interaction
2 Possibly significant interaction
3 Interaction of relatively little significance
4 Reported interaction that does not in fact exist or is insignificant

Trimethoprim (Proloprim, Trimpex) is commonly combined with sulfamethoxazole (Gantanol) for an antibiotic combination (called TMP-SMZ for short) that delivers a "one-two punch" against bacteria. Because both antibiotics interfere with the B vitamin folate, they are effective against bacteria that must produce their own folate. The sulfamethoxazole makes it hard for invading bacteria to manufacture folate,[1] and the trimethoprim makes it hard for bacteria to use folate.[2] The net effect is to starve the bacteria of this necessary vitamin. (See also **Antibiotics, page 19.**)

NEGATIVE INTERACTIONS

PABA: Possible Harmful Interaction

2 NEGATIVE PABA (para-aminobenzoic acid), a nutrient found primarily in grains and meat, is probably best known as the active ingredient in sunscreens.

One step in the manufacture of folate by bacteria requires PABA. Because sulfamethoxazole destroys bacteria by blocking this step,[3,4] PABA supplementation may make TMP-SMZ less effective.

Therefore, if you are being treated with this antibiotic, do not take PABA except on medical advice.

Potassium: Possible Harmful Interaction

 Trimethoprim-sulfamethoxazole might increase levels of potassium in the body. Of 80 people treated with TMP-SMZ, more than half developed high potassium blood levels, with several individuals having severely high levels.[5]

Symptoms of high potassium levels (hyperkalemia) might include irregular heart rhythm, muscle weakness, nausea, vomiting, irritability, and diarrhea.

If you are on long-term treatment with this antibiotic, you should not take potassium supplements except on the advice of a physician. Besides potassium supplements, other sources of potassium to avoid are high-potassium diets and salt substitutes containing potassium.

St. John's Wort, Dong Quai: Possible Harmful Interaction

3 NEGATIVE St. John's wort (*Hypericum perforatum*) is primarily used to treat mild to moderate depression.

The herb dong quai (*Angelica sinensis*) is often recommended for menstrual disorders such as dysmenorrhea, PMS, and irregular menstruation.

Sulfamethoxazole, a sulfa drug, can cause increased sensitivity to the sun, amplifying the risk of sunburn or skin rash. Because St. John's wort and dong quai may also cause this problem, taking these herbal supplements during sulfamethoxazole therapy might add to the risk.

It may be a good idea to wear a sunscreen or protective clothing during sun exposure if you take one of these herbs while using sulfamethoxazole.

POSITIVE INTERACTIONS

Folate: Supplementation Probably Helpful

1 POSITIVE Folate (aka folic acid) is a B vitamin that plays an important role in many vital aspects of health, including preventing neural tube birth defects and possibly reducing the risk of heart disease. Because inadequate intake of folate is widespread, if you are taking any medication that depletes or impairs folate even slightly, you may need supplementation.

Since trimethoprim and sulfamethoxazole work by interfering with folate in bacteria, there may be concern that these agents might exert similar effects in humans. Fortunately, humans and other mammals are much less affected by the anti-folate action of these antibiotics than are bacteria, due to the different way we process folate. However, trimethoprim can still interfere to some extent in your body's ability to utilize this essential nutrient.

For this reason, folate supplementation may be helpful if you take this antibiotic for a long period of time (to prevent urinary tract infections, for example).[6]

Please see Appendix D, Safety Issues, for more information.

N-acetyl cysteine (NAC): Interaction Unlikely or Probably Insignificant

4
POSITIVE N-acetyl cysteine (NAC) is a specially modified form of the dietary amino acid cysteine that has various proposed uses.

It has been suggested that NAC might help prevent side effects caused by long term use of TMP-SMX. However, two double-blind studies found that NAC did not significantly decrease adverse reactions to TMP-SMX compared to placebo.[7,8]

Please see Appendix D, Safety Issues, for more information.

VALPROIC ACID

Trade Names: Depakene, Depakote

Interactions	Rating*
Negative Interactions	
Ginkgo	3
Glutamine	4
Kava, Valerian, Passionflower, Hops	2
St. John's Wort, Dong Quai	3
Vitamin A	3
Mixed Interactions	
Biotin	3
Folate	2

Interactions	Rating*
Positive Interactions	
Calcium	2
Carnitine	2
Vitamin D	2
Vitamin K	2

*Rating Key

1 Significant interaction
2 Possibly significant interaction
3 Interaction of relatively little significance
4 Reported interaction that does not in fact exist or is insignificant

Valproic acid is an anticonvulsant agent used primarily to prevent seizures in conditions such as epilepsy.

Other anticonvulsant agents include **carbamazepine** (see page 54), **phenobarbital** (see page 134), **phenytoin** (see page 140), and **primidone** (see page 146). In some cases, combination therapy with two or more anticonvulsant drugs may be used.

NEGATIVE INTERACTIONS

Ginkgo: Possible Harmful Interaction

3 NEGATIVE The herb ginkgo (*Ginkgo biloba*) has been used to treat Alzheimer's disease and ordinary age-related memory loss, among many other uses.

This interaction involves potential contaminants in ginkgo, not ginkgo itself.

A recent study found that a natural nerve toxin present in the seeds of *Ginkgo biloba* made its way into standardized ginkgo extracts prepared from the leaves.[1] This toxin has been associated with convulsions and death in laboratory animals.[2,3,4]

Fortunately, the detected amounts of this toxic substance are considered harmless.[5] However, given the lack of satisfactory standardization of herbal formulations in the United States, it is possible that some batches of

Valproic Acid

product might contain higher contents of the toxin depending on the season of harvest.

In light of these findings, taking a ginkgo product that happened to contain significant levels of the nerve toxin might theoretically prevent an anticonvulsant from working as well as expected.

Glutamine: Possible Harmful Interaction

4 NEGATIVE The amino acid glutamine is converted to glutamate in the body. Glutamate is thought to act as a neurotransmitter (a chemical that enables nerve transmission). Because anticonvulsants work (at least in part) by blocking glutamate pathways in the brain, high dosages of the amino acid glutamine might theoretically diminish an anticonvulsant's effect and increase the risk of seizures.

Kava, Valerian, Passionflower, Hops: Possible Harmful Interaction

2 NEGATIVE The herb kava (*Piper methysticum*) has a sedative effect and is used for anxiety and insomnia.

Combining kava with anticonvulsants, which possess similar depressant effects, could result in "add-on" or excessive physical depression, sedation, and impairment. In one case report, a 54-year-old man was hospitalized for lethargy and disorientation, side effects attributed to his having taken the combination of kava and the antianxiety agent alprazolam (Xanax) for 3 days.[6]

Other herbs having a sedative effect that might cause problems when combined with anticonvulsants include ashwagandha (*Withania somnifera*), calendula (*Calendula officinalis*), catnip (*Nepeta cataria*), hops (*Humulus lupulus*), lady's slipper (*Cypripedium* species), lemon balm (*Melissa officinalis*), passionflower (*Passiflora incarnata*), sassafras (*Sassafras officinale*), skullcap (*Scutellaria lateriflora*), valerian (*Valeriana officinalis*), and yerba mansa (*Anemopsis californica*).

Because of the potentially serious consequences, you should avoid combining these herbs with anticonvulsants or other drugs that also have sedative or depressant effects, unless advised by your physician.

St. John's Wort, Dong Quai: Possible Harmful Interaction

3 NEGATIVE St. John's wort (*Hypericum perforatum*) is primarily used to treat mild to moderate depression.

The herb dong quai (*Angelica sinensis*) is often recommended for menstrual disorders such as dysmenorrhea, PMS, and irregular menstruation.

The anticonvulsant agents valproic acid, carbamazepine, and phenobarbital have been reported to cause increased sensitivity to the sun, amplifying the risk of sunburn or skin rash. Because St. John's wort and dong quai may also cause this problem, taking them during treatment with these drugs might add to this risk.

It may be a good idea to wear a sunscreen or protective clothing during sun exposure if you take one of these herbs while using these anticonvulsants.

Vitamin A: Possible Harmful Interaction

3 NEGATIVE Although the research on this subject is slim, some evidence suggests that valproic acid may interfere with the body's ability to safely handle vitamin A.[7] For this reason, vitamin A supplements should be taken with caution (if at all) by those on valproic acid. Taking beta carotene, which is converted into vitamin A in the body, may not present a problem.

MIXED INTERACTIONS

Biotin: Supplementation Possibly Helpful, but Take at a Different Time of Day

3 MIXED Anticonvulsants may deplete biotin, an essential water-soluble B vitamin, possibly by competing with it for absorption in the intestine. It is not clear, however, whether this effect is great enough to be harmful.

Blood levels of biotin were found to be substantially lower in 404 people with epilepsy on long-term treatment with anticonvulsants compared to 112 untreated people with epilepsy.[8] The effect occurred with phenytoin, carbamazepine, phenobarbital, and primidone. Valproic acid appears to affect biotin to a lesser extent than other anticonvulsants.

A test tube study suggested that anticonvulsants might lower biotin levels by interfering with the way biotin is transported in the intestine.[9]

Biotin supplementation may be beneficial if you are on long-term anticonvulsant therapy. To avoid a potential interaction, take the supplement 2 to 3 hours apart from the drug. It has been suggested that the action of anticonvulsant drugs may be at least partly related to their effect of reducing biotin levels. For this reason, it may be desirable to take enough biotin to prevent a deficiency, but not an excessive amount.

Please see Appendix D, Safety Issues, for more information.

Folate: Supplementation Possibly Helpful

2 MIXED Folate (also known as folic acid) is a B vitamin that plays an important role in many vital aspects of health, including preventing neural tube birth defects and possibly reducing the risk of heart disease. Because inadequate intake of folate is widespread, if you are taking any medication that depletes or impairs folate even slightly, you may need supplementation.

Valproic acid appears to decrease the body's absorption of folate,[10] and other antiseizure drugs can also reduce levels of folate in the body.[11–15]

The low serum folate caused by anticonvulsants can raise homocysteine levels, a condition believed to increase the risk of heart disease.[16]

Adequate folate intake is also necessary to prevent neural tube birth defects such as spina bifida and anencephaly. Because anticonvulsant drugs deplete folate, babies born to women taking anticonvulsants are at increased risk for such birth defects. Anticonvulsants may also play a more direct role in the development of birth defects.[17]

However, the case for taking extra folate during anticonvulsant therapy is not as simple as it might seem. It is possible that folate supplementation might itself impair the effectiveness of anticonvulsant drugs, and physician supervision is necessary.

Please see Appendix D, Safety Issues, for more information.

POSITIVE INTERACTIONS

Calcium: Supplementation Probably Helpful, but Take at a Different Time of Day

2 POSITIVE Anticonvulsant drugs may impair calcium absorption and in this way increase the risk of osteoporosis and other bone disorders.

Calcium absorption was compared in 12 people on anticonvulsant therapy with various drugs and 12 people receiving no treatment.[18] Calcium absorption was found to be 27% lower in the treated participants.

An observational study found low calcium blood levels in 48% of 109 people taking anticonvulsants.[19] Other findings in this study suggested that anticonvulsants might also reduce calcium levels by directly interfering with parathyroid hormone, a substance that helps keep calcium levels in proper balance.

A low blood level of calcium can itself trigger seizures, and this might reduce the effectiveness of anticonvulsants.[20]

Calcium supplementation may be beneficial for people taking anticonvulsant drugs. However, some studies indicate that antacids containing calcium carbonate may interfere with the absorption of phenytoin and perhaps other anticonvulsants.[21,22] For this reason, take calcium supplements and anticonvulsant drugs several hours apart if possible.

Please see Appendix D, Safety Issues, for more information.

Carnitine: Supplementation Possibly Helpful

2 POSITIVE Carnitine is an amino acid that has been used for heart conditions, Alzheimer's disease, and intermittent claudication (a possible complication of atherosclerosis in which impaired blood circulation causes severe pain in calf muscles during walking or exercising).

Long-term therapy with anticonvulsant agents, particularly valproic acid, is associated with low levels of carnitine.[23] However, it isn't clear whether the anticonvulsants cause the carnitine deficiency or whether it occurs for other reasons. It has been hypothesized that low carnitine levels may contribute to valproic acid's damaging effects on the liver.[24,25] The risk of this liver damage increases in children younger than 24 months,[26] and carnitine supplementation does seem to be protective.[27] However, in one double-blind crossover study, carnitine supplementation produced no real improvement in "well-being" as assessed by parents of children receiving either valproic acid or carbamazepine.[28]

L-carnitine supplementation may be advisable in certain cases, such as in infants and young children (especially those younger than 2 years) who have neurologic disorders and are receiving valproic acid and multiple anticonvulsants.[29]

Please see Appendix D, Safety Issues, for more information.

Vitamin D: Supplementation Possibly Helpful

2 POSITIVE Anticonvulsant drugs may interfere with the activity of vitamin D. As proper handling of calcium by the body depends on vitamin D, this may be another way that these drugs increase the risk of osteoporosis and related bone disorders (see the previous Calcium topic).

Anticonvulsants appear to speed up the body's normal breakdown of vitamin D, decreasing the amount of the vitamin in the blood.[30] A survey of 48 people taking both phenytoin and phenobarbital found significantly lower levels of calcium and vitamin D in many of them as compared to 38 untreated individuals.[31] Similar but lesser changes were seen in 13 people taking phenytoin or phenobarbital alone. This effect may be apparent only after several weeks of treatment. Though valproic acid was not studied, in some cases it may be used in combination therapy with these other drugs.

Another study found decreased blood levels of one form of vitamin D but normal levels of another.[32] Because there are two primary forms of vitamin D circulating in the blood, the body might be able to adjust in some cases to keep vitamin D in balance, at least for a time, despite the influence of anticonvulsants.[33]

Adequate sunlight exposure may help overcome the effects of anticonvulsants on vitamin D by stimulating the skin to manufacture the vitamin.[34] Of 450 people on anticonvulsants residing in a Florida facility, none were found to have low blood levels of vitamin D or evidence of bone disease. This suggests that environments providing regular sun exposure may be protective.

Individuals regularly taking anticonvulsants, especially those taking combination therapy and those with limited exposure to sunlight, may benefit from vitamin D supplementation.

Please see Appendix D, Safety Issues, for more information.

Vitamin K: Supplementation Possibly Helpful for Pregnant Women

2 POSITIVE Phenytoin, carbamazepine, phenobarbital, and primidone speed up the normal breakdown of vitamin K into inactive byproducts, thus depriving the body of active vitamin K. This can lead to bone problems such as osteoporosis. Also, use of these anticonvulsants can lead to a vitamin K deficiency in babies born to mothers taking the drugs, resulting in bleeding disorders or facial bone abnormalities in the newborns.[35,36] Because valproic acid may be used in combination therapy with these other drugs, this interaction is something to keep in mind.

Mothers who take these anticonvulsants may need vitamin K supplementation during pregnancy to prevent these conditions in their newborns.

Please see Appendix D, Safety Issues, for more information.

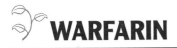

WARFARIN

Trade Name: Coumadin

Interactions	Rating*
Negative Interactions	
Alfalfa	2
Asian Ginseng	2
Coenzyme Q_{10} (CoQ_{10})	2
Danshen	2
Devil's Claw	2
Dong Quai	2
Feverfew	2
Garlic	1
Ginger	2
Ginkgo	1
Green Tea	2
Ipriflavone	1
Papain, Bromelain	3
Policosanol	1
St. John's Wort	2

Interactions	Rating*
Negative Interactions *(cont.)*	
Vinpocetine	3
Vitamin A	3
Vitamin C	3
Vitamin E	2
Vitamin K	1
White Willow	3
Other Herbs and Supplements	3

*Rating Key

1 Significant interaction
2 Possibly significant interaction
3 Interaction of relatively little significance
4 Reported interaction that does not in fact exist or is insignificant

Warfarin (Coumadin) is an anticoagulant used to thin the blood and prevent it from clotting. It is a somewhat dangerous drug that can be affected by many substances, including foods. If you are taking warfarin, we don't recommend taking any herb or supplement except on a physician's advice.

Similar blood-thinning drugs are anisindione (Miradon) and dicumarol.

NEGATIVE INTERACTIONS

Alfalfa: Possible Harmful Interaction

2 NEGATIVE The herb alfalfa (*Medicago sativa*) is promoted for a variety of conditions. The high vitamin K content in alfalfa could, in theory, reduce the effectiveness of warfarin. Vitamin K directly counteracts warfarin's blood-thinning effects.

As a precaution, avoid alfalfa supplements during warfarin therapy except under medical supervision.

Warfarin

Asian Ginseng: Possible Harmful Interaction

 The herb Asian ginseng (*Panax ginseng*) is promoted as an adaptogen, a treatment that helps the body adapt to stress and resist illness in general.

According to one case report, Asian ginseng might decrease warfarin's blood-thinning effects.[1]

For this reason, if you are taking warfarin, you should not use ginseng without consulting a physician.

Coenzyme Q_{10} (CoQ$_{10}$): Possible Harmful Interaction

Coenzyme Q_{10} is a vitamin-like substance that plays a fundamental role in the body's energy production.[2,3]

Coenzyme Q_{10} (CoQ$_{10}$) is somewhat similar in structure to vitamin K, and reportedly, it too can reduce the therapeutic effects of warfarin.[4] In three case reports, CoQ$_{10}$ was found to interfere with warfarin's blood-thinning effects.[5]

If you take warfarin, avoid CoQ$_{10}$ supplementation except under a physician's supervision.

Danshen: Possible Harmful Interaction

The herb danshen, the root of *Salvia miltorrhiza*, is used for treating heart disease in traditional Chinese medicine.

Preliminary evidence,[6] including one case report,[7] suggests that danshen might increase the effects of warfarin, though it does not appear to have blood-thinning effects itself.[8] This could potentially cause abnormal bleeding problems.

It is probably best not to combine danshen and warfarin except under a physician's supervision.

Devil's Claw: Possible Harmful Interaction

 The herb devil's claw (*Harpogophytum procumbens*) is used for various types of arthritis and digestive problems.

According to one case report, devil's claw might increase the risk of abnormal bleeding when taken with warfarin.[9]

As a precaution, you should probably not combine devil's claw and warfarin except under a physician's supervision.

Dong Quai: Possible Harmful Interaction

2 NEGATIVE The herb dong quai (*Angelica sinensis*) is used for menstrual disorders.

According to one case report, dong quai may add to the blood-thinning effects of warfarin, thus increasing the risk of abnormal bleeding.[10]

You should probably avoid combining dong quai and warfarin without medical supervision.

Feverfew: Possible Harmful Interaction

2 NEGATIVE The herb feverfew (*Tanacetum parthenium*) is primarily used for the prevention and treatment of migraine headaches.

In vitro studies suggest that feverfew thins the blood by interfering with the ability of blood platelets to clump together.[11–14] This raises the concern that feverfew might increase the risk of abnormal bleeding when combined with warfarin. However, there is as yet no evidence that the blood-thinning effect of feverfew is significant in humans.[15]

Though an additive effect of feverfew and warfarin appears to be theoretical at this time, it may be best to avoid this combination except under medical supervision.

Garlic: Possible Harmful Interaction

1 NEGATIVE The herb garlic (*Allium sativum*) is taken to lower cholesterol, among many other proposed uses.

One of the possible side effects of garlic is an increased tendency to bleed.[16,17] This blood-thinning effect has been demonstrated in a double-blind trial of garlic in 60 volunteers,[18] as well as in other studies[19,20] and a case report.[21]

According to two other case reports, the blood-thinning effects of warfarin were greatly enhanced in individuals taking garlic.[22] This could amplify the risk of bleeding problems.

Based on these findings, you should avoid combining garlic and warfarin except under a physician's supervision.

Ginger: Possible Harmful Interaction

2 NEGATIVE The herb ginger (*Zingiber officianale*) is used for nausea associated with motion sickness, morning sickness in pregnancy, and the postsurgical period.

Ginger appears to thin the blood by interfering with the ability of blood platelets to clump together.[23,24] As with feverfew, this raises the concern that ginger might increase the risk of abnormal bleeding when taken with warfarin. However, there is no evidence at present that the blood-thinning effect of ginger is significant in humans.[25,26,27]

Though an additive effect of ginger and warfarin appears to be theoretical based on current evidence, it may be best to avoid this combination except under medical supervision. Ginger flavored drinks should not present a problem, but candies containing whole dried ginger are potentially of concern.

Ginkgo: Possible Harmful Interaction

1 NEGATIVE The herb ginkgo (*Ginkgo biloba*) has been used to treat Alzheimer's disease and ordinary age-related memory loss, among many other uses.

Ginkgo appears to reduce the ability of platelets (blood-clotting cells) to stick together.[28] Several case reports suggest that this blood-thinning effect of ginkgo may be associated with an increased risk of serious abnormal bleeding episodes in individuals taking the herb.[29,30,31] These findings raise the additional concern that ginkgo might add to the blood-thinning effects of warfarin, and there is one report of abnormal bleeding in an individual who had been taking the herb and drug together.[32]

Because of this risk, you should not combine ginkgo and warfarin without physician supervision.

Green Tea: Possible Harmful Interaction

2 NEGATIVE Green tea contains strong antioxidant substances and may have cancer-preventive effects.

Because green tea (*Camellia sinensis*) contains vitamin K, which directly interferes with warfarin's blood-thinning action, drinking large amounts of it might reduce the therapeutic effects of the drug.[33]

Ipriflavone: Possible Harmful Interaction

1 NEGATIVE Ipriflavone, a synthetic isoflavone that slows bone breakdown, is used to treat osteoporosis.

Warfarin use increases the risk of osteoporosis. Because ipriflavone has been found to help prevent osteoporosis in certain circumstances, you might be tempted to consider taking this supplement while you use warfarin. However, some evidence indicates that ipriflavone might interfere with the body's normal breakdown of warfarin.[34] This could raise the levels of warfarin in your body and increase the risk of abnormal bleeding.

If you try this combination, you need to do so under physician supervision.

Papain, Bromelain: Possible Harmful Interaction

 One case report suggests that papain, a digestive enzyme found in papaya extract (*Carica papaya*), might add to warfarin's blood-thinning effect.[35] Additionally, other proteolytic digestive enzymes such as bromelain (from the fruit and stem of pineapple, *Ananas comosus*) have at least the potential to damage membranes lining the digestive tract and cause bleeding in this way.

Because papain or bromelain might increase the risk of abnormal bleeding when taken with warfarin, this combination should be avoided. Papaya fruit might present risk, but pineapple fruit probably does not contain enough bromelain to cause any problems.

Policosanol: Possible Harmful Interaction

 Policosanol, derived from sugar cane, has been taken for hyperlipidemia and intermittent claudication.

Human trials suggest that policosanol makes blood platelets more slippery, an action that could potentiate the blood-thinning effects of warfarin, possibly causing a risk of abnormal bleeding episodes.[36] A 30-day double-blind placebo-controlled trial of 27 individuals with high cholesterol levels found that policosanol at 10 mg daily markedly reduced the ability of blood platelets to clump together.[37] Another double-blind placebo-controlled study of 37 healthy volunteers found evidence that the blood-thinning effect of policosanol increased as the dose was increased—the larger the policosanol dose, the greater the effect.[38] Yet another double-blind placebo-controlled study of 43 healthy volunteers compared the effects of policosanol (20 mg daily), the blood-thinner aspirin (100 mg daily), and policosanol and aspirin combined at these same doses.[39] The results again showed that policosanol substantially reduced the ability of blood platelets to stick together, and that the combined therapy exhibited additive effects.

Based on these findings, you should not combine warfarin and policosanol except under medical supervision.

St. John's Wort: Possible Harmful Interaction

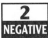 The herb St. John's wort (*Hypericum perforatum*) is primarily used to treat mild to moderate depression.

Evidence suggests that St. John's wort may interfere with warfarin, possibly requiring an increased dosage of the drug to maintain the proper therapeutic effect.[40,41,42] Seven cases have been reported in which the blood-thinning effects of warfarin have been impaired in individuals taking St. John's wort.[43]

A "hidden" risk lies in this type of interaction. Suppose your physician has raised the warfarin dose to take into account the effect of St. John's wort in holding down drug levels. If you then stop taking the herbal product, it would be like releasing the brakes, and your warfarin levels could surge dangerously high.

For these reasons, if you take warfarin, avoid St. John's wort except under a physician's supervision.

Vinpocetine: Possible Harmful Interaction

3 NEGATIVE The substance vinpocetine is sold as a dietary supplement for the treatment of age-related memory loss and impaired mental function.

Vinpocetine might impair the effectiveness of warfarin,[44] according to a 24-day study with 18 individuals. However, the observed effects appeared to be small and clinically unimportant, and factors other than vinpocetine use might have influenced the findings.

Even so, you probably should avoid this combination unless supervised by a physician.

Vitamin A: Possible Harmful Interaction

3 NEGATIVE Supplemental vitamin A might increase the blood-thinning effects of warfarin, and this could potentially lead to an increased risk of abnormal bleeding.[45]

For this reason, it may be best to avoid combining vitamin A with warfarin unless supervised by a physician.

Vitamin C: Possible Harmful Interaction

3 NEGATIVE Vitamin C taken in high dosages (more than 1,000 mg daily) has been reported to reduce the blood-thinning effect of warfarin.[46–49] In one case, the person was taking 1,000 mg of vitamin C daily; another involved huge megadoses (about 16,000 mg daily).

As a precaution, if you take warfarin, consult with your physician before taking high-dose vitamin C supplements.

Vitamin E: Possible Harmful Interaction

2 NEGATIVE On the basis that vitamin E "thins" the blood,[50] it has been suggested not to combine vitamin E with warfarin. However, a 4-week double-blind study of 25 individuals taking warfarin found no additive effect.[51] None of the participants taking vitamin E at a daily dose of 800 or 1,200 IU (international units) showed an increased risk for abnormal bleeding.

In contrast, a case report indicated that vitamin E (800 IU daily) added to the effects of warfarin and resulted in abnormal bleeding.[52] Because this effect did not become apparent until the fourth week, it is possible that problems might take longer to develop than the 4-week period covered by the double-blind study, or that certain individuals might be more prone to an interaction. An unpublished 30-day study of three volunteers taking a warfarin-like drug also found an additive effect with only 42 IU of vitamin E daily.[53]

Though the evidence supporting a possible interaction is scanty, it is best not to risk serious bleeding problems. Avoid combining vitamin E with warfarin except under the supervision of a physician.

Vitamin K: Possible Harmful Interaction

1 NEGATIVE Vitamin K is an antidote to warfarin—it directly counteracts warfarin's blood-thinning effects. This is true for both supplemental vitamin K and foods high in vitamin K. For this reason, eating more vitamin K–rich vegetables can decrease warfarin's therapeutic effect, and eating less of these foods can increase the drug's effect.[54,55] Either situation can lead to potential life-threatening complications.

Therefore, once you are established on a certain dose of warfarin, you should not change your usual intake of vitamin K without medical supervision.

White Willow: Possible Harmful Interaction

3 NEGATIVE The herb white willow (*Salix alba*), also known as willow bark, is used to treat pain and fever. White willow contains a substance that is converted by the body into a salicylate similar to the blood-thinner aspirin.

Because white willow, like aspirin, may enhance the blood-thinning effects of warfarin, this combination should be avoided unless medically supervised.

Other Herbs and Supplements: Possible Harmful Interaction

3 NEGATIVE Based on their known effects or the effects of their constituents, the following herbs and supplements might not be safe to combine with warfarin, though this has not been proven: chamomile (*Matricaria recutita*), *Coleus forskohlii*, ginger (*Zingiber officinale*), horse chestnut (*Aesculus hippocastanum*), papaya (*Carica papaya*), red clover (*Trifolium pratense*), and reishi (*Ganoderma lucidum*); aortic glycosaminoglycans (GAGs), fish oil, OPCs (oligomeric proanthocyanidins), and phosphatidylserine.

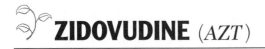

ZIDOVUDINE (AZT)

Trade Name: Retrovir

Interactions	Rating*
Positive Interactions	
L-Carnitine	3
Zinc, Copper and Vitamin B$_{12}$	2

*Rating Key

1   Significant interaction

2   Possibly significant interaction

3   Interaction of relatively little significance

4   Reported interaction that does not in fact exist or is insignificant

Zidovudine (AZT) is used to manage HIV infection. The drug works by interfering with a DNA compound (reverse transcriptase) needed by the virus to replicate itself. AZT's potential side effects include anemia, muscle damage, and possible depletion of certain nutrients.

POSITIVE INTERACTIONS

L-Carnitine: Supplementation Possibly Helpful

3 POSITIVE   Carnitine is an amino acid that has been used for heart conditions, Alzheimer's disease, and intermittent claudication (a possible complication of atherosclerosis in which impaired blood circulation causes severe pain in calf muscles during walking or exercising).

Carnitine has also been proposed as a treatment for AZT side effects. Based on early evidence, carnitine may have a preventive effect against AZT-induced muscle damage[1] and may enhance immune functioning in people with HIV infection.[2,3]

Carnitine supplementation might be beneficial for HIV-infected individuals whether or not they are taking AZT or similar drugs, but you should consult with your physician before taking it for this purpose. Only the "L" form of carnitine (L-carnitine) is safe to take.

Please see Appendix D, Safety Issues, for more Information.

Zinc, Copper, and Vitamin B$_{12}$: Supplementation Possibly Helpful

2 POSITIVE   AZT may deplete the body of zinc, copper, and vitamin B$_{12}$.

A 1991 study found significantly decreased blood levels of zinc and copper in a large proportion of AZT-treated participants compared to untreated controls.[4] The zinc depletion occurred despite adequate zinc intake. The findings also suggested that zinc levels were particularly important in maintaining immune function in the drug-treated group. Furthermore, since AZT requires a zinc-dependent enzyme for conversion to its active form, zinc deficiency may diminish drug effectiveness.

A more recent study (1995) found that zinc sulfate supplementation decreased the number of opportunistic infections in HIV-infected persons treated with AZT.[5] The zinc supplement was given orally for 1 month at a dose of 200 mg daily. During the 2-year follow-up, 12 infections occurred in the zinc-supplemented groups (29 participants) compared to 38 infections in the groups not receiving zinc supplementation (28 participants).

However, zinc supplementation may also carry risk. An observational study linked higher zinc intake to more rapid development of AIDS in HIV-positive individuals.[6] In another observational study of HIV-positive individuals, those with higher zinc intake or those taking zinc supplements in any dosage had a greater risk of death within the following 8 years.[7] These preliminary findings suggest that zinc intake at levels above the RDA may exhibit harmful effects in people with HIV infection, and more research is needed to determine optimal levels of intake.

AZT may also reduce vitamin B_{12} levels. One study found low B_{12} blood levels in 61 of 200 HIV-infected persons, particularly in those taking AZT.[8]

HIV infection may adversely affect the absorption of many nutrients, and adequate nutrition in general is important. Supplementation with zinc, copper, and vitamin B_{12} at standard nutritional doses may be advisable in individuals taking AZT. However, until more is known, supplementation at higher doses may not be advisable.

Please see Appendix D, Safety Issues, for more information.

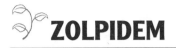

ZOLPIDEM

Trade Name: Ambien

Interactions	Rating*
Negative Interactions	
5-HTP (5-Hydroxytryptophan), L-Tryptophan, St. John's Wort	2
Kava, Valerian, Passionflower, Hops	2

*Rating Key

1   Significant interaction

2   Possibly significant interaction

3   Interaction of relatively little significance

4   Reported interaction that does not in fact exist or is insignificant

Zolpidem (Ambien) is a hypnotic (sleeping pill) prescribed for the short-term treatment of insomnia.

NEGATIVE INTERACTIONS

5-HTP (5-Hydroxytryptophan), L-Tryptophan, St. John's Wort: Possible Harmful Interaction

2 NEGATIVE Supplemental forms of 5-hydroxytryptophan (5-HTP) and the amino acid L-tryptophan have been used for treating depression, sleep disorders, and other conditions.

The herb St. John's wort (*Hypericum perforatum*) is primarily used to treat mild to moderate depression.

The risk of zolpidem-induced visual hallucinations appears to be increased when the drug is combined with agents that boost activity of the neuro-transmitter serotonin.

Of 10 reports of zolpidem-induced hallucinations, nine of the individuals were also taking serotonin-enhancing antidepressant drugs.[1] In some cases, the hallucinations were prolonged, lasting up to 7 hours. Interestingly, zolpidem itself has no known effect on serotonin.

It is possible that the supplements 5-HTP and L-tryptophan might also increase the risk of zolpidem-induced visual hallucinations, since the body can use both compounds to manufacture serotonin. The herb St. John's wort, which is thought to raise serotonin levels, might also cause problems.

Based on this evidence, you should not combine these supplements with zolpidem.

Zolpidem

Kava, Valerian, Passionflower, Hops: Possible Harmful Interaction

2 NEGATIVE The herb kava (*Piper methysticum*) has a sedative effect and is used for anxiety and insomnia. Combining kava with zolpidem, which possesses similar depressant effects, could result in "add-on" or excessive physical depression, sedation, and impairment. Other herbs with a sedative effect that might cause problems when combined with zolpidem include ashwagandha (*Withania somnifera*), calendula (*Calendula officinalis*), catnip (*Nepeta cataria*), hops (*Humulus lupulus*), lady's slipper (*Cypripedium* species), lemon balm (*Melissa officinalis*), passionflower (*Passiflora incarnata*), sassafras (*Sassafras officinale*), skullcap (*Scutellaria lateriflora*), valerian (*Valeriana officinalis*), and yerba mansa (*Anemopsis californica*).

Because of the potentially serious consequences, you should avoid combining these herbs with zolpidem or other drugs that have sedative or depressant effects unless advised by your physician.

Appendices

APPENDIX A
INTERACTIONS BY HERB OR SUPPLEMENT

This appendix is arranged by supplement name rather than drug name. This makes it easy to find out which drugs may interact with a particular supplement. For each supplement listed, interacting drugs or drug families are listed alphabetically according to interaction type: Negative, Mixed, and Positive. Refer to the main text of this book for detailed information on a particular interaction.

RATING KEY

1   Significant interaction

2   Possibly significant interaction

3   Interaction of relatively little significance

4   Reported interaction that does not in fact exist or is insignificant

5-HTP (5-HYDROXYTRYPTOPHAN)

NEGATIVE

Possible Harmful Interaction:

Levodopa	2
Levodopa/Carbidopa	2
MAO Inhibitors	2
Selective Serotonin-Reuptake Inhibitors (SSRIs)	2
Tramadol	2
Tricyclic Antidepressants	2
Zolpidem	2

ACIDOPHILUS AND OTHER PROBIOTICS

POSITIVE

Probable Helpful Interaction:

Antibiotics	2

Appendix A

ALFALFA

NEGATIVE

Possible Harmful Interaction:

Warfarin   2

ALOE

POSITIVE

Possible Benefits and Risks:

Antidiabetic Agents   3

*Possibly Helpful When Applied
With Hydrocortisone:*

Corticosteroids   3

ALUMINUM (IN ANTACIDS)

NEGATIVE

Take at a Different Time of Day:

Tetracyclines   2

ANDROSTENEDIONE

NEGATIVE

Possible Harmful Interaction:

Estrogen   3
Oral Contraceptives   3

AORTIC GLYCOSAMINOGLYCANS

NEGATIVE

Possible Harmful Interaction:

Heparin   3
Nonsteroidal Anti-Inflammatory   3
   Drugs (NSAIDs)
Pentoxifylline   3
Warfarin   3

ARGININE

NEGATIVE

Possible Harmful Interaction:

ACE Inhibitors	3
Amiloride	3
Nonsteroidal Anti-Inflammatory Drugs (NSAIDs)	3
Spironolactone	3
Triamterene	3

ASHWAGANDHA

NEGATIVE

Possible Harmful Interaction:

Antipsychotic Agents	2
Benzodiazepines	2
Carbamazepine	2
Phenobarbital	2
Phenytoin	2
Primidone	2
Valproic Acid	2
Tricyclic Antidepressants	2
Zolpidem	2

BCAAs

NEGATIVE

Possible Harmful Interaction:

Levodopa	2
Levodopa/Carbidopa	2

BILBERRY

POSITIVE

Possible Benefits and Risks:

Antidiabetic Agents	3

BIOTIN

MIXED

*Supplementation Possibly Helpful,
but Take at a Different Time of Day:*

Anticonvulsant Agents	3
Carbamazepine	3
Phenobarbital	3
Phenytoin	3
Primidone	3
Valproic Acid	3

BISMUTH SUBSALICYLATE

NEGATIVE

Take at a Different Time of Day:

Tetracyclines	2

POSITIVE

Supplementation Possibly Helpful:

Cisplatin	3

BITTER MELON

POSITIVE

Possible Benefits and Risks:

Antidiabetic Agents	3

BITTER ORANGE PEEL

NEGATIVE

Possible Harmful Interaction:

Antipsychotic Agents	3
Nonsteroidal Anti-Inflammatory Drugs (NSAIDs)	3

BORON

NEGATIVE

Possible Harmful Interaction:

Estrogen	3

BROMELAIN

NEGATIVE

Possible Harmful Interaction:

Heparin	3
Pentoxifylline	3
Warfarin	3

POSITIVE

Supplementation Possibly Helpful:

Amoxicillin	2

BURDOCK

POSITIVE

Possible Benefits and Risks:

Antidiabetic Agents	3

CALCIUM

NEGATIVE

Possible Harmful Interaction:

Antacids	3
Calcium-Channel Blockers	3
Thiazide Diuretics	1

Take at a Different Time of Day:

Beta Blockers	3
Bisphosphonates	3
Fluoroquinolones	2
Tetracyclines	2
Thyroid Hormone	2

Appendix A

POSITIVE

Supplementation Probably Helpful, but Take at a Different Time of Day:

Anticonvulsant Agents	2
Carbamazepine	2
Corticosteroids	2
Estrogen	1
Phenobarbital	2
Phenytoin	2
Primidone	2
Valproic Acid	2

Supplementation Possibly Helpful:

Antidiabetic Agents	2
Bile Acid Sequestrants	3
Digoxin	3

CALCIUM CITRATE

NEGATIVE

Possible Harmful Interaction:

Antidiabetic Agents	2
Methotrexate	3
Nonsteroidal Anti-Inflammatory Drugs (NSAIDs)	2
Tetracyclines	2

CALENDULA

NEGATIVE

Possible Harmful Interaction:

Antipsychotic Agents	2
Benzodiazepines	2
Carbamazepine	2
Phenobarbital	2
Phenytoin	2

Primidone	2
Tricyclic Antidepressants	2
Valproic Acid	2
Zolpidem	2

CARNITINE

POSITIVE

Supplementation Possibly Helpful:

Anticonvulsant Agents	2
Carbamazepine	2
Phenobarbital	2
Phenytoin	2
Primidone	2
Valproic Acid	2
Zidovudine	3

Possible Benefits and Risks:

Antidiabetic Agents	3

CATNIP

NEGATIVE

Possible Harmful Interaction:

Antipsychotic Agents	2
Benzodiazepines	2
Carbamazepine	2
Phenobarbital	2
Phenytoin	2
Primidone	2
Tricyclic Antidepressants	2
Valproic Acid	2
Zolpidem	2

CAYENNE

NEGATIVE

Possible Harmful Interaction:

Theophylline   2

POSITIVE

Supplementation Possibly Helpful:

Nonsteroidal Anti-Inflammatory   3
Drugs (NSAIDs)

CELERY

NEGATIVE

Possible Harmful Interaction:

Antipsychotic Agents   3

Nonsteroidal Anti-Inflammatory   3
Drugs (NSAIDs)

CHAMOMILE

NEGATIVE

Possible Harmful Interaction:

Heparin   3
Pentoxifylline   3
Warfarin   3

CHAPARREL

NEGATIVE

Possible Harmful Interaction:

Acetaminophen   2
Amiodarone   2
Statin Drugs   2

CHASTEBERRY

NEGATIVE

Possible Harmful Interaction:

Bromocriptine   3

CHROMIUM

MIXED

Possible Benefits and Risks:

Antidiabetic Agents	2
Corticosteroids	2

POSITIVE

Supplementation Possibly Helpful,
but Take at a Different Time of Day:

Antacids	3

Supplementation Possibly Helpful:

Beta Blockers	3

COCCINIA INDICA

POSITIVE

Possible Benefits and Risks:

Antidiabetic Agents	3

COENZYME Q$_{10}$ (CoQ$_{10}$)

NEGATIVE

Possible Harmful Interaction:

Warfarin	2

POSITIVE

Supplementation Possibly Helpful:

Acetaminophen	3
Anthracyclines	2
Antidiabetic Agents	3
Antihypertensive Agents	3
Antipsychotic Agents	3
Beta Blockers	2
Tricyclic Antidepressants	3

POSITIVE

Supplementation Probably Helpful:

Statin Drugs	2

COLEUS FORSKOHLII

NEGATIVE

Possible Harmful Interaction:

Beta Blockers	4
Heparin	3
Hydralazine	4
Pentoxifylline	3
Warfarin	3

COLOSTRUM

POSITIVE

Supplementation Possibly Helpful:

Nonsteroidal Anti-Inflammatory Drugs (NSAIDs)	3

COMFREY

NEGATIVE

Possible Harmful Interaction:

Acetaminophen	2
Amiodarone	2
Statin Drugs	2

COLTSFOOT

NEGATIVE

Possible Harmful Interaction:

Acetaminophen	2
Amiodarone	2
Statin Drugs	2

COPPER

NEGATIVE

Possible Harmful Interaction:

Oral Contraceptives	3
Penicillamine	1

POSITIVE

Supplementation Possibly Helpful:

Ethambutol	3
Zidovudine	2

DANDELION

POSITIVE

Possible Benefits and Risks:

Antidiabetic Agents	3

DANSHEN

NEGATIVE

Possible Harmful Interaction:

Heparin	3
Pentoxifylline	3
Warfarin	2

DEVIL'S CLAW

NEGATIVE

Possible Harmful Interaction:

Heparin	3
Warfarin	2

DHEA (DEHYDROEPIANDROSTERONE)

POSITIVE

Supplementation Possibly Helpful:

Corticosteroids	3

DONG QUAI

NEGATIVE

Possible Harmful Interaction:

ACE Inhibitors	3
Anticonvulsant Agents	3
Antidiabetic Agents	3
Amiodarone	3
Antipsychotic Agents	3
Carbamazepine	3
Fluoroquinolones	3
Heparin	3
Isotretinoin	3
Loop Diuretics	3
Methotrexate	3
Methyldopa	3
Nonsteroidal Anti-Inflammatory Drugs (NSAIDs)	3
Oral Contraceptives	3
Pentoxifylline	3
Phenobarbital	3
Primidone	3
Tetracyclines	3
Thiazide Diuretics	3
Tricyclic Antidepressants	3
Trimethoprim-Sulfamethoxazole	3
Valproic Acid	3
Warfarin	2

Interaction Unlikely or Probably Insignificant:

Estrogen	4

EPHEDRA

NEGATIVE

Harmful Interaction:

MAO Inhibitors	1

FENUGREEK

POSITIVE

Possible Benefits and Risks:

Antidiabetic Agents	3

FEVERFEW

NEGATIVE

Possible Harmful Interaction:

Heparin	3
Nonsteroidal Anti-Inflammatory Drugs (NSAIDs)	2
Pentoxifylline	3
Warfarin	2

FISH OIL

NEGATIVE

Possible Harmful Interaction:

Heparin	3
Nonsteroidal Anti-Inflammatory Drugs (NSAIDs)	3
Pentoxifylline	3
Warfarin	3

FOLATE

MIXED

Supplementation Possibly Helpful:

Anticonvulsant Agents	2
Carbamazepine	2
Phenobarbital	2
Phenytoin	2
Primidone	2
Valproic Acid	2

POSITIVE

Interaction Unlikely or Probably Insignificant:

Oral Contraceptives	4

Supplementation Possibly Helpful:

Antacids	3
H2 Antagonist	3
Methotrexate	1
Nitrous Oxide	1
Nonsteroidal Anti-Inflammatory Drugs (NSAIDs)	2
Proton Pump Inhibitors	3
Triamterene	3

Supplementation Probably Helpful:

Bile Acid Sequestrants	2
Trimethoprim-Sulfamethoxazole	1

GAMMA LINOLENIC ACID (GLA)

POSITIVE

Supplementation Possibly Helpful:

Tamoxifen	2

GARLIC

NEGATIVE

Possible Harmful Interaction:

Heparin	1
Nonsteroidal Anti-Inflammatory Drugs (NSAIDs)	2
Pentoxifylline	2
Warfarin	1

POSITIVE

Possible Benefits and Risks:

Antidiabetic Agents	3

GINGER

NEGATIVE

Possible Harmful Interaction:

Heparin	3
Nonsteroidal Anti-Inflammatory Drugs (NSAIDs)	3
Pentoxifylline	3
Warfarin	2

GINKGO

NEGATIVE

Possible Harmful Interaction:

Anticonvulsant Agents	3
Carbamazepine	3
Phenobarbital	3
Phenytoin	3
Primidone	3
Valproic Acid	3
Heparin	1
Nonsteroidal Anti-Inflammatory Drugs (NSAIDs)	2
Pentoxifylline	2
Warfarin	1

POSITIVE

Supplementation Possibly Helpful:

Antipsychotic Agents	3
Cisplatin	3
Selective Serotonin-Reuptake Inhibitors (SSRIs)	2

GINSENG, ASIAN

NEGATIVE

Possible Harmful Interaction:

MAO Inhibitors	2
Warfarin	2

MIXED

Possible Benefits and Risks:

Antidiabetic Agents	3

POSITIVE

Supplementation Probably Helpful:

Influenza Vaccine	3

GINSENG, SIBERIAN

NEGATIVE

Possible Harmful Interaction:

Digoxin	1

GLUTAMINE

NEGATIVE

Possible Harmful Interaction:

Anticonvulsant Agents	4
Carbamazepine	4
Phenobarbital	4
Phenytoin	4
Primidone	4
Valproic Acid	4

GLUTATHIONE

POSITIVE

Supplementation Possibly Helpful:

Anthracyclines	3
Cisplatin	3

GRAPEFRUIT JUICE

NEGATIVE

Possible Harmful Interaction:

Anticonvulsant Agents	1
Azole Antifungal Agents	2
Benzodiazepines	3
Calcium-Channel Blockers	1
Carbamazepine	1
Cyclosporine	2
Estrogen	2
Itraconazole	2
Protease Inhibitors	1
Statin Drugs	1

MIXED

Possible Benefits and Risks:

Tricyclic Antidepressants	2

GREEN TEA

NEGATIVE

Possible Harmful Interaction:

MAO Inhibitors	2
Warfarin	2

GYMNEMA

POSITIVE

Possible Benefits and Risks:

Antidiabetic Agents	3

HAWTHORN

NEGATIVE

Possible Harmful Interaction:

Digoxin	3

HOPS

NEGATIVE

Possible Harmful Interaction:

Anticonvulsant Agents	2
Antipsychotic Agents	2
Benzodiazepines	2
Carbamazepine	2
Phenobarbital	2
Phenytoin	2
Primidone	2
Tricyclic Antidepressants	2
Valproic Acid	2
Zolpidem	2

HORSE CHESTNUT

NEGATIVE

Possible Harmful Interaction:

Heparin	3
Nonsteroidal Anti-Inflammatory Drugs (NSAIDs)	3
Pentoxifylline	3
Warfarin	3

HORSETAIL

NEGATIVE

Possible Harmful Interaction:

Digoxin	3

IPRIFLAVONE

NEGATIVE

Possible Harmful Interaction:

Anticonvulsant Agents	2

Antidiabetic Agents	3
Carbamazepine	2
Phenytoin	2
Theophylline	1
Warfarin	1

MIXED

Possible Benefits and Risks:

Estrogen	2

IRON

NEGATIVE

Take at a Different Time of Day:

ACE Inhibitors	2
Fluoroquinolones	2
Levodopa	1
Levodopa/Carbidopa	1
Methyldopa	1
Penicillamine	1
Tetracyclines	2
Thyroid Hormone	1

POSITIVE

Supplementation Possibly Helpful,
but Take at a Different Time of Day:

Antacids	3

Supplementation Possibly Helpful:

Bile Acid Sequestrants	3
H_2 Antagonists	3
Proton Pump Inhibitors	3

KAVA

NEGATIVE

Possible Harmful Interaction:

Anticonvulsant Agents	2
Antipsychotic Agents	2
Benzodiazepines	2
Carbamazepine	2
Levodopa	2
Levodopa/Carbidopa	2
Phenobarbital	2
Phenytoin	2
Primidone	2
Tricyclic Antidepressants	2
Valproic Acid	2
Zolpidem	2

LACTOBACILLUS ACIDOPHILUS

POSITIVE

Supplementation Probably Helpful:

Antibiotics	2

LADY'S SLIPPER

NEGATIVE

Possible Harmful Interaction:

Antipsychotic Agents	2
Benzodiazepines	2
Carbamazepine	2
Phenobarbital	2
Phenytoin	2
Primidone	2
Tricyclic Antidepressants	2
Valproic Acid	2
Zolpidem	2

LEMON BALM

NEGATIVE

Possible Harmful Interaction:

Antipsychotic Agents	2
Benzodiazepines	2
Carbamazepine	2
Phenobarbital	2
Phenytoin	2
Primidone	2
Tricyclic Antidepressants	2
Valproic Acid	2
Zolpidem	2

LICORICE

NEGATIVE

Possible Harmful Interaction:

ACE Inhibitors	2
Amiloride	1
Corticosteroids	1
Digoxin	2
Loop Diuretics	2
Oral Contraceptives	2
Spironolactone	1
Thiazide Diuretics	2
Triamterene	1

POSITIVE

*Possibly Helpful When Applied
with Hydrocortisone:*

Corticosteroids	3

Supplementation Possibly Helpful:

Nonsteroidal Anti-Inflammatory Drugs (NSAIDs)	3

LIPOIC ACID

POSITIVE

Possible Benefits and Risks:

Antidiabetic Agents   3

L-TRYPTOPHAN

NEGATIVE

Possible Harmful Interaction:

Zolpidem   2

MAGNESIUM

NEGATIVE

Possible Harmful Interaction:

Amiloride   3

Spironolactone   3

Triamterene   3

Take at a Different Time of Day:

H_2 Antagonists   3

Nitrofurantoin   3

Penicillamine   2

Tetracyclines   2

MIXED

Possible Benefits and Risks:

Antidiabetic Agents   3

POSITIVE

*Supplementation Possibly Helpful,
but Take at a Different Time of Day:*

Antacids   3

Digoxin   3

Supplementation Possibly Helpful:

Estrogen   3

Oral Contraceptives   3

Supplementation Probably Helpful:

Cisplatin	1
Loop Diuretics	2
Thiazide Diuretics	2

MAGNESIUM CITRATE

NEGATIVE

Possible Harmful Interaction:

Antidiabetic Agents	2
Methotrexate	3
Nonsteroidal Anti-Inflammatory Drugs (NSAIDs)	2
Tetracyclines	2

MANGANESE

POSITIVE

Supplementation Possibly Helpful, but Take at a Different Time of Day:

Antacids	3

MELATONIN

POSITIVE

Supplementation Possibly Helpful:

Benzodiazepines	3

METHIONINE

POSITIVE

Supplementation Possibly Helpful:

Acetaminophen	3

MILK THISTLE

NEGATIVE

Possible Harmful Interaction:

Oral Contraceptives	3

POSITIVE

Supplementation Possibly Helpful:

Acetaminophen   3

Antipsychotic Agents   2

MOTHERWORT

NEGATIVE

Possible Harmful Interaction:

Antipsychotic Agents   3

Nonsteroidal Anti-Inflammatory   3
Drugs (NSAIDs)

MYRHH ONION

POSITIVE

Possible Benefits and Risks:

Antidiabetic Agents   3

N-ACETYL CYSTEINE (NAC)

MIXED

Possible Benefits and Risks:

Nitroglycerin   3

POSITIVE

Interaction Unlikely or Probably Insignificant:

Trimethoprim   4

Supplementation Possibly Helpful:

Cisplatin   3

NIACIN

NEGATIVE

Possible Harmful Interaction:

Statin Drugs   2

POSITIVE

Supplementation Possibly Helpful:

Isoniazid   2

NICOTINAMIDE

NEGATIVE

Possible Harmful Interaction:

Anticonvulsant Agents   3
Carbamazepine   3
Phenobarbital   3
Primidone   3

OPCS (OLIGOMERIC PROANTHOCYANIDINS)

NEGATIVE

Possible Harmful Interaction:

Heparin   3
Nonsteroidal Anti-Inflammatory   3
  Drugs (NSAIDs)
Pentoxifylline   3
Warfarin   3

PABA (PARA-AMINOBENZOIC ACID)

NEGATIVE

Possible Harmful Interaction:

Trimethoprim-Sulfamethoxazole   2

PAPAIN

NEGATIVE

Possible Harmful Interaction:

Warfarin   3

PAPAYA

NEGATIVE

Possible Harmful Interaction:

Heparin	3
Pentoxifylline	3
Warfarin	3

PARSLEY

NEGATIVE

Possible Harmful Interaction:

Antipsychotic Agents	3
Nonsteroidal Anti-Inflammatory Drugs (NSAIDs)	3

PASSIONFLOWER

NEGATIVE

Possible Harmful Interaction:

Anticonvulsant Agents	2
Antipsychotic Agents	2
Benzodiazepines	2
Carbamazepine	2
Phenobarbital	2
Phenytoin	2
Primidone	2
Tricyclic Antidepressants	2
Valproic Acid	2
Zolpidem	2

PEPPERMINT

NEGATIVE

Possible Harmful Interaction:

Antipsychotic Agents	3
Nonsteroidal Anti-Inflammatory Drugs (NSAIDs)	3

PHENYLALANINE

NEGATIVE

Possible Harmful Interaction:

Antipsychotic Agents	3

PHOSPHATIDYLSERINE

NEGATIVE

Possible Harmful Interaction:

Heparin	3
Warfarin	3

PHOSPHORUS

POSITIVE

Supplementation Possibly Helpful,
but Take at a Different Time of Day:

Antacids	3

POLICOSANOL

NEGATIVE

Possible Harmful Interaction:

Heparin	1
Nonsteroidal Anti-Inflammatory Drugs (NSAIDs)	2
Pentoxifylline	2
Warfarin	1

POTASSIUM

NEGATIVE

Possible Harmful Interaction:

ACE Inhibitors	1
Amiloride	1
Spironolactone	1
Triamterene	1
Trimethoprim-Sulfamethoxazole	2

POSITIVE

Supplementation Probably Helpful:

Cisplatin	1
Loop Diuretics	1
Thiazide Diuretics	1

POTASSIUM CITRATE

NEGATIVE

Possible Harmful Interaction:

Antidiabetic Agents	2
Methotrexate	3
Nonsteroidal Anti-Inflammatory Drugs (NSAIDs)	2
Tetracyclines	2

PROBIOTICS

POSITIVE

Supplementation Probably Helpful:

Antibiotics	2

PTEROCARPUS

POSITIVE

Possible Benefits and Risks:

Antidiabetic Agents	3

RED CLOVER

NEGATIVE

Possible Harmful Interaction:

Heparin	3
Nonsteroidal Anti-Inflammatory Drugs (NSAIDs)	3
Pentoxifylline	3
Warfarin	3

RED YEAST RICE

NEGATIVE

Possible Harmful Interaction:

Statin Drugs	2

REISHI

NEGATIVE

Possible Harmful Interaction:

Heparin	3
Warfarin	3

SACCHAROMYCES BOULARDII

POSITIVE

Supplementation Possibly Helpful:

Antibiotics	2

SALT BUSH

POSITIVE

Possible Benefits and Risks:

Antidiabetic Agents	3

SAME (S-ADENOSYLMETHIONINE)

NEGATIVE

Possible Harmful Interaction:

MAO Inhibitors	2
Selective Serotonin-Reuptake Inhibitors (SSRIs)	2
Tramadol	2
Tricyclic Antidepressants	2

MIXED

Possible Benefits and Risks:

Levodopa	3
Levodopa/Carbidopa	3

SASSAFRAS

NEGATIVE

Possible Harmful Interaction:

Antipsychotic Agents	2
Benzodiazepines	2
Carbamazepine	2
Phenobarbital	2
Phenytoin	2
Primidone	2
Tricyclic Antidepressants	2
Valproic Acid	2
Zolpidem	2

SCOTCH BROOM

NEGATIVE

Harmful Interaction:

MAO Inhibitors	1

SELENIUM

POSITIVE

Supplementation Possibly Helpful:

Anthracyclines	3
Cisplatin	2

SILIBININ

POSITIVE

Supplementation Possibly Helpful:

Cisplatin	3

SKULLCAP

NEGATIVE

Possible Harmful Interaction:

Antipsychotic Agents	2
Benzodiazepines	2
Carbamazepine	2

Phenobarbital	2
Phenytoin	2
Primidone	2
Tricyclic Antidepressants	2
Valproic Acid	2
Zolpidem	2

SOY

NEGATIVE

Possible Harmful Interaction:

Thyroid Hormone	2

POSITIVE

Interaction Unlikely or Probably Insignificant:

Oral Contraceptives	4

ST. JOHN'S WORT

NEGATIVE

Possible Harmful Interaction:

ACE Inhibitors	3
Amiodarone	3
Anticonvulsant Agents	3
Antidiabetic Agents	3
Antipsychotic Agents	2
Carbamazepine	3
Cyclosporine	2
Digoxin	1
Etoposide	2
Fluoroquinolones	3
Isotretinoin	3
Loop Diuretics	3
MAO Inhibitors	2
Methotrexate	3
Methyldopa	3
Nonsteroidal Anti-Inflammatory Drugs (NSAIDs)	3

Appendix A

Oral Contraceptives	2
Phenobarbital	3
Primidone	3
Protease Inhibitors	1
Proton Pump Inhibitors	2
Selective Serotonin-Reuptake Inhibitors (SSRIs)	2
Tetracyclines	3
Theophylline	2
Thiazide Diuretics	3
Tramadol	2
Tricyclic Antidepressants	2
Trimethoprim-Sulfamethoxazole	3
Valproic Acid	3
Warfarin	2
Zolpidem	2

TANGERETIN

NEGATIVE

Possible Harmful Interaction:

Tamoxifen	3

VALERIAN

NEGATIVE

Possible Harmful Interaction:

Anticonvulsant Agents	2
Antipsychotic Agents	2
Benzodiazepines	2
Carbamazepine	2
Phenobarbital	2
Phenytoin	2
Primidone	2
Tricyclic Antidepressants	2
Valproic Acid	2
Zolpidem	2

VANADIUM

MIXED

Possible Benefits and Risks:

Antidiabetic Agents   3

VINPOCETINE

NEGATIVE

Possible Harmful Interaction:

Warfarin   3

VITAMIN A

NEGATIVE

Possible Harmful Interaction:

Anticonvulsant Agents   3
Isotretinoin   1
Valproic Acid   3
Warfarin   3

POSITIVE

Supplementation Possibly Helpful:

Bile Acid Sequestrants   3

VITAMIN B$_1$

POSITIVE

Supplementation Probably Helpful:

Loop Diuretics   2

VITAMIN B$_2$

POSITIVE

Supplementation Possibly Helpful:

Oral Contraceptives   3

VITAMIN B₃

NEGATIVE

Possible Harmful Interaction:

Statin Drugs	2

POSITIVE

Supplementation Possibly Helpful:

Isoniazid	2

VITAMIN B₆

NEGATIVE

Possible Harmful Interaction:

Levodopa	1

POSITIVE

Interaction Unlikely or Probably Insignificant:

Oral Contraceptives	4

Supplementation Possibly Helpful:

Penicillamine	3

Supplementation Probably Helpful:

Hydralazine	1
Isoniazid	1
MAO Inhibitors	2
Theophylline	2

VITAMIN B₁₂

POSITIVE

Interaction Unlikely or Probably Insignificant:

Oral Contraceptives	4

Supplementation Possibly Helpful:

Antidiabetic Agents	3
Bile Acid Sequestrants	3
Colchicine	3

Nitrous Oxide	1
Zidovudine	2

Supplementation Probably Helpful:

H_2 Antagonists	2
Proton Pump Inhibitors	2

VITAMIN C

NEGATIVE

Possible Harmful Interaction:

Acetaminophen	3
Heparin	3
Warfarin	3

POSITIVE

Supplementation Possibly Helpful:

Anthracyclines	3
Cisplatin	3
Nonsteroidal Anti-Inflammatory Drugs (NSAIDs)	3
Nitroglycerin	3
Oral Contraceptives	3

VITAMIN D

POSITIVE

Supplementation Possibly Helpful:

Anticonvulsant Agents	2
Carbamazepine	2
H_2 Antagonist	3
Heparin	1
Isoniazid	3
Phenobarbital	2
Phenytoin	2
Primidone	2
Rifampin	3
Valproic Acid	2

Appendix A

Supplementation Probably Helpful:

Corticosteroids	2
Estrogen	1

VITAMIN E

NEGATIVE

Possible Harmful Interaction:

Heparin	3
Nonsteroidal Anti-Inflammatory Drugs (NSAIDs)	2
Pentoxifylline	3
Warfarin	2

MIXED

Possible Benefits and Risks:

Antidiabetic Agents	3

POSITIVE

Supplementation Possibly Helpful:

Amiodarone	2
Anthracyclines	3
Antipsychotic Agents	3
Bile Acid Sequestrants	3
Cisplatin	2

VITAMIN K

NEGATIVE

Possible Harmful Interaction:

Warfarin	1

POSITIVE

Supplementation Possibly Helpful:

Antibiotics	3
Bile Acid Sequestrants	3
Cephalosporins	3

*Supplementation Possibly Helpful
for Pregnant Women:*

Anticonvulsant Agents	2
Carbamazepine	2
Phenobarbital	2
Phenytoin	2
Primidone	2
Valproic Acid	2

WHITE WILLOW

NEGATIVE

Possible Harmful Interaction:

Anticonvulsant Agents	3
Heparin	2
Methotrexate	2
Nonsteroidal Anti-Inflammatory Drugs (NSAIDs)	3
Pentoxifylline	3
Phenytoin	3
Spironolactone	3
Warfarin	3

WORMWOOD

NEGATIVE

Possible Harmful Interaction:

Antipsychotic Agents	3
Nonsteroidal Anti-Inflammatory Drugs (NSAIDs)	3

YERBA MANSA

NEGATIVE

Possible Harmful Interaction:

Antipsychotic Agents	2
Benzodiazepines	2
Carbamazepine	2

Phenobarbital	2
Phenytoin	2
Primidone	2
Tricyclic Antidepressants	2
Valproic Acid	2
Zolpidem	2

YOHIMBE

NEGATIVE

Possible Harmful Interaction:

Antipsychotic Agents	3
Clonidine	2

ZINC

NEGATIVE

Take at a Different Time of Day:

Fluoroquinolones	2
Tetracyclines	2

POSITIVE

*Supplementation Possibly Helpful,
but Take at a Different Time of Day:*

Antacids	3

Supplementation Possibly Helpful:

ACE Inhibitors	2
Ethambutol	3
H_2 Antagonists	3
Oral Contraceptives	3
Proton Pump Inhibitors	3
Thiazide Diuretics	3
Zidovudine	2

APPENDIX B
NUTRIENT DEPLETIONS

This appendix lists nutrient depletion interactions in summary form. Use it to quickly find out which nutrients may be adversely affected by a particular medication.

Numerous medications can deplete the body of necessary nutrients. Some drugs may interfere with the body's absorption or synthesis of nutrients, or increase their excretion. Other drugs may block the natural activation of nutrients for use in the body or hamper their action.

In such cases, there may be benefit in taking extra nutrients to balance the effect of certain drugs. Since nutrient supplementation may help, depletion interactions are termed *Positive*.

Each entry includes a significance rating and any special instructions that might apply. Refer to the main text of this book for detailed information on these interactions.

RATING KEY

1   Significant interaction

2   Possibly significant interaction

3   Interaction of relatively little significance

4   Reported interaction that does not in fact exist or is insignificant

ACE INHIBITORS

POSITIVE

Supplementation Possibly Helpful:

Zinc	2

ANTACIDS

POSITIVE

Supplementation Possibly Helpful, but Take at a Different Time of Day:

Chromium	3
Folate	3

Iron	3
Magnesium	3
Manganese	3
Phosphorus	3
Zinc	3

ANTHRACYCLINES

POSITIVE

Supplementation Possibly Helpful:

Coenzyme Q_{10} (CoQ_{10})   2

ANTIBIOTICS

POSITIVE

Supplementation Possibly Helpful:

Vitamin K   3

Supplementation Probably Helpful:

Lactobacillus acidophilus and Other   2
"Friendly Bacteria"

ANTICONVULSANT AGENTS

MIXED

Supplementation Possibly Helpful,
but Take at a Different Time of Day:

Biotin   3

Note: Although anticonvusants may deplete biotin, there are also concerns that taking extra biotin might interfere with the effectiveness of these drugs, potentially increasing the risk of seizures. See the full topic for more information.

Supplementation Possibly Helpful:

Folate   2

Note: Although anticonvusants may deplete folate, there are also concerns that taking extra folate might possibly interfere with the effectiveness of these drugs, potentially increasing the risk of seizures. See the full topic for more information.

POSITIVE

Supplementation Probably Helpful, but Take at a Different Time of Day:

Calcium   2

Supplementation Possibly Helpful:

Carnitine   2

Vitamin D   2

Supplementation Possibly Helpful: for Pregnant Women

Vitamin K   2

ANTIDIABETIC AGENTS

POSITIVE

Supplementation Possibly Helpful:

Coenzyme Q_{10} (CoQ_{10})   3

Vitamin B_{12} 3

ANTIHYPERTENSIVE AGENTS

POSITIVE

Supplementation Possibly Helpful:

Coenzyme Q_{10} 3

ANTIPSYCHOTIC AGENTS

POSITIVE

Supplementation Possibly Helpful:

Coenzyme Q_{10} (CoQ_{10})   3

BETA BLOCKERS

POSITIVE

Supplementation Possibly Helpful:

Chromium   3

Coenzyme Q_{10} (CoQ_{10})   2

BILE ACID SEQUESTRANTS

POSITIVE

Supplementation Possibly Helpful:

Calcium	3
Iron	3
Vitamin A	3
Vitamin B_{12}	3
Vitamin E	3
Vitamin K	3

Supplementation Probably Helpful:

Folate	2

CARBAMAZEPINE

MIXED

Supplementation Possibly Helpful,
but Take at a Different Time of Day:

Biotin	3

Supplementation Possibly Helpful:

Folate	2
Carnitine	2
Vitamin D	2

POSITIVE

Supplementation Possibly Helpful:
for Pregnant Women

Vitamin K	2

Supplementation Probably Helpful,
but Take at a Different Time of Day:

Calcium	2

CEPHALOSPORINS

POSITIVE

Supplementation Possibly Helpful:

Vitamin K   3

CISPLATIN

POSITIVE

Supplementation Possibly Helpful:

Glutathione   3

Supplementation Probably Helpful:

Magnesium   1

Potassium   1

COLCHICINE

POSITIVE

Supplementation Possibly Helpful:

Vitamin B_{12} 3

CORTICOSTEROIDS

POSITIVE

Supplementation Probably Helpful:

Calcium   2

Vitamin D   2

DIGOXIN

POSITIVE

Supplementation Possibly Helpful:

Calcium   3

*Supplementation Possibly Helpful,
but Take at a Different Time of Day:*

Magnesium   3

Appendix B

ESTROGEN

POSITIVE

Supplementation Possibly Helpful:

Magnesium   3

ETHAMBUTOL

POSITIVE

Supplementation Possibly Helpful:

Copper   3
Zinc   3

H$_2$ ANTAGONISTS

POSITIVE

Supplementation Possibly Helpful:

Folate   3
Iron   3
Vitamin D   3
Zinc   3

Supplementation Probably Helpful:

Vitamin B$_{12}$ 2

HEPARIN

POSITIVE

Supplementation Possibly Helpful:

Vitamin D   1

HYDRALAZINE

POSITIVE

Supplementation Probably Helpful:

Vitamin B$_6$ 1

ISONIAZID

POSITIVE

Supplementation Possibly Helpful:

Niacin (Vitamin B_3)	2
Vitamin D	3

Supplementation Probably Helpful:

Vitamin B_6	1

LEVODOPA

MIXED

Possible Benefits and Risks:

S-Adenosylmethionine (SAMe)	3

LEVODOPA/CARBIDOPA

MIXED

Possible Benefits and Risks:

S-Adenosylmethionine (SAMe)	3

LOOP DIURETICS

POSITIVE

Supplementation Probably Helpful:

Magnesium	2
Potassium	1
Vitamin B_1 (Thiamin)	2

MAO INHIBITORS

POSITIVE

Supplementation Probably Helpful:

Vitamin B_6 (Pyridoxine)	2

Appendix B

METHOTREXATE

POSITIVE

Supplementation Possibly Helpful:

Folate   1

Note: See the full topic for more information.

NITROUS OXIDE

POSITIVE

Supplementation Possibly Helpful:

Vitamin B_{12} 1
Folate   1

NONSTEROIDAL ANTI-INFLAMMATORY DRUGS

POSITIVE

Supplementation Possibly Helpful:

Folate   2
Vitamin C   3

ORAL CONTRACEPTIVES

POSITIVE

Interaction Unlikely or Probably Insignificant:

Folate   4
Vitamin B_6 4
Vitamin B_{12} 4

Supplementation Possibly Helpful:

Magnesium   3
Vitamin B_2 (Riboflavin)   3
Vitamin C   3
Zinc   3

PENICILLAMINE

POSITIVE

Supplementation Possibly Helpful:

Vitamin B_6 (Pyridoxine)   3

PHENOBARBITAL

MIXED

Supplementation Possibly Helpful,
but Take at a Different Time of Day:

Biotin   3

Supplementation Possibly Helpful:

Folate   2

POSITIVE

Supplementation Probably Helpful,
but Take at a Different Time of Day:

Calcium   2

Supplementation Possibly Helpful:

Carnitine   2

Vitamin D   2

Supplementation Possibly Helpful
for Pregnant Women:

Vitamin K   2

PHENYTOIN

MIXED

Supplementation Possibly Helpful,
but Take at a Different Time of Day:

Biotin   3

Supplementation Possibly Helpful:

Folate   2

POSITIVE

*Supplementation Probably Helpful,
but Take at a Different Time of Day:*

Calcium   2

Supplementation Possibly Helpful:

Carnitine   2

Vitamin D   2

*Supplementation Possibly Helpful:
for Pregnant Women*

Vitamin K   2

PRIMIDONE

MIXED

*Supplementation Possibly Helpful,
but Take at a Different Time of Day:*

Biotin   3

Supplementation Possibly Helpful:

Folate   2

POSITIVE

*Supplementation Probably Helpful,
but Take at a Different Time of Day:*

Calcium   2

Supplementation Possibly Helpful:

Carnitine   2

Vitamin D   2

*Supplementation Possibly Helpful
for Pregnant Women:*

Vitamin K   2

PROTON PUMP INHIBITORS

POSITIVE

Supplementation Possibly Helpful:

Folate	3
Iron	3
Zinc	3

Supplementation Probably Helpful:

Vitamin B_{12}	2

RIFAMPIN

POSITIVE

Supplementation Possibly Helpful:

Vitamin D	3

STATIN DRUGS

POSITIVE

Supplementation Probably Helpful:

Coenzyme Q_{10} (CoQ_{10})	2

THEOPHYLLINE

POSITIVE

Supplementation Probably Helpful:

Vitamin B_6 (Pyridoxine)	2

THIAZIDE DIURETICS

POSITIVE

Supplementation Possibly Helpful:

Zinc	3

Supplementation Probably Helpful:

Magnesium	2
Potassium	1

TRIAMTERENE

POSITIVE

Supplementation Possibly Helpful:

Folate   3

TRICYCLIC ANTIDEPRESSANTS

POSITIVE

Supplementation Possibly Helpful:

Coenzyme Q_{10} (CoQ_{10})   3

TRIMETHOPRIM-SULFAMETHOXAZOLE (TMP-SMZ)

POSITIVE

Supplementation Probably Helpful:

Folate   1

VALPROIC ACID

MIXED

Supplementation Possibly Helpful,
but Take at a Different Time of Day:

Biotin   3

Supplementation Possibly Helpful:

Folate   2

POSITIVE

Supplementation Probably Helpful,
but Take at a Different Time of Day:

Calcium   2

Supplementation Possibly Helpful:

Carnitine   2

Vitamin D   2

Supplementation Possibly Helpful:
for Pregnant Women

    Vitamin K   2

ZIDOVUDINE

POSITIVE

Supplementation Possibly Helpful:

Copper	2
Vitamin B$_{12}$	2
Zinc	2

Note: There are concerns that zinc supplementation may also carry risk. See the full topic for more information.

APPENDIX C
HERB AND DRUG INTERACTIONS THAT MIGHT CAUSE EXCESS SEDATION

Add-on depressant interactions can occur when drugs that cause central nervous system depression or sedation are combined. *Add-on* means that the actions of each medication add together to increase the depressant effects significantly beyond that of any one agent alone.

Such interactions are potentially the most common type of drug-to-drug interaction, since drugs causing depressant effects are widely used and some are available in nonprescription products.

The result can be excessive central nervous system depression with drowsiness, dizziness, and loss of muscle coordination, making it hazardous to drive or engage in other activities requiring complete alertness; in severe cases, there may be failure of blood circulation and breathing functions causing coma and death. For this reason, add-on depressant interactions can be among the most dangerous.

Just as the effects of sedative drugs can add to each other, herbs with depressant or sedative properties can add to the effects of depressant drugs. This appendix, by providing detailed lists of herbs and drugs with these effects, is designed to help you identify and prevent potential problems. Please note, however, that no such lists can be completely comprehensive.

HERBS THAT MAY PRODUCE SEDATIVE EFFECTS

Baikal skullcap (*Scutellaria baicalensis*)

ashwagandha (*Withania somnifera*)

calamus (*Acorus calamus*)

calendula (*Calendula officinalis*)

California poppy (*Eschscholzia californica*)

capsicum (*Capsicum frutescens*)

catnip (*Nepeta cataria*)

celery (*Apium graveolens*)

couch grass (*Agropyron repens*)

elecampane (*Inula helenium*)

German chamomile (*Matricaria recutita*)

goldenseal (*Hydrastis canadensis*)

gotu kola (*Centella asiatica*)

hops (*Humulus lupulus*)

Jamaican dogwood (*Piscidia piscipula*)

kava (*Piper methysticum*)

lady's slipper (*Cypripedium pubescens*)

lemon balm (*Melissa officinalis*)

passionflower (*Passiflora incarnata*)

sage (*Salvia officinalis; Salvia lavandulaefolia*)

sassafras (*Sassifras officinale*)

shepherd's purse (*Capsella bursa-pastoris*)

Siberian ginseng (*Eleutherococcus senticosus*)

skullcap (*Scutellaria lateriflora*)

St. John's wort (*Hypericum perforatum*)

stinging nettle (*Urtica dioica; Urtica urens*)

valerian (*Valeriana officinalis*)

wild carrot (*Daucus carota*)

wild lettuce (*Lactuca virosa*)

withania (*Withania somnifera*)

yerba mansa (*Anemopsis californica*)

and others

HERB AND DRUG DEPRESSANT INTERACTIONS

Be aware of potentially dangerous add-on depressant interactions when you combine the previously listed herbs with drugs in any of the following depressant drug classes:

alcohol (ethanol, beer, liquor, wine, etc.)

antianxiety agents

anticholinergics

anticonvulsant agents

antidepressants

antihistamines

antihypertensive agents (certain types)

antipsychotic agents

muscle relaxants

narcotic analgesics

sedatives/hypnotics

ANTIANXIETY AGENTS

Antianxiety agents are used for anxiety disorders and for the short-term relief of the symptoms of anxiety.

alprazolam (Xanax)

busipirone (BuSpar) (may not interact)

chlordiazepoxide (Librium)

clorazepate (Tranxene)

diazepam (Valium)

doxepin (Adapin, Sinequan)

halazepam (Paxipam)

hydroxyzine (Atarax, Vistaril)

lorazepam (Ativan)

meprobamate (Equanil, Equagesic, Micrainin, Miltown, Neuramate)

oxazepam (Serax)

ANTICHOLINERGICS

Anticholinergics are used primarily for stomach and digestive tract disorders and to control tremors resulting from Parkinson's disease or from treatment with antipsychotic drugs.

atropine

atropine/scopolamine/hyoscyamine (e.g., Barbidonna, Donnatal, Hyosophen)

belladonna

benztropine (Cogentin)

biperiden (Akineton)

clidinium (Quarzan)

dicyclomine (Bentyl)

glycopyrrolate (Robinul)

hyoscyamine (Anaspaz, Levsin)

methantheline (Banthine)

orphenadrine (Norflex)

oxybutynin (Ditropan)

procyclidine (Kemadrin)

propantheline (Pro-Banthine)

scopolamine (Scopace, Transderm-Scop)

tridihexethyl chloride (Pathilon)

trihexyphenidyl HCl (Artane)

ANTICONVULSANT AGENTS

Anticonvulsant agents are used for seizure disorders such as epilepsy.

carbamazepine (Atretol, Carbatrol, Epitol, Tegretol)

clonazepam (Klonopin)

clorazepate (Tranxene)

diazepam (Valium, Valrelease)

ethosuximide (Zarontin)

ethotoin (Peganone)

felbamate (Felbatol)

gabapentin (Neurontin)

lamotrigine (Lamictal)

levetiracetam (Keppra)

mephenytoin (Mesantoin)

methsuximide (Celontin)

oxcarbazepine (Trileptal)

phenobarbital

phensuximide (Milontin)

phenytoin (Dilantin)

primidone (Mysoline)

tiagabine (Gabitril)

trimethadione (Tridione)

valproic acid (Depakene)

ANTIDEPRESSANTS

Antidepressants are used for clinical depression.

amitriptyline (Elavil)

amoxapine (Asendin)

bupropion (Wellbutrin, Zyban)

citalopram (Celexa)

clomipramine (Anafranil)

desipramine (Norpramin)

doxepine (Sinequan)

fluoxetine (Prozac, Sarafem)

fluvoxamine (Luvox)

imipramine (Tofranil)

maprotiline (Ludiomil)

mirtazapine (Remeron)

nefazodone (Serzone)

nortriptyline (Aventyl, Pamelor)

paroxetine (Paxil)

protriptyline (Vivactil)

sertraline (Zoloft)

trazodone (Desyrel)

trimipramine (Surmontil)

venlafaxine (Effexor)

ANTIHISTAMINES

Antihistamines are used to relieve the symptoms of allergies and for various other conditions. Newer antihistamines, which appear less likely to cause sedative effects, include astemizole, cetirizine, loratadine, and fexofenadine.

astemizole (Hismanal)

azatadine (Optimine)

azelastine (Astelin)

brompheniramine (Dimetapp Allergy)

cetirizine (Zyrtec)

chlorpheniramine (e.g., Chlor-Trimeton)

clemastine (e.g., Tavist)

cyproheptadine (Periactin)

dexchlorpheniramine (Polaramine)

diphenhydramine (e.g., Benadryl)

fexofenadine (Allegra)

hydroxyzine (Atarax, Vistaril)

loratadine (Claritin)

phenindamine (Nolahist)

promethazine (Phenergan)

tripelennamine (PBZ)

ANTIHYPERTENSIVE AGENTS

Antihypertensive agents are used to lower elevated blood pressure. The following drugs, which may also be included in combination products for high blood pressure, are most likely to cause drowsiness or sedation.

clonidine (Catapres)

doxazosin (Cardura)

guanabenz (Wytensin)

guanadrel (Hylorel)

guanethidine (Ismelin)

guanfacine (Tenex)

methyldopa (Aldomet)

prazosin (Minipress)

reserpine (included in various combination products)

tamsulosin (Flomax)

terazosin (Hytrin)

ANTIPSYCHOTIC AGENTS

Antipsychotic agents are used for psychotic disorders such as schizophrenia and manic-depressive illness, as well as for other conditions.

chlorpromazine (Thorazine)

clozapine (Clozaril)

fluphenazine (Permitil, Prolixin)

haloperidol (Haldol)

lithium (Eskalith, Lithane, Lithotabs, Lithobid, Cibalith-S)

loxapine (Loxitane)

mesoridazine (Serentil)

molindone (Moban)

olanzapine (Zyprexa)

perphenazine (Trilafon)

pimozide (Orap)

prochlorperazine (Compazine)

promazine (Sparine)

quetiapine (Seroquel)

risperidone (Risperdal)

thioridazine (Mellaril)

thiothixene (Navane)

trifluoperazine (Stelazine)

triflupromazine (Vesprin)

MUSCLE RELAXANTS

Muscle relaxants are used to relieve the discomfort associated with acute, painful musculoskeletal conditions.

baclofen (Lioresal)

carisoprodol (Soma)

chlorphenesin (Maolate)

chlorzoxazone (Paraflex, Remular-S)

cyclobenzaprine (Flexeril)

dantrolene (Dantrium)

diazepam (Valium)

metaxalone (Skelaxin)

methocarbamol (Robaxin, Robaxisal)

orphenadrine (e.g., Norflex, Norgesic)

NARCOTIC ANALGESICS

Narcotic analgesics are used to relieve pain. Some of these drugs are also useful for cough or diarrhea.

butorphanol (Stadol)

codeine (e.g., Empirin w/Codeine, Fioricet w/Codeine, Fiorinal w/Codeine, Phenaphen w/Codeine, Tylenol w/Codeine)

dihydrocodeine (Synalgos-DC)

fentanyl (e.g., Actiq, Duragesic)

hydrocodone (e.g., Anexia, Lorcet, Lortab, Vicodin, Zydone)

hydromorphone (Dilaudid)

levomethadyl (Orlaam)

levorphanol (Levo-Dromoran)

meperidine (Demerol, Mepergan)

methadone (Dolophine)

morphine (e.g., MS-Contin)

opium (Paregoric)

oxycodone (e.g., Percocet, Percodan, Percolone, Percodan-Demi, Roxicet, Roxicodone, Tylox)

oxymorphone (Numorphan)

pentazocine (Talacen, Talwin)

propoxyphene (e.g., Darvocet-N, Darvon, Darvon Compound-65, Darvon-N, Propacet, Wygesic)

tramadol (Ultram) [non-narcotic pain reliever]

SEDATIVES / HYPNOTICS

These drugs are used for sedation and to induce sleep. This class includes both barbiturates and non-barbiturates.

acetylcarbromal (Paxarel)

amobarbital (Tuinal)

aprobarbital (Alurate)

butabarbital (Butisol)

butalbital (used in various combination pain-relieving products)

chloral hydrate

estazolam (ProSom)

ethchlorvynol (Placidyl)

flurazepam (Dalmane)

glutethimide

mephobarbital (Mebaral)

midazolam (Versed)

paraldehyde (Paral)

pentobarbital (Nembutal)

phenobarbital (Bellatal, Solfoton)

primidone (Mysoline)

quazepam (Doral)

secobarbital (Seconal, Tuinal)

temazepam (Restoril)

triazolam (Halcion)

zaleplon (Sonata)

zolpidem (Ambien)

nonprescription sleep aids (these products contain antihistamines such as diphenhydramine and doxylamine, and include Aspirin Free Anacin P.M., Compoz, Dormin, Excedrine P.M., Extra Strength Tylenol PM, Midol PM, Miles Nervine, Nighttime Pamprin, Nytol, Sleep-eze, Sominex, and Unisom)

APPENDIX D
SAFETY ISSUES

This appendix covers safety issues for herbs and supplements given positive or mixed interaction ratings in the main body of the book. If you are considering using one of those substances, you can find relevant safety considerations here.

For dosage information, see the *Natural Health Bible, Second Edition*, Prima, 2000.

ACIDOPHILUS AND OTHER PROBIOTICS

There are no known safety problems with the use of acidophilus or other probiotics. Occasionally, some people notice a temporary increase in digestive gas.

ALOE

Other than occasional allergic reactions, no serious problems have been reported with aloe gel, whether used internally or externally. However, comprehensive safety studies are lacking. Safety in young children, pregnant or nursing women, or those with severe liver or kidney disease has not been established.

In addition, keep in mind that if aloe is successful as a treatment for diabetes, blood sugar levels could fall too low, necessitating a reduction in medication dosage.

BILBERRY

Bilberry fruit is a food and as such is quite safe. Enormous quantities have been administered to rats without toxic effects.[1,2] One study of 2,295 people given bilberry extract found a 4% incidence of side effects such as mild digestive distress, skin rashes, and drowsiness.[3] Although safety in pregnancy has not been proven, clinical trials have enrolled pregnant women.[4] Safety in young children, nursing women, or those with severe liver or kidney disease is not known. There are no known drug interactions. Bilberry does not appear to interfere with blood clotting.[5]

Little is known about the safety of bilberry leaf. Based on animal evidence that it can reduce blood sugar levels in people with diabetes, it is possible that use of bilberry leaf by diabetics could require a reduction in drug dosage.[6]

References

1. Lietti A, Cristoni A, Picci M. Studies on *Vaccinium myrtillus* anthocyanosides. I. Vasoprotective and antiinflammatory activity. *Arzneimittelforschung*. 1976;26:829–832.

2. Lietti A, Forni G. Studies on *Vaccinium myrtillus* anthocyanosides. II. Aspects of anthocyanin pharmacokinetics in the rat. *Arzneimittelforschung*. 1976;26:832–835.

3. Eandi M. Post marketing investigation on Tegens® preparation with respect to side effects. Unpublished results. Cited by: Morazzoni P, Bombardelli E. *Vaccinium myrtillus. Fitoterapia*. 1996;67:3–29.

4. Grismondi GL. Treatment of phlebopathies caused by stasis in pregnancy [translated from Italian]. *Minerva Ginecol*. 1981;33:221–230.

5. Scharrer A, Ober M. Anthocyanosides in the treatment of retinopathies [translated from German]. *Klin Monatsbl Augenheilkd*. 1981;178:386–389.

6. Cignarella A, Nastasi M, Cavalli E, et al. Novel lipid-lowering properties of *Vaccinium myrtillus* L. leaves, a traditional antidiabetic treatment, in several models of rat dyslipidaemia: a comparison with ciprofibrate. *Thromb Res*. 1996;84:311–322.

BIOTIN

Biotin appears to be quite safe. However, maximum safe dosages for young children, pregnant or nursing women, or those with severe liver or kidney disease have not been established.

BITTER MELON

As a widely eaten food in Asia, bitter melon is generally regarded as safe. It can cause diarrhea and stomach pain if taken in excessive amounts, but the main risk of bitter melon comes from the fact that it may work! Combining it with standard drugs may reduce blood sugar too well, possibly leading to dangerously low levels.[1,2] For this reason, if you already take drugs for diabetes, you should add bitter melon to your diet only with a physician's supervision. And definitely don't stop your medication and substitute bitter melon instead. It is not as powerful as insulin or other conventional treatments.

Safety in young children, pregnant or nursing women, or those with severe liver or kidney disease has not been established.

References

1. Leatherdale BA, Panesar RK, Singh G, et al. Improvement in glucose tolerance due to *Momordica charantia* (karela). *Br Med J (Clin Res Ed)*. 1981;282:1823–1824.

2. Aslam M, Stockley IH. Interaction between curry ingredient (karela) and drug (chlorpropamide). *Lancet*. 1979;1:607.

BROMELAIN

Bromelain appears to be essentially nontoxic, and it seldom causes side effects other than occasional mild gastrointestinal distress or allergic reactions.[1]

However, because bromelain "thins the blood" to some extent, it shouldn't be combined with drugs such as Coumadin (warfarin) without a doctor's supervision.

According to one small animal study, bromelain might interact with sedative medications, increasing their effect.[2] As noted above, it might also increase blood levels of various antibiotics, which could present risks in some cases. Safety in young children, pregnant or nursing women, or those with liver or kidney disease has not been established.

References

1. Blumenthal M, ed. *The Complete German Commission E Monographs, Therapeutic Guide to Herbal Medicines*. Boston, Mass: Integrative Medicine Communications; 1998:94.

2. Moss JN, Frazier CV, Martin GJ. Bromelains. The pharmacology of the enzymes. *Arch Int Pharmacodyn Ther.* 1963;145:166–188.

BURDOCK

As a food commonly eaten in Japan (it is often found in sukiyaki), burdock root is believed to be safe. However, in 1978, the *Journal of the American Medical Association* caused a brief scare by publishing a report of burdock poisoning. Subsequent investigation showed that the herbal product involved was actually contaminated with the poisonous chemical atropine from an unknown source.[1] Safety in young children, pregnant or nursing women, or those with severe liver or kidney disease is not established.

References

1. Bryson PD, Watanabe AS, Rumack BH, et al. Burdock root tea poisoning. Case report involving a commercial preparation. *JAMA*. 1978; 239:2157.

CALCIUM

In general, it's safe to take up to 2,000 mg of calcium daily, although this is more than you need.[1] Greatly excessive intake of calcium can cause numerous side effects, including dangerous or painful deposits of calcium within the body.

If you have cancer, hyperparathyroidism, or sarcoidosis, you should take calcium only under a physician's supervision.

People with kidney stones or a history of kidney stones are also often warned not to take supplemental calcium. The reason for this caution is that kidney stones are commonly made of calcium oxalate crystals. However, studies have found that increased intake of calcium from food actually reduces the risk of kidney stones.[2,3] Calcium supplements, on the other hand, might increase kidney stone risk, especially if they are not taken with meals.[4] The bottom line: Restriction of calcium—whether supplemental or dietary—may still be appropriate for certain people.[5] Ask your physician for advice specific to you.

Large observational studies have found that higher intakes of calcium are associated with a greatly increased risk of prostate cancer.[6,7,8] This seems to be the case whether the calcium comes from milk or from calcium supplements. However, without further research it is difficult to tell whether this is a cause-and-effect relationship or simply an accidental correlation.

Calcium supplements combined with high doses of vitamin D might interfere with some of the effects of calcium channel–blockers.[9] It is very important that you consult your physician before trying this combination.

Concerns have been raised that the aluminum in some antacids may not be good for you.[10] Since there is some evidence that calcium citrate supplements might increase the absorption of aluminum,[11–15] it might not be a good idea to take calcium citrate at the same time of day as aluminum-containing antacids. Another option is to use other forms of calcium, or to avoid antacids containing aluminum.

When taken over the long term, thiazide diuretics tend to increase levels of calcium in the body, by decreasing the amount excreted by the body.[16–19] It's not likely that this will cause a problem. However, since greatly increased calcium levels in the body can cause side effects such as calcium deposits, if you are using thiazide diuretics, you should consult with your physician on the proper doses of calcium and vitamin D for you.

Finally, calcium may interfere with the absorption of antibiotics in the tetracycline and fluoroquinolone families as well as thyroid hormone. If you are taking any of these drugs you should take your calcium supplements at least 2 hours before or after your medication dose.[20–25]

References

1. [No authors listed]. Optimal calcium intake. Sponsored by National Institutes of Health Continuing Medical Education. *Nutrition*. 1995;11:409–417.

2. Curhan GC, Willett WC, Speizer FE, et al. Comparison of dietary calcium with supplemental calcium and other nutrients as factors affecting the risk for kidney stones in women. *Ann Intern Med*. 1997;126:497–504.

3. Curhan GC, Willett WC, Rimm EB, et al. A prospective study of dietary calcium and other nutrients and the risk of symptomatic kidney stones. *N Engl J Med*. 1993;328:833–838.

4. Curhan GC, Willett WC, Speizer FE, et al. Comparison of dietary calcium with supplemental calcium and other nutrients as factors affecting the risk for kidney stones in women. *Ann Intern Med*. 1997;126:497–504.

5. Parivar F, Low RK, Stoller ML. The influence of diet on urinary stone disease. *J Urol*. 1996;155:432–440.

6. Giovannucci E, Rimm EB, Wolk A, et al. Calcium and fructose intake in relation to risk of prostate cancer. *Cancer Res*. 1998;58:442–447.

7. Chan JM, Giovannucci E, Andersson SO, et al. Dairy products, calcium, phosphorous, vitamin D, and risk of prostate cancer (Sweden). *Cancer Causes Control*. 1998;9:559–566.

8. Giovannucci E. Dietary influences of 1,25(OH)2 vitamin D in relation to prostate cancer: a hypothesis. *Cancer Causes Control*. 1998;9:567–582.

9. Bar-Or D, Gasiel Y. Calcium and calciferol antagonise effect of verapamil in atrial fibrillation. *Br Med J (Clin Res Ed)*. 1981;282:1585–1586.

10. Gaby AR. Aluminum: The ubiquitous poison. *Nutr Healing*. 1997;4:3–4, 11.

11. Walker JA, Sherman RA, Cody RP. The effect of oral bases on enteral aluminum absorption. *Arch Intern Med*. 1990;150:2037–2039.

12. [No authors listed]. Preliminary findings suggest calcium citrate supplements may raise aluminum levels in blood, urine. *Fam Pract News.* 1992;22:74–75.

13. Weberg R, Berstad A. Gastrointestinal absorption of aluminium from single doses of aluminium containing antacids in man. *Eur J Clin Invest.* 1986;16:428–432.

14. Nolan CR, Califano JR, Butzin CA. Influence of calcium acetate or calcium citrate on intestinal aluminum absorption. *Kidney Int.* 1990;38:937–941.

15. Slanina P, Frech W, Bernhardson A, et al. Influence of dietary factors on aluminium absorption and retention in the brain and bone of rats. *Acta Pharmacol Toxicol (Copenh).* 1985;56:331–336.

16. Riis B, Christiansen C. Actions of thiazide on vitamin D metabolism: a controlled therapeutic trial in normal women early in the postmenopause. *Metabolism.* 1985;34:421–424.

17. Lemann J Jr, Gray RW, Maierhofer WJ, et al. Hydrochlorothiazide inhibits bone resorption in men despite experimentally elevated serum 1,25-dihydroxyvitamin D concentrations. *Kidney Int.* 1985;28:951–958.

18. Crowe M, Wollner L, Griffiths RA. Hypercalcaemia following vitamin D and thiazide therapy in the elderly. *Practitioner.* 1984;228:312–313.

19. Gora ML, Seth SK, Bay WH, et al. Milk–alkali syndrome associated with use of chlorothiazide and calcium carbonate. *Clin Pharm.* 1989;8:227–229.

20. Neuvonen PJ, Kivisto KT, Lehto P. Interference of dairy products with the absorption of ciprofloxacin. *Clin Pharmacol Ther.* 1991;50:498–502.

21. Minami R, Inotsume N, Nakano M, et al. Effect of milk on absorption of norfloxacin in healthy volunteers. *J Clin Pharmacol.* 1993;33:1238–1240.

22. Lehto P, Kivisto KT. Different effects of products containing metal ions on the absorption of lomefloxacin. *Clin Pharmacol Ther.* 1994;56:477–482.

23. Dudley MN, Marchbanks CR, Flor SC, et al. The effect of food or milk on the absorption kinetics of ofloxacin. *Eur J Clin Pharmacol.* 1991;41:569–571.

24. Flor S, Guay DR, Opsahl JA, et al. Effects of magnesium-aluminum hydroxide and calcium carbonate antacids on bioavailability of ofloxacin. *Antimicrob Agents Chemother.* 1990;34:2436–2438.

25. Butner LE, Fulco PP, Feldman G. Calcium carbonate-induced hypothyroidism. *Ann Intern Med.* 2000;132:595.

Appendix D

CARNITINE

L-carnitine in its three forms appears to be safe, even when taken with medications. Individuals should take care, however, not to use forms of the supplement known as "D-carnitine" or "DL-carnitine," as these can cause angina, muscle pain, and loss of muscle function (probably by interfering with L-carnitine).

The maximum safe dosages for young children, pregnant or nursing women, or those with severe liver or kidney disease have not been established.

CAYENNE

As a commonly used food, cayenne is generally recognized as safe. Contrary to some reports, cayenne does not appear to aggravate stomach ulcers.[1]

References

1. Graham DY, Smith JL, Opekun AR. Spicy food and the stomach. Evaluation by videoendoscopy. *JAMA*. 1988;260:3473–3475.

CHROMIUM

Chromium appears to be safe when taken at a dosage of 50 to 200 mcg daily.[1] Side effects appear to be rare.

However, chromium is a heavy metal and might conceivably build up and cause problems if taken to excess. Recently, there have been a few reports of kidney damage in people who took a relatively high dosage of chromium: 1,200 mcg or more daily for several months.[2,3]

For this reason, the dosage found most effective for individuals with type 2 diabetes—1,000 mcg daily—might present some health risks. It would be advisable to seek medical supervision if you want to take more than 200 mcg daily.

Also, keep in mind that if you have diabetes and chromium is effective, you may need to cut down your dosage of any medication you take for diabetes.[4] Medical supervision is advised.

There has been one report of a severe skin reaction caused by chromium picolinate.[5]

Concerns have also been raised over the use of the picolinate form of chromium in individuals suffering from affective or psychotic disorders, because picolinic acids can change the levels of neurotransmitters.[6] There are also concerns, still fairly theoretical, that chromium picolinate could cause adverse effects on DNA.[7]

The maximum safe dosages of chromium for young children, women who are pregnant or nursing, or those with severe liver or kidney disease have not been established.

References

1. Anderson RA, Bryden NA, Polansky MM. Lack of toxicity of chromium chloride and chromium picolinate in rats. *J Am Coll Nutr*. 1997;16:273–279.

2. Cerulli J, Grabe DW, Gauthier I, et al. Chromium picolinate toxicity. *Ann Pharmacother*. 1998;32:428–431.

3. Wasser WG, Feldman NS, D'Agati VD. Chronic renal failure after ingestion of over-the-counter chromium picolinate [letter]. *Ann Intern Med*. 1997;126:410.

4. Ravina A, Slezack L. Chromium in the treatment of clinical diabetes mellitus [translated from Hebrew]. *Harefuah*. 1993;125:142–145.

5. Young PC, Turiansky GW, Bonner MW, et al. Acute generalized exanthematous pustulosis induced by chromium picolinate. *J Am Acad Dermatol*. 1999;41(5 Pt 2):820–823.

6. Reading SA. Chromium picolinate. *J Fla Med Assoc*. 1996;83:29–31.

7. Speetjens JK, Collins RA, Vincent JB, et al. The nutritional supplement chromium(III) tris(picolinate) cleaves DNA. *Chem Res Toxicol*. 1999;12:483–487.

COENZYME Q$_{10}$

CoQ$_{10}$ appears to be extremely safe. No significant side effects have been found, even in studies that lasted a year.[1] However, individuals with severe heart disease should not take CoQ$_{10}$ (or any other supplement) except under a doctor's supervision.

One study suggests that CoQ$_{10}$ might reduce blood sugar levels in people with diabetes.[2] While this could potentially be helpful for treatment of diabetes, it might present a risk as well: Diabetics using CoQ$_{10}$ might inadvertently push their blood sugar levels dangerously low. However, another trial in people with diabetes found no effect on blood sugar control.[3] The bottom line: If you have diabetes, make sure to track your blood sugar closely if you start taking CoQ$_{10}$ (or, indeed, any herb or supplement).

Finally, CoQ$_{10}$ might interfere with the anticoagulant effects of Coumadin (warfarin).[4] If you are taking Coumadin, you should not take CoQ$_{10}$ unless under a doctor's supervision.

The maximum safe dosages of CoQ_{10} for young children, pregnant or nursing women, or those with severe liver or kidney disease have not been determined.

References

1. Lampertico M, Comis S. Italian multicenter study on the efficacy and safety of coenzyme Q_{10} as adjuvant therapy in heart failure. *Clin Investig.* 1993;71(8 suppl):S129–S133.

2. Singh RB, Niaz MA, Rastogi SS, et al. Effect of hydrosoluble coenzyme Q_{10} on blood pressures and insulin resistance in hypertensive patients with coronary artery disease. *J Human Hypertens.* 1999;13:203–208.

3. Eriksson JG, Forsen TJ, Mortensen SA, et al. The effect of coenzyme Q_{10} administration on metabolic control in patients with type 2 diabetes mellitus. *Biofactors.* 1999;9:315–318.

4. Spigset O. Reduced effect of warfarin caused by ubidecarenone [letter]. *Lancet.* 1994;344:1372–1373.

COLOSTRUM

Colostrum does not seem to cause any significant side effects. However, comprehensive safety studies have not been performed. Safety in young children or women who are pregnant or nursing has not been established.

COPPER

Copper is safe when taken at nutritional dosages, but these should not be exceeded. As little as 10 mg of copper daily produces nausea, and 60 mg may cause vomiting.

Oral contraceptives might increase levels of copper in the body. Women taking oral contraceptives should consult a physician before taking copper supplements.[1,2,3]

Maximum safe dosages of copper for young children, pregnant or nursing women, or those with severe liver or kidney disease have not been determined.

References

1. Berg G, Kohlmeier L, Brenner H. Effect of oral contraceptive progestins on serum copper concentration. *Eur J Clin Nutr.* 1998;52:711–715.

Appendix D

2. Milne DB, Johnson PE. Assessment of copper status: effect of age and gender on reference ranges in healthy adults. *Clin Chem.* 1993;39:883–887.

3. Newhouse IJ, Clement DB, Lai C. Effects of iron supplementation and discontinuation on serum copper, zinc, calcium, and magnesium levels in women. *Med Sci Sports Exerc.* 1993;25:562–571.

DANDELION

Dandelion root and leaves are believed to be quite safe, with no side effects or likely risks other than rare allergic reactions.[1–4] It is on the FDA's GRAS (generally recognized as safe) list and approved for use as a food flavoring by the Council of Europe.

However, based on dandelion root's effect on bile secretion, Germany's Commission E has recommended that it not be used at all by individuals with obstruction of the bile ducts or other serious diseases of the gallbladder, and only under physician supervision by those with gallstones.[5]

Some references state that dandelion root can cause hyperacidity and thereby increase ulcer pain, but this concern has been disputed.[6]

Because the leaves contain so much potassium, they probably resupply any potassium lost due to dandelion's mild diuretic effect, although this has not been proven.

People with known allergies to related plants, such as chamomile and yarrow, should use dandelion with caution.

There are no known drug interactions with dandelion. However, based on what we know about dandelion root's effects, there might be some risk when combining it with pharmaceutical diuretics or drugs that reduce blood sugar levels.

Safety in young children, pregnant or nursing women, or those with severe liver or kidney disease has not been established.

References

1. Newall C, Anderson LA, Phillipson JD. *Herbal Medicines: A Guide for Health-Care Professionals*. London, England: Pharmaceutical Press; 1996:96.

2. European Scientific Cooperative on Phytotherapy. *Taraxaci radix* (dandelion). Exeter, UK: ESCOP; 1996–1997:2. Monographs on the Medicinal Uses of Plant Drugs, Fascicule 2.

3. *Review of Natural Products*. St. Louis, Mo: Facts and Comparisons; 1998: Dandelion monograph.

4. Hirono I, Mori H, Kato K, et al. Saftey examination of some edible plants, part 2. *J Environ Pathol Toxicol*. 1978;1:71–74.

5. Blumenthal M, ed. *The Complete German Commission E Monographs, Therapeutic Guide to Herbal Medicines*. Boston, Mass: Integrative Medicine Communications; 1998:119–120.

6. McGuffin M, ed. *American Herbal Products Association's Botanical Safety Handbook*. Boca Raton, Fla: CRC Press; 1997:114.

DHEA

DHEA appears to be safe when taken in therapeutic doses, at least in the short term. One study found no significant side effects in 50 women who took up to 200 mg daily for up to 1 year.[1]

However, DHEA, even at the low dose of 25 mg per day, may decrease levels of HDL ("good") cholesterol.[2,3] In addition, DHEA may cause acne and male pattern hair growth.[4,5]

Concerns have been raised by one study in rats and another in trout that linked DHEA to liver cancer.[6,7] However, at least four other animal studies suggest that DHEA may have some anticancer effects.[8,9]

A 15-year human observational trial looking for a connection between naturally occurring DHEA levels and breast cancer found no relationship, either positive or negative.[10] However, another study found a relationship between higher levels of DHEA and ovarian cancer.[11] Overall, the long-term safety of DHEA supplements remains unknown. This is the case with many supplements, but because there are animal studies suggesting that DHEA might increase the risk of liver cancer, caution is warranted. Estrogen is one example of a hormone that increases the risk for certain forms of cancer, and it took years for researchers to discover that risk. Keep in mind also that the body converts DHEA into other hormones, including estrogen and testosterone. This could be dangerous for women with hormone-influenced diseases such as breast cancer.

The safety of DHEA in young children, pregnant or nursing women, and individuals with severe liver or kidney disease has not been established. We also don't know whether DHEA interacts with other hormone treatments, such as estrogen, although it certainly stands to reason that it might.

References

1. van Vollenhoven RF, Morabito LM, Engleman EG, et al. Treatment of systemic lupus erythematosus with dehydroepiandrosterone: 50 patients treated up to 12 months. *J Rheumatol*. 1998;25:285–289.

2. Casson PR, Santoro N, Elkind-Hirsch K, et al. Postmenopausal dehydroepiandrosterone administration increases free insulin-like growth factor-I and decreases high-density lipoprotein: a six-month trial. *Fertil Steril*. 1998;70:107–110.

3. Mease PJ, Merrill JT, Lahita R, et al. GL701 (prasterone, dehydroepiandrosterone) improves or stabilizes disease activity in systemic lupus erythematosus. Poster presented at: The Endocrine Society's 82nd annual meeting; June 21–24, 2000; Toronto, Ontario.

4. Mease PJ, Merrill JT, Lahita R, et al. GL701 (prasterone, dehydroepiandrosterone) improves or stabilizes disease activity in systemic lupus erythematosus. Poster presented at: The Endocrine Society's 82nd annual meeting; June 21–24, 2000; Toronto, Ontario.

5. van Vollenhoven RF, Engleman EG, McGuire JL. Dehydroepiandrosterone in systemic lupus erythematosus. Results of a double-blind, placebo-controlled, randomized clinical trial. *Arthritis Rheum*. 1995;38:1826–1831.

6. Gatto V, Aragno M, Gallo M, et al. Dehydroepiandrosterone inhibits the growth of DMBA-induced rat mammary carcinoma via the androgen receptor. *Oncol Rep*. 1998;5:241–243.

7. Orner GA, Mathews C, Hendricks JD, et al. Dehydroepiandrosterone is a complete hepatocarcinogen and potent tumor promoter in the absence of peroxisome proliferation in rainbow trout. *Carcinogenesis*. 1995;16:2893–2898.

8. Shibata M, Hasegawa R, Imaida K, et al. Chemoprevention by dehydroepiandrosterone and indomethacin in a rat multiorgan carcinogenesis model. *Cancer Res*. 1995;55:4870–4874.

9. Simile M, Pascale RM, De Miglio MR, et al. Inhibition by dehydroepiandrosterone of growth and progression of persistent liver nodules in experimental rat liver carcinogenesis. *Int J Cancer*. 1995;62:210–215.

10. Barrett-Connor E, Friedlander NJ, Khaw K-T. Dehydroepiandrosterone sulfate and breast cancer risk. *Cancer Res*. 1990;50:6571–6574.

11. Helzlsouer KJ, Alberg AJ, Gordon GB, et al. Serum gonadotropins and steroid hormones and the development of ovarian cancer. *JAMA*. 1995;274:1926–1930.

Appendix D

FENUGREEK

As a commonly eaten food, fenugreek is generally regarded as safe. The only common side effect is mild gastrointestinal distress when it is taken in high doses.

Because fenugreek can lower blood sugar levels, it is advisable to seek medical supervision before combining it with diabetes medications.

Extracts made from fenugreek have been shown to stimulate uterine contractions in guinea pigs.[1] For this reason, pregnant women should not take fenugreek in dosages higher than is commonly used as a spice, perhaps 5 g daily. Besides concerns over pregnant women, safety in young children, nursing women, or those with severe liver or kidney disease has also not been established.

References

1. Leung AY, Foster S. *Encyclopedia of Common Natural Ingredients Used in Food, Drugs, and Cosmetics*. 2nd ed. New York, NY: Wiley; 1996:243–244.

FOLATE

Folate at nutritional doses is extremely safe. The only serious potential problem is that folate supplementation can mask the early symptoms of vitamin B_{12} deficiency (a special type of anemia), potentially allowing more irreversible symptoms of nerve damage to develop. For this reason, when taking more than 400 mcg daily, it is important to get your B_{12} level checked.

Very high dosages of folate, greater than 5 mg (5,000 mcg) daily, can cause digestive upset. Maximum safe dosages have not been established for young children or pregnant or nursing women.

As mentioned previously, the antiseizure drug phenytoin may interfere with folate absorption. Conversely, folate may reduce the effectiveness of phenytoin.[1-6] If you are taking phenytoin, you should consult with a physician about the proper dosage of folate for you.

Contrary to some reports, individuals who are taking the drug methotrexate for rheumatoid arthritis, juvenile rheumatoid arthritis, or psoriasis can safely take folate supplements at the same time.[7,8,9] In fact, supplemental folate may actually be helpful under these conditions.[10,11] However, if you are taking methotrexate for any other purpose, do not take folate except on the advice of a physician.

References

1. Butterworth CE Jr, Tamura T. Folic acid safety and toxicity: a brief review. *Am J Clin Nutr*. 1989;50:353–358.

2. Lewis DP, Van Dyke DC, Willhite LA, et al. Phenytoin-folic acid interaction. *Ann Pharmacother*. 1995;29:726–735.

3. Berg MJ, Stumbo PJ, Chenard CA, et al. Folic acid improves phenytoin pharmacokinetics. *J Am Diet Assoc*. 1995;95:352–356.

4. Ono H, Sakamoto A, Eguchi T, et al. Plasma total homocysteine concentrations in epileptic patients taking anticonvulsants. *Metabolism*. 1997;46:959–962.

5. Kishi T, Fujita N, Eguchi T, et al. Mechanism for reduction of serum folate by antiepileptic drugs during prolonged therapy. *J Neurol Sci*. 1997;145:109–112.

6. Lewis DP, Van Dyke DC, Stumbo PJ, et al. Drug and environmental factors associated with adverse pregnancy outcomes. Part I: Antiepileptic drugs, contraceptives, smoking, and folate. *Ann Pharmacother*. 1998;32:802–817.

7. Morgan SL, Baggott JE, Vaughn WH, et al. Supplementation with folic acid during methotrexate therapy for rheumatoid arthritis. A double-blind, placebo-controlled trial. *Ann Intern Med*. 1994;121:833–841.

8. Duhra P. Treatment of gastrointestinal symptoms associated with methotrexate therapy for psoriasis. *J Am Acad Dermatol*. 1993;28:466–469.

9. Hunt PG, Rose CD, McIlvain-Simpson G, et al. The effects of daily intake of folic acid on the efficacy of methotrexate therapy in children with juvenile rheumatoid arthritis. A controlled study. *J Rheumatol*. 1997;24:2230–2232.

10. Jackson RC. Biological effects of folic acid antagonists with antineoplastic activity. *Pharmacol Ther*. 1984;25:61–82.

11. Omer A, Mowat AG. Nature of anaemia in rheumatoid arthritis. IX. Folate metabolism in patients with rheumatoid arthritis. *Ann Rheum Dis*. 1968;27:414–424.

GARLIC

As a commonly used food, garlic is on the FDA's GRAS (generally recognized as safe) list. Rats have been fed gigantic doses of aged garlic (2,000 mg per kilogram body weight) for 6 months without any signs of negative effects.[1] Unfortunately, there do not appear to be any animal toxicity studies on the most commonly used form of garlic—powdered garlic standardized to alliin content.

The only common side effect of garlic is unpleasant breath odor. Even "odorless garlic" produces an offensive smell in up to 50% of those who use it.[2]

Other side effects occur only rarely. For example, a study that followed 1,997 people who were given a normal dose of deodorized garlic daily over a 16-week period showed a 6% incidence of nausea, a 1.3% incidence of dizziness on standing (perhaps a sign of low blood pressure), and a 1.1% incidence of allergic reactions.[3] These are very low percentages in comparison to those usually reported in drug studies. There were also a few reports of bloating, headaches, sweating, and dizziness.

When raw garlic is taken in excessive doses, it can cause numerous symptoms, such as stomach upset, heartburn, nausea, vomiting, diarrhea, flatulence, facial flushing, rapid pulse, and insomnia.

Topical garlic can cause skin irritation, blistering, and even third-degree burns, so be very careful about applying garlic directly to the skin.[4]

Since garlic "thins" the blood, it is not a good idea to take high-potency garlic pills immediately prior to or after surgery or labor and delivery, due to the risk of excessive bleeding.[5] Similarly, garlic should not be combined with blood-thinning drugs, such as Coumadin (warfarin), heparin, aspirin, or Trental (pentoxifylline). In addition, garlic could conceivably interact with natural products with blood-thinning properties, such as ginkgo or high-dose vitamin E.

Garlic may also combine poorly with certain HIV medications. Two people with HIV experienced severe gastrointestinal toxicity from the HIV drug ritonavir after taking garlic supplements.[6]

Garlic is presumed to be safe for pregnant women (except just before and immediately after delivery) and nursing mothers, although this has not been proven.

References

1. Sumiyoshi H, Kanezawa A, Masamoto K, et al. Chronic toxicity test of garlic extract in rats [in Japanese; English abstract]. *J Toxicol Sci.* 1984;9:61–75.

2. Schulz V, Hansel R, Tyler VE. *Rational Phytotherapy: A Physicians' Guide to Herbal Medicine.* 3rd ed. Berlin, Germany: Springer-Verlag; 1998:121.

3. Schulz V, Hansel R, Tyler VE. *Rational Phytotherapy: A Physicians' Guide to Herbal Medicine.* 3rd ed. Berlin, Germany: Springer-Verlag; 1998:121.

4. Garty BZ. Garlic burns. *Pediatrics.* 1993;91:658–659.

5. Burnham BE. Garlic as a possible risk for postoperative bleeding. *Plast Reconstr Surg.* 1995;95:213.

6. Piscatelli SC. Use of complementary medicines by patients with HIV: Full sail into uncharted waters. Medscape HIV/AIDS. 2000;6.

GINKGO

Ginkgo appears to be safe. Extremely high doses have been given to animals for long periods of time without serious consequences.[1] Safety in young children, pregnant or nursing women, or those with severe liver or kidney disease, however, has not been established.

In all the clinical trials of ginkgo up through 1991 combined, involving a total of almost 10,000 participants, the incidence of side effects produced by ginkgo extract was extremely small. There were 21 cases of gastrointestinal discomfort, and even fewer cases of headaches, dizziness, and allergic skin reactions.[2]

One study found that when high concentrations of ginkgo were placed in a test tube with hamster sperm and ova, the sperm were less able to penetrate the ova.[3] However, since we have no idea whether this much ginkgo can actually come into contact with sperm and ova when they are in the body rather than a test tube, these results may not be meaningful in real life.

Contact with live ginkgo plants can cause severe allergic reactions, and ingestion of ginkgo seeds can be dangerous.

German medical authorities do not believe that ginkgo possesses any serious drug interactions.[4] However, because of ginkgo's "blood-thinning" effects, some experts warn that it should not be combined with blood-thinning drugs such as Coumadin (warfarin), heparin, aspirin, and Trental (pentoxifylline), and use of such drugs was prohibited in most of the double-blind trials of ginkgo. It is also possible that ginkgo could cause bleeding problems if combined with natural blood thinners, such as garlic and high-dose vitamin E. There have been two case reports in highly regarded journals of subdural hematoma (bleeding in the skull) and hyphema (spontaneous bleeding into the iris chamber) in association with ginkgo use.[5,6]

References

1. DeFeudis FV. Ginkgo biloba *Extract (EGb 761): Pharmacological Activities and Clinical Applications*. Paris, France: Elsevier Science; 1991:143–146.

2. DeFeudis FV. Ginkgo biloba *Extract (EGb 761): Pharmacological Activities and Clinical Applications*. Paris, France: Elsevier Science; 1991:143–146.

3. Ondrizek RR, Chan PJ, Patton WC, et al. An alternative medicine study of herbal effects on the penetration of zona-free hamster oocytes and the integrity of sperm deoxyribonucleic acid. *Fertil Steril.* 1999;71:517–522.

4. Schulz V, Hansel R, Tyler VE. *Rational Phytotherapy: A Physicians' Guide to Herbal Medicine*. 3rd ed. Berlin, Germany: Springer-Verlag; 1998:247.

5. Rosenblatt M, Mindel J. Spontaneous hyphema associated with ingestion of *Ginkgo biloba* extract. *N Engl J Med.* 1997;336:1108.

6. Rowin J, Lewis SL. Spontaneous bilateral subdural hematomas associated with chronic *Ginkgo biloba* ingestion. *Neurology.* 1996;46:1775–1776.

GINSENG

The various forms of ginseng appear to be nontoxic, both in the short and long term, according to the results of studies in mice, rats, chickens, and dwarf pigs.[1–4] Ginseng also does not seem to be carcinogenic.

Side effects are rare. Occasionally women report menstrual abnormalities and/or breast tenderness when they take ginseng. However, a large double-blind trial found no estrogen-like effects.[5]

Unconfirmed reports suggest that highly excessive doses of ginseng can cause insomnia, raise blood pressure, increase heart rate, and possibly cause other significant effects. Whether some of these cases were actually caused by caffeine mixed in with ginseng remains unclear. Ginseng allergy can also occur, as can allergy to any other substance.

In 1979, an article was published in the *Journal of the American Medical Association* claiming that people can become addicted to ginseng and develop blood pressure elevation, nervousness, sleeplessness, diarrhea, and hypersexuality.[6] This report has since been thoroughly discredited and should no longer be taken seriously.[7,8]

However, there is some evidence that ginseng can interfere with drug metabolism, specifically drugs processed by an enzyme called "CYP 3A4."[9] Ask your physician or pharmacist whether you are taking any medications of this type. There have also been specific reports of ginseng interacting with MAO inhibitor drugs[10] and also with a test for digitalis,[11] although again it is not clear whether it was the ginseng or a contaminant that caused the problem. There has also been one report of ginseng reducing the anti-coagulant effects of Coumadin (warfarin).[12]

Safety in young children, pregnant or nursing women, or people with severe liver or kidney disease has not been established. Interestingly, Chinese tradition suggests that ginseng should not be used by pregnant or nursing mothers.

References

1. Baldwin CA, Anderson LA, Phillipson JD. What pharmacists should know about ginseng. *Pharm J.* 1986;237:583–586.

2. Hess FG, Parent RA, Cox GE, et al. Reproduction study in rats on ginseng extract G115. *Food Chem Toxicol.* 1982;20:189–192.

3. Newall C, Anderson LA, Phillipson JD. *Herbal Medicines: A Guide for Health-Care Professionals.* London, England: Pharmaceutical Press; 1996:143, 148.

4. Sonnenborn U, Proppert Y. Ginseng (*Panax ginseng* C.A. Meyer). *Br J Phytother.* 1991;2:3–14.

5. Wiklund IK, Mattsson LA, Lindgren R, et al. Effects of a standardized ginseng extract on quality of life and physiological parameters in symptomatic postmenopausal women: a double-blind, placebo-controlled trial. *Int J Clin Pharmacol Res.* 1999;19:89–99.

6. Siegel RK. Ginseng abuse syndrome. Problems with the panacea. *JAMA.* 1979;241:1614–1615.

7. Tyler VE. *Herbs of Choice: The Therapeutic Use of Phytomedicinals.* New York, NY: Pharmaceutical Products Press; 1994.

8. Schulz V, Hansel R, Tyler VE. *Rational Phytotherapy: A Physicians' Guide to Herbal Medicine.* 3rd ed. Berlin, Germany: Springer-Verlag; 1998.

9. Kroll D, University of Colorado School of Pharmacy. Unpublished communication, 1998.

10. Jones BD, Runikis AM. Interaction of ginseng with phenelzine. *J Clin Psychopharmacol.* 1987;7:201–202.

11. McRae S. Elevated serum digoxin levels in a patient taking digoxin and Siberian ginseng. *Can MedAssocJ.* 1996;155:293–295.

12. Janetzky K, Morreale AP. Probable interaction between warfarin and ginseng. *Am J Health Syst Pharm.* 1997;54:692–693.

GLA (GAMMA-LINOLENIC ACID)

Most of the safety information we have regarding GLA comes from experience with evening primrose oil. Animal studies suggest that evening primrose oil is completely nontoxic and noncarcinogenic.[1] Over 4,000 people have taken GLA or evening primrose oil in scientific studies, and no significant adverse effects have ever been noted. Early reports suggested the possibility that GLA might worsen temporal lobe epilepsy, but there has been no later confirmation.[2] The maximum safe dosage of GLA for young children, pregnant or nursing women, or those with severe liver or kidney disease has not been established.

References

1. Horrobin DF. Nutritional and medical importance of gamma-linolenic acid. *Prog Lipid Res*. 1992;31:163–194.

2. Vaddadi KS. The use of gamma-linolenic acid and linoleic acid to differentiate between temporal lobe epilepsy and schizophrenia. *Prostaglandins Med*. 1981;6:375–379.

GYMNEMA

When used in appropriate dosages, gymnema appears to be fairly safe, although extensive studies have not been performed. One obvious risk is that if gymnema is successful, it may lower blood sugar levels too far, causing a dangerous hypoglycemic reaction. For this reason, medical supervision is essential. Safety in young children, pregnant or nursing women, or those with severe kidney or liver disease has not been established.

IPRIFLAVONE

About 3,000 people have used ipriflavone in clinical studies, and, in all but two, no significant adverse effects were seen.[1,2] However, these trials found worrisome evidence that ipriflavone can reduce levels of white blood cells called lymphocytes. For this reason, anyone taking ipriflavone long term should have periodic measurements of white blood cell count. In addition, ipriflavone should not be used by anyone with immune deficiencies, such as HIV, or by those who take drugs that suppress the immune system, except under physician supervision. Because ipriflavone is metabolized by the kidneys, individuals with severe kidney disease should have their ipriflavone dosage monitored by a physician.[3] Individuals with ulcers should also avoid ipriflavone.[4]

Also, although ipriflavone itself does not affect tissues outside of bone, some evidence suggests that if it is combined with estrogen, estrogen's effects on the uterus are increased.[5,6] This might mean that risk of uterine cancer would be elevated over taking estrogen alone. It should be possible to overcome this risk, by taking progesterone along with estrogen, which is standard medical practice in any case. However, this finding does make one wonder whether ipriflavone–estrogen combinations raise the risk of breast cancer too, an estrogen side effect that has no easy solution.

Additionally, ipriflavone may interfere with certain drugs by affecting the way they are processed in the liver. For example, it may raise blood levels of the older asthma drug theophylline.[7,8,9] It could also raise levels of caffeine. Ipriflavone could also interact with tolbutamide (a drug for diabetes), phenytoin (used for epilepsy), and Coumadin (a blood thinner).[10] Such interactions are potentially dangerous, especially since phenytoin and warfarin cause osteoporosis, and some people might be tempted to try taking ipriflavone at the same time.

References

1. Agnusdei D, Bufalino L. Efficacy of ipriflavone in established osteoporosis and long-term safety. *Calcif Tissue Int*. 1997;61(suppl 1):S23–S27.

2. Alexandersen P, Toussaint A, Christiansen C, et al. Ipriflavone in the treatment of postmenopausal osteoporosis: a randomized controlled trial. *JAMA*. 2001;285:1482–1488.

3. Agnusdei D, Bufalino L. Efficacy of ipriflavone in established osteoporosis and long-term safety. *Calcif Tissue Int*. 1997;61 (suppl 1):S23–S27.

4. Matsuoka M, Yoshida Y, Hayakawa K, et al. Gastrojejunal fistula caused by gastric ulcer. *J Gastroenterol*. 1998;33:267–271.

5. Petilli M, Fiorelli G, Benvenuti U, et al. Interactions between ipriflavone and the estrogen receptor. *Calcif Tissue Int*. 1995;56:160–165.

6. Cecchini MG, Fleisch H, Muhibauer RC. Ipriflavone inhibits bone resorption in intact and ovariectomized rats. *Calcif Tissue Int*. 1997;61(suppl 1):S9–S11.

7. Takahashi J, Kawakatsu K, Wakayama T, et al. Elevation of serum theophylline levels by ipriflavone in a patient with chronic obstructive pulmonary disease [letter]. *Eur J Clin Pharmacol*. 1992;43:207–208.

8. Monostory K, Vereczkey L. Interaction of theophylline and ipriflavone at the cytochrome P450 level. *Eur J Drug Metab Pharmacokinet*. 1995;20:43–47.

9. Monostory K, Vereczkey L. The effect of ipriflavone and its main metabolites on theophylline biotransformation. *Eur J Drug Metab Pharmacokinet*. 1996;21:61–66.

10. Monostory K, Vereczkey L, Levai F, et al. Ipriflavone as an inhibitor of human cytochrome P450 enzymes. *Br J Pharmacol*. 1998;123:605–610.

IRON

At the recommended dosage, iron is quite safe. Excessive dosages, however, can be toxic—damaging the intestines and liver, and possibly resulting in death. Iron poisoning in children is a surprisingly common problem, so make sure to keep your iron supplements out of their reach. Mildly excessive levels of iron may be unhealthy for another reason: it acts as an oxidant (the opposite of an antioxidant), perhaps increasing the risk of cancer and heart disease. Elevated levels of iron may also play a role in brain injury caused by stroke.[1] In addition, excess iron appears to increase complications of pregnancy.[2] Simultaneous use of iron and high-dose vitamin C can cause excessive iron absorption.[3–10]

References

1. Davolos A, Castillo J, Marrugat J, et al. Body iron stores and early neurologic deterioration in acute cerebral infarction. *Neurology*. 2000;54:1568–1574.

2. Lao TT, Tam K, Chan LY. Third trimester iron status and pregnancy outcome in non-anaemic women; pregnancy unfavourably affected by maternal iron excess. *Hum Reprod*. 2000;15:1843–1848.

3. Maskos Z, Koppenol WH. Oxyradicals and multivitamin tablets. *Free Radic Biol Med*. 1991;11:609–610.

4. Conrad ME, Schade SG. Ascorbic acid chelates in iron absorption: a role for hydrochloric acid and bile. *Gastroenterology*. 1968;55:35–45.

5. Brise H, Hallberg L. Effect of ascorbic acid on iron absorption. *Acta Med Scand*. 1962;171(suppl 376):51.

6. Lynch SR, Cook JD. Interaction of vitamin C and iron. *Ann N Y Acad Sci*. 1980;355:32–44.

7. Hunt JR, Gallagher SK, Johnson LK. Effect of ascorbic acid on apparent iron absorption by women with low iron stores. *Am J Clin Nutr*. 1994;59:1381–1385.

8. Diplock AT. Safety of antioxidant vitamins and beta-carotene. *Am J Clin Nutr*. 1995;62(suppl 6):1510S–1516S.

9. Hoffman KE, Yanelli K, Bridges KR. Ascorbic acid and iron metabolism: alterations in lysosomal function. *Am J Clin Nutr*. 1991;54(suppl 6):1188S–1192S.

Appendix D

10. Siegenberg D, Baynes RD, Bothwell TH, et al. Ascorbic acid prevents the dose-dependent inhibitory effects of polyphenols and phytates on nonheme-iron absorption. *Am J Clin Nutr.* 1991;53:537–541.

LICORICE

Due to its aldosterone-like effects, whole licorice can cause fluid retention, high blood pressure, and potassium loss when taken at dosages exceeding 3 g daily for more than 6 weeks. These effects can be especially dangerous if you take digitalis, or if you have high blood pressure, heart disease, diabetes, or kidney disease.

Licorice may also reduce testosterone levels in men.[1] For this reason, men with impotence, infertility, or decreased libido may wish to avoid this herb. Licorice may also increase both the positive and negative effects of treatment with corticosteroids, such as prednisone.[2,3,4]

DGL is believed to be safe, although extensive safety studies have not been performed. Side effects are rare.

Safety for either form of licorice in young children, pregnant or nursing women, or those with severe liver or kidney disease has not been established. According to one report, licorice possesses significant estrogenic activity and, as such, shouldn't be taken by women who have had breast cancer.[5]

References

1. Armanini D, Palermo M. Reduction of serum testosterone in men by licorice. *N Engl J Med.* 1999;341:1158.

2. Brinker F. *Herb Contraindications and Drug Interactions: with Appendices Addressing Specific Conditions and Medicines.* 2nd ed. Sandy, Ore: Eclectic Medical Publications; 1998:92.

3. Kumagai A, Nanaboshi M, Asanuma Y, et al. Effects of glycyrrhizin on thymolytic and immunosupressive action of cortisone. *Endocrinol Jpn.* 1967;14:39–42.

4. Tamura Y, Nishikawa T, Yamada K, et al. Effects of glycyrrhetinic acid and its derivatives on delta-4-5-alpha- and 5-beta-reductase in rat liver. *Arzneimittelforschung.* 1979;29:647–649.

5. Zava DT, Dollbaum CM, Blen M. Estrogen and progestin bioactivity of foods, herbs and spices. *Proc Soc Exp Biol Med.* 1998;217:369–378.

LIPOIC ACID

Lipoic acid appears to have no significant side effects at dosages up to 1,800 mg daily.[1]

Safety for young children, women who are pregnant or nursing, or those with severe liver or kidney disease has not been established.

References

1. Ziegler D, Hanefeld M, Ruhnau KJ, et al. Treatment of symptomatic diabetic polyneuropathy with the antioxidant alpha-lipoic acid: a 7-month multicenter randomized controlled trial (ALADIN III Study). ALADIN III Study Group. *Diabetes Care.* 1999;22:1296–1301.

MAGNESIUM

In general, magnesium appears to be quite safe when taken at recommended dosages. The most common complaint is loose stools. However, people with severe kidney or heart disease should not take magnesium (or any other supplement) except on the advice of a physician. Maximum safe dosages have not been established for young children or women who are pregnant or nursing. There has been one case of death caused by excessive use of magnesium supplements in a developmentally and physically disabled child.[1]

Magnesium can interfere with the absorption of antibiotics in the tetracycline family.[2] Also, when combined with oral diabetes drugs in the sulfonylurea family (Tolinase, Micronase, Orinase, Glucotrol, Diabinese, DiaBeta), magnesium may cause blood sugar levels to fall more than expected.[3]

References

1. McGuire JK, Kulkarni MS, Baden HP. Fatal hypermagnesemia in a child treated with megavitamin/megamineral therapy. *Pediatrics.* 2000;105:E18.

2. Tatro D, ed. *Drug Interaction Facts.* St. Louis, Mo: Facts and Comparisons;1999.

3. *Drug Evaluations Annual.* Vol 2. Milwaukee, Wis: American Medical Association;1994.

MANGANESE

Manganese appears to be safe when taken at the usual recommended dosage of 6 mg or less daily. However, the safety of higher doses is not known. Very high exposure to manganese (due either to environmental pollution or manganese mining) has resulted in a serious psychiatric disorder known as "manganese madness."

MELATONIN

Melatonin is probably safe for occasional use, but its safety when used on a regular basis remains unknown. Keep in mind that melatonin is not truly a food supplement but a hormone.

As we know from other hormones used in medicine, such as estrogen and cortisone, harmful effects can take years to appear. Hormones are powerful substances that have many subtle effects in the body, and we're far from understanding them fully.

Because melatonin promotes sleep, you should not drive or operate machinery for several hours after taking it. In addition, melatonin may impair balance.[1] Also, based on theoretical ideas of how melatonin works, some authorities specifically recommend against using it in people with depression, schizophrenia, autoimmune diseases, and other serious illnesses. Maximum safe dosages for young children, pregnant or nursing women, or those with serious liver or kidney disease have not been established.

References

1. Fraschini F, Cesarani A, Alpini D, et al. Melatonin influences human balance. *Biol Signals Recept.* 1999;8:111–119.

METHIONINE

Methionine is thought to be generally safe. However, the maximum safe dosages for young children, pregnant or nursing women, or those with serious liver or kidney disease have not been established.

Like other amino acids, methionine may interfere with the absorption or action of the drug levodopa which is used for Parkinson's disease.[1]

References

1. Nutt JG, Woodward WR, Hammerstad JP, et al. The "on-off" phenomenon in Parkinson's disease. Relation to levodopa absorption and transport. *N Engl J Med.* 1984;310:483–488.

MILK THISTLE

Milk thistle is believed to possess very little toxicity. Animal studies have not shown any negative effects even when high doses were administered over a long period of time.[1]

A study of 2,637 participants reported in 1992 showed a low incidence of side effects, limited mainly to mild gastrointestinal disturbance.[2] However, on rare occasions severe abdominal discomfort may occur.[3]

On the basis of its extensive use as a food, milk thistle is believed to be safe for pregnant or nursing women and researchers have enrolled pregnant women in studies.[4] However, safety in young children, pregnant or nursing women, and individuals with severe renal disease has not been formally established.

No drug interactions are known. However, one report has noted that silibinin (a constituent of silymarin) can inhibit a bacterial enzyme called beta-glucuronidase, which plays a role in the activity of certain drugs, such as oral contraceptives.[5] This could reduce their effectiveness.

References

1. Awang D. Milk thistle. *Can Pharm J*. 1993;126:403–404.

2. Albrecht M, Frerick H, Kuhn U, et al. Therapy of toxic liver pathologies with Legalon [in German]. *Z Klin Med*. 1992;47:87–92.

3. Adverse Drug Reactions Advisory Committee. An adverse reaction to the herbal medication milk thistle (*Silybum marianum*). *Med J Aust*. 1999;170:218–219.

4. Giannola C, Buogo F, Forestiere G, et al. A two-center study on the effects of silymarin in pregnant women and adult patients with so-called minor hepatic insufficiency [in Italian; English abstract]. *Clin Ter*. 1985;114:129–135.

5. Kim DH, Jin YH, Park JB, et al. Silymarin and its components are inhibitors of beta-glucuronidase. *Biol Pharm Bull*. 1994;17:443–445.

N-ACETYL CYSTEINE (NAC)

NAC appears to be a very safe supplement when taken alone, although one study in rats suggests that 60 to 100 times the normal dose can cause liver injury.[1]

As mentioned earlier, the combination of nitroglycerin and NAC causes severe headaches. Safety in young children, women who are pregnant or nursing, and individuals with severe liver or kidney disease has not been established.

Appendix D

References

1. Badawy AH, Abdel Aal SF, Samour SA. Liver injury associated with N-acetylcysteine administration. *J Egypt Soc Parasitol*. 1989;19:563–571.

POTASSIUM

As an essential nutrient, potassium is safe when taken at appropriate dosages. If you take a bit too much, your body will simply excrete it in the urine. However, people who have severe kidney disease cannot excrete potassium normally, and should consult a physician before taking a potassium supplement. Similarly, individuals taking potassium-sparing diuretics (such as spironolactone), ACE inhibitors (such as captopril),[1–5] or trimethoprim/sulfomethoxazole[6] should also not take potassium supplements except under doctor supervision.

Potassium pills can cause injury to the esophagus if they get stuck on the way down, so make sure to take them with plenty of water.

References

1. Stoltz ML, Andrews CE Jr. Severe hyperkalemia during very-low-calorie diets and angiotensin converting enzyme use. *JAMA*. 1990;264:2737–2738.

2. Good CB, McDermott L, McCloskey B. Diet and serum potassium in patients on ACE inhibitors. *JAMA*. 1995;274:538.

3. Warren SE, O'Conner DT. Hyperkalemia resulting from captopril administration. *JAMA*. 1980;244:2551–2552.

4. Grossman A, Eckland D, Price P, et al. Captopril: reversible renal failure with severe hyperkalaemia. *Lancet*. 1980;1:712.

5. Burnakis TG, Mioduch HJ. Combined therapy with captopril and potassium supplementation: a potential for hyperkalemia. *Arch Intern Med*. 1984;144:2371–2372.

6. Alappan R, Perazella MA, Buller GK. Hyperkalemia in hospitalized patients treated with trimethoprim-sulfamethoxazole. *Ann Intern Med*. 1996;124:316–320.

SALT BUSH

As a plant food commonly consumed by animals and humans, salt bush appears to be relatively safe. However, no comprehensive safety testing of salt bush has been performed. For this reason, it should not be used by young children, pregnant or nursing women, or people with severe liver or kidney disease.

Keep in mind that if salt bush is effective, the result might be excessive lowering of blood sugar levels. For this reason, people with diabetes who take salt bush should do so only under a physician's supervision.[1,2]

References

1. Stern E. Successful use of Atriplex halimus in the treatment of type 2 diabetic patients: a preliminary study. Zamenhoff Medical Center, Tel Aviv, 1989.

2. Earon G, Stern E, and Lavosky H. Successful use of Atriplex halimus in the treatment of type 2 diabetic patients. Controlled clinical research report on the subject of Atriplex. Unpublished study conducted at the Hebrew University, Jerusalem, 1989.

SAMe

SAMe appears to be quite safe, according to both human and animal studies.[1–4] The most common side effect is mild digestive distress. However, SAMe does not actually damage the stomach.[5]

Like other substances with antidepressant activity, SAMe might trigger a manic episode in those with bipolar disease (manic-depressive illness).[6–11]

Safety in young children, pregnant or nursing women, or those with severe liver or kidney disease has not been established.

SAMe might interfere with the action of the Parkinson's drug levodopa.[12] In addition, there may also be risks involved in combining SAMe with standard antidepressants.[13] For this reason, you shouldn't try either combination except under physician supervision.

References

1. Cozens DD, Barton SJ, Clark R, et al. Reproductive toxicity studies of ademetionine. *Arzneimittelforschung*. 1988;38:1625–1629.

2. Berger R, Nowak H. A new medical approach to the treatment of osteoarthritis: Report of an open phase IV study with ademetionine (Gumbaral). *Am J Med*. 1987;83(5A):84–88.

3. Konig B. A long-term (two years) clinical trial with S-adenosylmethionine for the treatment of osteoarthritis. *Am J Med*. 1987;83(5A):89–94.

Appendix D

4. Caruso I, Peitrogrande V. Italian double-blind multicenter study comparing S-adenosylmethionine, naproxen and placebo in the treatment of degenerative joint disease. *Am J Med*. 1987;83(5A):66–71.

5. di Padova C. S-adenosylmethionine in the treatment of osteoarthritis. Review of the clinical studies. *Am J Med*. 1987;83(5A):60–65.

6. Carney MW, Chary TK, Bottiglieri T, et al. The switch mechanism and the bipolar/unipolar dichotomy. *Br J Psychiatry*. 1989;154:48–51.

7. Carney MW, Chary TK, Bottiglieri T, et al. Switch and S-adenosylmethionine. *Ala J Med Sci*. 1988;25:316–319.

8. Kagan BL, Sultzer DL, Rosenlicht N, et al. Oral S-adenosylmethionine in depression: a randomized, double-blind placebo-controlled trial. *Am J Psychiatry*. 1990;147:591–595.

9. Bressa GM. S-adenosyl-l-methionine (SAMe) as antidepressant: Meta-analysis of clinical studies. *Acta Neurol Scand Suppl*. 1994;154:7–14.

10. Cerutti R, Sichel MP, Perin M, et al. Psychological distress during puerperium: a novel therapeutic approach to using S-adenosylmethionine. *Curr Ther Res*. 1993;53:707–716.

11. Mato JM, Camara J, Fernandez de Paz J, et al. S-adenosylmethionine in alcoholic liver cirrhosis: a randomized, placebo-controlled, double-blind multicenter clinical trial. *J Hepatol*. 1999;30:1081–1089.

12. Liu X, Lamango N, Charlton C. L-dopa depletes S-adenosylmethionine and increases S-adenosyl homocysteine: relationship to the wearing-off effects [abstract]. *Abstr Soc Neurosci*. 1998;24:1469.

13. Iruela LM, Minguez L, Merino J, et al. Toxic interaction of S-adenosyl-methionine and clomipramine [letter]. *Am J Psychiatry*. 1993;150:522.

SELENIUM

Selenium is safe when taken at the recommended dosages. However, very high selenium dosages, above 850 mcg daily, are known to cause selenium toxicity. Signs of selenium toxicity include depression, nervousness, emotional instability, nausea, vomiting, and in some cases loss of hair and fingernails.

SOY

Studies in animals have found soy isoflavones essentially nontoxic.[1]

However, the isoflavones in soy could conceivably have some potentially harmful hormonal effects in certain specific situations. There is some evidence that although soy generally seems to reduce the risk of breast cancer, it also may cause some influences in the opposite direction.[2] For this and other reasons, we don't know if high doses of soy are safe for women who have already had breast cancer. There are also concerns that intensive use of soy products by pregnant women could exert a hormonal effect that impacts unborn fetuses.[3,4] Finally, fears have been expressed by some experts that soy might interfere with the action of oral contraceptives. However, one study of 40 women suggests that such concerns are groundless.[5] Another trial found that soy does not interfere with the action of estrogen-replacement therapy in menopausal women.[6]

Soy may impair thyroid function or reduce absorption of thyroid medication, at least in children.[7,8,9] For this reason, individuals with impaired thyroid function should use soy with caution.

Soy also may reduce the absorption of the nutrients zinc, iron, and calcium.[10–14] To avoid absorption problems, you should probably take these vitamins at least 2 hours apart from eating soy.

References

1. Crowell JA, Levine BS, Page JG, et al. Preclinical safety studies of isoflavones [abstract]. *J Nutr.* 2000;130(suppl):677S.

2. Petrakis NL, Barnes S, King EB, et al. Stimulatory influence of soy protein isolate on breast secretion in pre- and post-menopausal women. *Cancer Epidemiol Biomarkers Prev.* 1996;5:785–794.

3. [No authors listed]. 3rd International Symposium on the Role of Soy in Preventing and Treating Chronic Disease. Washington DC, USA. October 31–November 3, 1999. Proceedings and abstracts. *J Nutr.* 2000;130(3):653S–711S.

4. Hilakivi-Clarke L, Cho E, Onojafe I, et al. Maternal exposure to genistein during pregnancy increases carcinogen-induced mammary tumorigenesis in female rat offspring. *Oncol Rep.* 1999;6:1089–1095.

5. Martini MC, Dancisak BB, Haggans CJ, et al. Effects of soy intake on sex hormone metabolism in premenopausal women. *Nutr Cancer.* 1999;34:133–139.

6. Scambia G, Mango D, Signorile PG, et al. Clinical effects of a standardized soy extract in postmenopausal women: a pilot study. *Menopause.* 2000;7:105–111.

7. Divi RL, Chang HC, Doerge DR. Anti-thyroid isoflavones from soybean: isolation, characterization, and mechanisms of action. *Biochem Pharmacol.* 1997;54:1087–1096.

8. Chorazy PA, Himelhoch S, Hopwood NJ, et al. Persistent hypothyroidism in an infant receiving a soy formula: case report and review of the literature. *Pediatrics.* 1995;96(1 pt 1):148–150.

Appendix D

9. Jabbar MA, Larrea J, Shaw RA. Abnormal thyroid function tests in infants with congenital hypothyroidism: the influence of soy-based formula. *J Am Coll Nutr.* 1997;16:280–282.

10. Navert B, Sandstrom B, Cederblad A. Reduction of the phytate content of bran by leavening in bread and its effect on zinc absorption in man. *Br J Nutr.* 1985;53:47–53.

11. Hallberg L, Rossander L, Skanberg AB. Phytates and the inhibitory effects of bran on iron absorption in man. *Am J Clin Nutr.* 1987;45:988–996.

12. Heaney RP, Weaver CM, Fitzsimmons ML. Soybean phytate content: effect on calcium absorption. *Am J Clin Nutr.* 1991;53:745–747.

13. Vohra P, Gray GA, Kratzer FH. Phytic acid-metal complexes. *Proc Soc Exp Biol Med.* 1965;120:447–449.

14. Evans GW. Normal and abnormal zinc absorption in man and animals: the tryptophan connection. *Nutr Rev.* 1980;38:137–141.

VANADIUM

Studies of diabetic rats suggest that, at high dosages, vanadium can accumulate in the body until it reaches toxic levels.[1–4] Based on these results, high dosages of vanadium can't be considered safe for human use. If you wish to take it, stick to 10 to 30 mcg a day.

References

1. Domingo JL, Gomez M, Llobet JM, et al. Oral vanadium administration to streptozotocin-diabetic rats has marked negative side-effects which are independent of the form of vanadium used. *Toxicology.* 1991;66:279–287.

2. Srivastava AK. Anti-diabetic and toxic effects of vanadium compounds. *Mol Cell Biochem.* 2000;206:177–182.

3. Sanchez DJ, Colomina MT, Domingo JL. Effects of vanadium on activity and learning in rats. *Physiol Behav.* 1998;63:345–350.

4. Domingo JL. Vanadium: a review of the reproductive and developmental toxicity. *Reprod Toxicol.* 1996;10:175–182.

VITAMIN A

Dosages of vitamin A above 50,000 IU per day taken for several years can cause liver injury, bone problems, fatigue, hair loss, headaches, and dry skin. If you already have liver disease, check with your doctor before taking vitamin A supplements, because even small doses may be harmful for you. Also, it is thought that people with diabetes may have trouble releasing vitamin A stored in the liver. This may mean that they are at greater risk for vitamin A toxicity. For different reasons, individuals who consume too much alcohol may also be at higher risk of vitamin A toxicity.[1] In addition, excessive intake of vitamin A may increase the risk of osteoporosis.[2]

Women should avoid supplementing with vitamin A during pregnancy, because at toxic levels it may increase the risk of birth defects. Pregnant women taking valproic acid may be even more at risk of vitamin A toxicity.[3]

Vitamin A may also increase the anticoagulant effects of warfarin.[4] You should not take supplementary vitamin A unless under a physician's supervision.

Warning: Be sure to store vitamin A supplements where children cannot reach them!

References

1. Leo MA, Lieber CS. Alcohol, vitamin A, and beta-carotene: adverse interactions, including hepatotoxicity and carcinogenicity. *Am J Clin Nutr.* 1999;69:1071–1085.

2. Melhus H, Michaelsson K, Kindmark A, et al. Excessive dietary intake of vitamin A is associated with reduced bone mineral density and increased risk for hip fracture. *Ann Intern Med.* 1998;129:770–778.

3. Nau H, Tzimas G, Mondry M, et al. Antiepileptic drugs alter endogenous retinoid concentrations: a possible mechanism of teratogenesis of anticonvulsant therapy. *Life Sci.* 1995;57:53–60.

4. Harris JE. Interaction of dietary factors with oral anticoagulants: review and applications. *J Am Diet Assoc.* 1995;95:580–584.

VITAMIN B₁

Vitamin B_1 appears to be quite safe even when taken in very high doses.

VITAMIN B₂

Riboflavin seems to be an extremely safe supplement.

VITAMIN B₃

When taken at a dosage of more than 100 mg daily, niacin frequently causes annoying skin flushing, especially in the face. This reaction may be accompanied by stomach distress, itching, and headache. In studies, as many as 43% of individuals taking niacin quit because of unpleasant side effects.[1]

A more dangerous effect of niacin is liver inflammation. Although most commonly seen with slow-release niacin, it can occur with any type of niacin when taken at a daily dose of more than 500 mg (usually 3 g or more). Regular blood tests to evaluate liver function are therefore mandatory when using high-dose niacin (or niacinamide or inositol hexaniacinate). This side effect almost always goes away when niacin is stopped.

If you have liver disease, ulcers (presently or in the past), gout, or diabetes, or drink too much alcohol,[2] do not take high-dose niacin except on medical advice.

Although there have been concerns that high-dose niacin in combination with statin drugs could cause muscle damage and kidney injury, recent studies suggest the risk may be slight, especially in those with normal kidney function.[3,4] Nonetheless, a doctor's supervision is recommended before trying this combination.

Another potential drug interaction involves the anticonvulsant drugs carbamazepine and primidone. Niacinamide might increase blood levels of these drugs, possibly requiring reduction in drug dosage.[5] Do not use this combination except under physician supervision.

Maximum safe dosages for young children and pregnant or nursing women have not been established.

References

1. Gibbons LW, Gonzalez V, Gordon N, at al. The prevalence of side effects with regular and sustained-release nicotinic acid. *Am J Med*. 1995;99:378–385.

2. *Physicians' Desk Reference*. Montvale, NJ: Medical Economics Co; 1999:1507.

3. Jacobson TA, Amorosa LF. Combination therapy with fluvastatin and niacin in hypercholesterolemia: a preliminary report on safety. *Am J Cardiol*. 1994;73:25D–29D.

4. Kashyap ML, Evans R, Simmons PD, et al. New combination niacin/statin formulation shows pronounced effects on major lipoproteins and is well tolerated. *J Am Coll Cardiol*. 2000;35(suppl A):326.

5. Bourgeois BFD, Dodson WE, Ferrendelli JA. Interactions between primidone, carbamazepine, and nicotinamide. *Neurology.* 1982;32:1122–1126.

VITAMIN B$_6$

Vitamin B$_6$ appears to be completely safe for adults at dosages up to 50 mg daily. However, at higher dosages (especially above 2 g daily) there is a very real risk of nerve damage. Nerve-related symptoms have even been reported at doses as low as 200 mg.[1] (This is a bit ironic, given that B$_6$ deficiency *also* causes nerve problems.) In some cases, very high doses of vitamin B$_6$ can cause or worsen acne symptoms.[2,3]

In addition, doses of vitamin B$_6$ over 5 mg may interfere with the effects of the drug levodopa when it is taken alone.[4,5,6] However, levodopa/carbidopa combinations are immune to this effect.

Maximum safe dosages for children, pregnant or nursing women, or those with severe liver or kidney disease have not been established.

References

1. Parry GJ, Bredesen DE. Sensory neuropathy with low-dose pyridoxine. *Neurology.* 1985;35:1466–1468.

2. Sherertz EF. Acneiform eruption due to "megadose" vitamins B6 and B12. *Cutis.* 1991;48:119–120.

3. Braun-Falco O, Lincke H. The problem of vitamin B6/B12 acne. A contribution on acne medicamentosa [in German; English abstract]. *MMW Munch Med Wochenschr.* 1976;118:155–160.

4. Lim D, McKay M. Food-drug interactions. *Drug Information Bulletin* (UCLA Dept. of Pharmaceutical Services). 1995;15(2).

5. Yahr MD, Duvoisin RC. Pyridoxine and levodopa in the treatment of Parkinsonism. *JAMA.* 1972;220:861.

6. Leon AS, Spiegel HE, Thomas G, et al. Pyridoxine antagonism of levodopa in parkinsonism. *JAMA.* 1971;218:1924–1927.

VITAMIN B$_{12}$

Vitamin B$_{12}$ appears to be extremely safe. However, in some cases very high doses of vitamin B$_{12}$ can cause or worsen acne symptoms.[1,2]

Appendix D

References

1. Sherertz EF. Acneiform eruption due to "megadose" vitamins B6 and B12. *Cutis*. 1991;48:119–120.

2. Braun-Falco O, Lincke H. The problem of vitamin B6/B12 acne. A contribution on acne medicamentosa [in German; English abstract]. *MMW Munch Med Wochenschr*. 1976;118:155–160.

VITAMIN C

Vitamin C is indisputably safe at dosages up to 500 mg daily in adults, and is probably safe for most individuals at significantly higher doses. In recognition of this, the U.S. government has issued recommendations regarding "tolerable upper intake levels" (ULs) for vitamin C. The UL can be thought of as the highest daily intake over a prolonged time known to pose no risks to most members of a healthy population. The ULs for vitamin C are as follows:

- Children 1–3 years, 400 mg
  4–8 years, 650 mg
  9–13 years, 1,200 mg
- Males and females 14–18 years, 1,800 mg
  19 years and older, 2,000 mg
- Pregnant women 2,000 mg (1,800 mg if under 19 years old)
- Nursing women 2,000 mg (1,800 mg if under 19 years old)

However, the maximum safe dosages of vitamin C for those with severe liver or kidney disease have not been determined.

Even within the safe intake range for vitamin C, some individuals may develop diarrhea. This side effect will likely go away with continued use of vitamin C, but you might have to cut down your dosage for a while and then gradually build up again.

In addition, vitamin C supplements can cause copper[1–4] deficiency and excessive iron[5–12] absorption.

There is also reason for concern that long-term vitamin C treatment can cause kidney stones.[13] However, in large-scale observational studies, individuals who consume large amounts of vitamin C have shown either no change or a decreased risk of kidney stone formation.[14,15,16] Still, there may be certain individuals who are particularly at risk for vitamin C–induced kidney stones.[17] People with a history of kidney stones and those with kidney failure who have a defect in vitamin C or oxalate metabolism should probably restrict vitamin C intake to approximately 100 mg daily. You should also avoid high-dose vitamin C if you have glucose-6-phosphate dehydrogenase deficiency, iron overload, or a history of intestinal surgery.

One study from the 1970s suggests that very high doses of vitamin C (3 g daily) might increase the levels of acetaminophen (e.g., Tylenol) in the body.[18] This could potentially put you at higher risk for acetaminophen toxicity. This interaction is probably relatively unimportant when acetaminophen is taken in single doses for pain and fever, or for a few days during a cold. However, if you use acetaminophen daily or have kidney or liver problems, simultaneous use of high-dose vitamin C is probably not advisable.

Finally, weak evidence suggests that vitamin C, when taken in high doses, might reduce the blood-thinning effects of Coumadin (warfarin) and heparin.[19–22]

References

1. Milne DB, Klevay LM, Hunt JR. Effects of ascorbic acid supplements and a diet marginal in copper on indices of copper nutriture in women. *Nutr Res.* 1988;8:865–873.

2. Finley EB, Cerklewski FL. Influence of ascorbic acid supplementation on copper status in young adult men. *Am J Clin Nutr.* 1983;37:553–556.

3. Jacob RA, Skala JH, Omaye ST, et al. Effect of varying ascorbic acid intakes on copper absorption and ceruloplasmin levels of young men. *J Nutr.* 1987;117:2109–2115.

4. Harris ED, Percival SS. A role for ascorbic acid in copper transport. *Am J Clin Nutr.* 1991;54(suppl 6):1193S–1197S.

5. Maskos Z, Koppenol WH. Oxyradicals and multivitamin tablets. *Free Radic Biol Med.* 1991;11:609–610.

6. Conrad ME, Schade SG. Ascorbic acid chelates in iron absorption: a role for hydrochloric acid and bile. *Gastroenterology.* 1968;55:35–45.

7. Brise H, Hallberg L. Effect of ascorbic acid on iron absorption. *Acta Med Scand.* 1962;171(suppl 376):51.

8. Lynch SR, Cook JD. Interaction of vitamin C and iron. *Ann N Y Acad Sci.* 1980;355:32–44.

9. Hunt JR, Gallagher SK, Johnson LK. Effect of ascorbic acid on apparent iron absorption by women with low iron stores. *Am J Clin Nutr.* 1994;59:1381–1385.

10. Diplock AT. Safety of antioxidant vitamins and beta-carotene. *Am J Clin Nutr.* 1995;62(suppl 6):1510S–1516S.

Appendix D

11. Hoffman KE, Yanelli K, Bridges KR. Ascorbic acid and iron metabolism: alterations in lysosomal function. *Am J Clin Nutr.* 1991;54(suppl 6):1188S–1192S.

12. Siegenberg D, Baynes RD, Bothwell TH, et al. Ascorbic acid prevents the dose-dependent inhibitory effects of polyphenols and phytates on nonheme-iron absorption. *Am J Clin Nutr.* 1991;53:537–541.

13. Auer BL, Auer D, Rodgers AL. Relative hyperoxaluria, crystalluria, and hematuria after mega-dose ingestion of vitamin C. *Eur J Clin Invest.* 1998;28:695–700.

14. Curhan GC, Willett WC, Speizer FE, et al. Intake of vitamins B_6 and C and the risk of kidney stones in women. *Am Soc Nephrol.* 1999;10:840–845.

15. Curhan GC, Willett WC, Rimm EB, et al. A prospective study of the intake of vitamins C B_6 and the risk of kidney stones in men. *J Urol.* 1996;155:1847–1851.

16. Simon JA, Hudes ES. Relation of serum ascorbic acid to serum vitamin B12, serum ferritin, and kidney stones in US adults. *Arch Intern Med.* 1999;159:619–624.

17. Auer BL, Auer D, Rodgers AL. Relative hyperoxaluria, crystalluria, and hematuria after mega-dose ingestion of vitamin C. *Eur J Clin Invest.* 1998;28:695–700.

18. Houston JB, Levy G. Drug biotransformation interactions in man VI: acetaminophen and ascorbic acid. *J Pharm Sci.* 1976;65:1218–1221.

19. Owen CA Jr, Tyce GM, Flock EV, et al. Heparin-ascorbic acid antagonism. *Mayo Clin Proc.* 1970;45:140-145.

20. Rosenthal G. Interaction of ascorbic acid and warfarin [letter]. *JAMA.* 1971;215:1671.

21. Harris JE. Interaction of dietary factors with oral anticoagulants: review and applications. *J Am Diet Assoc.* 1995;95:580–584.

22. Smith EC, Skalski RJ, Johnson GC, et al. Interaction of ascorbic acid and warfarin. *JAMA.* 1972;221:1166.

VITAMIN D

When taken at recommended dosages, vitamin D appears to be safe. However, when used at considerable excess, vitamin D can build up in the body and cause toxic symptoms. According to current recommendations, the maximum safe dosage of vitamin D, in the absence of sunlight or other sources, is 2,000 IU daily. However, the actual dosage at which intake becomes toxic is a matter of dispute.[1,2]

People with sarcoidosis or hyperparathyroidism should never take vitamin D without first consulting a physician.

Taking vitamin D and calcium supplements might interfere with some of the effects of calcium channel–blockers.[3] It is very important that you consult your physician before trying this combination.

The combination of calcium, vitamin D and thiazide diuretics can lead to excessive calcium levels in the body.[4,5,6] If you are taking thiazide diuretics, you should consult with a physician about the right doses of vitamin D and calcium for you.

References

1. Vieth R. Vitamin D supplementation, 25-hydroxyvitamin D concentrations, and safety. *Am J Clin Nutr*. 1999;69:842–856.

2. Moon JC. A brief history of vitamin D toxicity. *J Appl Nutr*. 1997;49:18–31.

3. Bar-Or D, Gasiel Y. Calcium and calciferol antagonise effect of verapamil in atrial fibrillation. *Br Med J (Clin Res Ed)*. 1981;282:1585–1586.

4. Riis B, Christiansen C. Actions of thiazide on vitamin D metabolism: a controlled therapeutic trial in normal women early in the postmenopause. *Metabolism*. 1985;34:421–424.

5. Lemann J Jr, Gray RW, Maierhofer WJ, et al. Hydrochlorothiazide inhibits bone resorption in men despite experimentally elevated serum 1,25-dihydroxyvitamin D concentrations. *Kidney Int*. 1985;28:951–958.

6. Crowe M, Wollner L, Griffiths RA. Hypercalcaemia following vitamin D and thiazide therapy in the elderly. *Practitioner*. 1984;228:312–313.

VITAMIN E

Vitamin E is generally regarded as safe when taken at the recommended therapeutic dosage of 400 to 800 IU daily. However, vitamin E does have a "blood-thinning" effect that could lead to problems in certain situations. In one study of 28,519 men, vitamin E supplementation at the low dose of about 50 IU synthetic vitamin E per day caused an increase in fatal hemorrhagic strokes, the kind of stroke caused by bleeding. (However, it reduced the risk of a more common type of stroke, and the two effects essentially canceled out.)[1] Based on its blood-thinning effects, there are concerns that vitamin E could cause problems if it is combined with medications that also thin the blood, such as Coumadin (warfarin), heparin, Trental (pentoxifylline), and aspirin. Theoretically, the net result could be to thin the blood *too* much, causing bleeding problems. A study that evaluated vitamin E plus aspirin did in fact find an additive effect.[2] In contrast, the results of a study on vitamin E and Coumadin found no evidence of interaction, but it would still not be advisable to combine these treatments except under a physician's supervision.[3]

There is also at least a remote possibility that vitamin E could also interact with herbs that possess a mild blood-thinning effect, such as garlic and ginkgo. Individuals with bleeding disorders such as hemophilia, and those about to undergo surgery or labor and delivery should also approach vitamin E with caution.

In addition, vitamin E might enhance the body's sensitivity to its own insulin in individuals with adult-onset diabetes.[4,5] This could lead to risk of blood sugar levels falling too low. If you are taking oral hypoglycemic medications, do not take high-dose vitamin E without first consulting your physician.

Finally, considerable controversy exists regarding whether it is safe or appropriate to combine vitamin E with standard chemotherapy drugs.[6] The reasoning behind this concern is that many chemotherapy drugs work in part by creating free radicals that destroy cancer cells. Antioxidants like vitamin E might interfere with this beneficial effect. However, there is also some evidence that vitamin E might help protect against the side effects of certain chemotherapy drugs without interfering with their action.[7] Nonetheless, in view of the high stakes involved, we strongly recommend that you do not take any supplements while undergoing cancer chemotherapy, except on the advice of a physician.

References

1. Leppala JM, Virtamo J, Fogelholm R, et al. Controlled trial of alpha-tocopherol and beta-carotene supplements on stroke incidence and mortality in male smokers. *Arterioscler Thromb Vasc Biol.* 2000;20:230–235.

2. Liede KE, Haukka JK, Saxen LM, et al. Increased tendency towards gingival bleeding caused by joint effect of alpha-tocopherol supplementation and acetylsalicylic acid. *Ann Med.* 1998;30:542–546.

3. Kim JM, White RH. Effect of vitamin E on the anticoagulant response to warfarin. *Am J Cardiol.* 1996;77:545–546.

4. Paolisso G, D'Amore A, Giugliano D, et al. Pharmacologic doses of vitamin E improve insulin action in healthy subjects and non-insulin-dependent diabetic patients. *Am J Clin Nutr.* 1993;57:650–656.

5. Paolisso G, D'Amore A, Galzerano D, et al. Daily vitamin E supplements improve metabolic control but not insulin secretion in elderly type II diabetic patients. *Diabetes Care.* 1993;16:1433–1437.

6. Labriola D, Livingston R. Possible interactions between dietary antioxidants and chemotherapy. *Oncology.* 1999;13:1003–1012.

7. Weijl NI, Cleton FJ, Osanto S. Free radicals and antioxidants in chemotherapy-induced toxicity. *Cancer Treat Rev.* 1997;23:209–240.

VITAMIN K

Vitamin K is probably quite safe at the recommended therapeutic dosages, since those quantities are easily obtained from food.

Vitamin K directly counters the effects of the anticoagulant warfarin. If you are taking warfarin, you should not take vitamin K supplements or alter your dietary intake of vitamin K without doctor supervision.[1,2]

Newborns are commonly given vitamin K_1 injections to prevent bleeding problems. Although some have suggested that this practice may increase the risk of cancer,[3] enormous observational studies have found no such connection (one such trial involved more than a million participants).[4,5]

Appendix D

References

1. Pederson FM, Hamberg O, Hess K, et al. The effect of dietary vitamin K on warfarin-induced anticoagulation. *J Intern Med.* 1991;229:517–520.

2. Chow WH, Chow TC, Tse TM, et al. Anticoagulation instability with life-threatening complication after dietary modification. *Postgrad Med J.* 1990;66: 855–857.

3. Golding J, Paterson M, and Kinlon LJ. Factors associated with childhood cancer in a national cohort study. *Br J Cancer.* 1990;62:304–308.

4. Ekelund H, Finnstrom O, Gunnerskog J, et al. Administration of vitamin K to newborn infants and childhood cancer. *BMJ.* 1993;305:109.

5. Klebanoff MA, Read JS, Mills JL, and Shiono PH. The risk of childhood cancer after neonatal exposure to vitamin K. *N Engl J Med.* 1993;329:905–908.

ZINC

Zinc seldom causes any immediate side effects other than occasional stomach upset, usually when it's taken on an empty stomach. Some forms do have an unpleasant metallic taste.

However, long-term use of zinc at dosages of 100 mg or more daily can cause a number of toxic effects, including severe copper deficiency, impaired immunity, heart problems, and anemia.[1,2,3]

Use of zinc can interfere with the absorption of penicillamine and antibiotics in the tetracycline or fluoroquinolone (Cipro, Floxin) families.[4–9]

The potassium-sparing diuretic amiloride was found to significantly reduce zinc excretion from the body.[10] This means that if you take zinc supplements at the same time as amiloride, zinc accumulation could occur. This could lead to toxic side effects. However, the potassium-sparing diuretic triamterene does not seem to cause this problem.[11]

References

1. Hoffman HN II, Phyliky RL, Fleming CR. Zinc-induced copper deficiency. *Gastroenterology.* 1988;94:508–512.

2. Sandstead HH. Requirements and toxicity of essential trace elements, illustrated by zinc and copper. *Am J Clin Nutr.* 1995;61(suppl 3):621S–624S.

3. Fosmire GJ. Zinc toxicity. *Am J Clin Nutr.* 1990;51:225–227.

4. Lim D, McKay M. Food-drug interactions. *Drug Information Bulletin* (UCLA Dept. of Pharmaceutical Services). 1995;15(2).

5. *Drug Evaluations Annual.* Vol 2. Milwaukee, Wis: American Medical Association; 1993.

6. Neuvonen PJ. Interactions with the absorption of tetracyclines. *Drugs.* 1976;11:45–54.

7. Mapp RK, McCarthy TJ. The effect of zinc sulphate and of bicitropeptide on tetracycline absorption. *S Afr Med J.* 1976;50:1829–1830.

8. Polk RE, Healy DP, Sahai J, et al. Effect of ferrous sulfate and multivitamins with zinc on absorption of ciprofloxacin in normal volunteers. *Antimicrob Agents Chemother.* 1989;33:1841–1844.

9. Campbell NR, Kara M, Hasinoff BB, et al. Norfloxacin interaction with antacids and minerals. *Br J Clin Pharmacol.* 1992;33:115–116.

10. Reyes AJ, Olhaberry JV, Leary WP, et al. Urinary zinc excretion, diuretics, zinc deficiency and some side-effects of diuretics. *S Afr Med J.* 1983;64:936–941.

11. Wester PO. Urinary zinc excretion during treatment with different diuretics. *Acta Med Scand.* 1980;208:209–212.

P A R T

THREE

Notes

✎ NOTES

ACE INHIBITORS

1. *AHFS Drug Information*. Bethesda, Md: American Society of Health-System Pharmacists; 2000:2306–2307.

2. Campbell NR, Hasinoff BB. Iron supplements: a common cause of drug interactions. *Br J Clin Pharmacol*. 1991;31:251–255.

3. Walker BR, Edwards CR. Licorice-induced hypertension and syndromes of apparent mineralocorticoid excess. *Endocrinol Metab Clin North Am*. 1994;23:359–377.

4. Wash LK, Bernard JD. Licorice-induced pseudoaldosteronism. *Am J Hosp Pharm*. 1975;32:73–74.

5. Blachley JD, Knochel JP. Tobacco chewer's hypokalemia: licorice revisited. *N Engl J Med*. 1980;302:784–785.

6. Good CB, McDermott L, McCloskey B. Diet and serum potassium in patients on ACE inhibitors [letter]. *JAMA*. 1995;274:538.

7. Warren SE, O'Connor DT. Hyperkalemia resulting from captopril administration. *JAMA*. 1980;244:2551–2552.

8. Grossman A, Eckland D, Price P, et al. Captopril: reversible renal failure with severe hyperkalaemia [letter]. *Lancet*. 1980;1:712.

9. Burnakis TG, Mioduch HJ. Combined therapy with captopril and potassium supplementation. A potential for hyperkalemia. *Arch Intern Med*. 1984;144:2371–2372.

10. Stoltz ML, Andrews CE Jr. Severe hyperkalemia during very-low-calorie diets and angiotensin converting enzyme use. *JAMA*. 1990;264:2737–2738.

11. Golik A, Modai D, Averbukh Z, et al. Zinc metabolism in patients treated with captopril versus enalapril. *Metabolism*. 1990;39:665–667.

12. Golik A, Zaidenstein R, Dishi V, et al. Effects of captopril and enalapril on zinc metabolism in hypertensive patients. *J Am Coll Nutr*. 1998;17:75–80.

ACETAMINOPHEN (APAP)

1. Alderman S, Kailas S, Goldfarb S, et al. Cholestatic hepatitis after ingestion of chaparral leaf: confirmation by endoscopic retrograde cholangiopancreatography and liver biopsy. *J Clin Gastroenterol.* 1994;19:242–247.

2. [No authors listed]. From the Centers for Disease Control and Prevention. Chaparral-induced toxic hepatitis—California and Texas, 1992. *JAMA.* 1992;268:3295, 3298.

3. Gordon DW, Rosenthal G, Hart J, et al. Chaparral ingestion. The broadening spectrum of liver injury caused by herbal medications. *JAMA.* 1995;273:489–490.

4. Katz M, Saibil F. Herbal hepatitis: subacute hepatic necrosis secondary to chaparral leaf. *J Clin Gastroenterol.* 1990;12:203–206.

5. Smith BC, Desmond PV. Acute hepatitis induced by ingestion of the herbal medication chaparral [letter]. *Aust N Z J Med.* 1993;23:526.

6. Sheikh NM, Philen RM, Love LA. Chaparral-associated hepatotoxicity. *Arch Intern Med.* 1997;157:913–919.

7. Houston JB, Levy G. Drug biotransformation interactions in man. VI: acetaminophen and ascorbic acid. *J Pharm Sci.* 1976;65:1218–1221.

8. Mortensen SA, Leth A, Agner E, et al. Dose-related decrease of serum coenzyme Q10 during treatment with HMG-CoA reductase inhibitors. *Mol Aspects Med.* 1997;18(suppl):S137–S144.

9. Ghirlanda G, Oradei A, Manto A, et al. Evidence of plasma CoQ10-lowering effect by HMG-CoA reductase inhibitors: a double-blind, placebo-controlled study. *J Clin Pharmacol.* 1993;33:226–229.

10. Li H, Chen HZ, Wu XZ, et al. Preventive effect of coenzyme Q_{10} on hepatic damage caused by overdosage of paracetamol in mice. *Chin J Pharmacol Toxicol.* 1997;11:278–280.

11. Neuvonen PJ, Tokola O, Toivonen ML, et al. Methionine in paracetamol tablets, a tool to reduce paracetamol toxicity. *Int J Clin Pharmacol Ther Toxicol.* 1985;23:497–500.

12. Luper S. A review of plants used in the treatment of liver disease: part 1. *Altern Med Rev.* 1998;3:410-421.

13. Muriel P, Garciapina T, Perez-Alvarez V, et al. Silymarin protects against paracetamol-induced lipid peroxidation and liver damage. *J Appl Toxicol.* 1992;12:439–442.

14. Li H, Chen HZ, Wu XZ, et al. Preventive effect of coenzyme Q_{10} on hepatic damage caused by overdosage of paracetamol in mice. *Chin J Pharmacol Toxicol.* 1997;11:278–280.

15. Muriel P, Garciapina T, Perez-Alvarez V, et al. Silymarin protects against paracetamol-induced lipid peroxidation and liver damage. *J Appl Toxicol.* 1992;12:439–442.

AMILORIDE

1. *AHFS Drug Information.* Bethesda, Md: American Society of Health-System Pharmacists; 2000:2306–2307.

2. Stewart PM, Wallace AM, Valentino R, et al. Mineralocorticoid activity of liquorice: 11-beta-hydroxysteroid dehydrogenase deficiency comes of age. *Lancet.* 1987;2:821–824.

3. Walker BR, Edwards CR. Licorice-induced hypertension and syndromes of apparent mineralocorticoid excess. *Endocrinol Metab Clin North Am.* 1994;23:359–377.

4. Wash LK, Bernard JD. Licorice-induced pseudoaldosteronism. *Am J Hosp Pharm.* 1975;32:73–74.

5. Bernardi M, D'Intino PE, Trevisani F, et al. Effects of prolonged ingestion of graded doses of licorice by healthy volunteers. *Life Sci.* 1994;55:863–872.

6. Salassa RM. Inhibition of the "mineralocorticoid" activity of licorice by spironolactone. *J Clin Endocrinol.* 1962;22:1156–1159.

7. Devane J, Ryan MP. The effects of amiloride and triamterene on urinary magnesium excretion in conscious saline-loaded rats. *Br J Pharmacol.* 1981;72:285–289.

8. Reyes AJ, Olhaberry JV, Leary WP, et al. Urinary zinc excretion, diuretics, zinc deficiency and some side-effects of diuretics. *S Afr Med J.* 1983;64:936–941.

9. Wester PO. Urinary zinc excretion during treatment with different diuretics. *Acta Med Scand.* 1980;208:209–212.

AMIODARONE

1. Alderman S, Kailas S, Goldfarb S, et al. Cholestatic hepatitis after ingestion of chaparral leaf: confirmation by endoscopic retrograde cholangiopancreatography and liver biopsy. *J Clin Gastroenterol.* 1994;19:242–247.

2. [No authors listed]. From the Centers for Disease Control and Prevention. Chaparral-induced toxic hepatitis—California and Texas, 1992. *JAMA.* 1992;268:3295, 3298.

3. Gordon DW, Rosenthal G, Hart J, et al. Chaparral ingestion. The broadening spectrum of liver injury caused by herbal medications. *JAMA.* 1995;273:489–490.

4. Katz M, Saibil F. Herbal hepatitis: subacute hepatic necrosis secondary to chaparral leaf. *J Clin Gastroenterol.* 1990;12:203–206.

5. Smith BC, Desmond PV. Acute hepatitis induced by ingestion of the herbal medication chaparral [letter]. *Aust N Z J Med.* 1993;23:526.

6. Sheikh NM, Philen RM, Love LA. Chaparral-associated hepatotoxicity. *Arch Intern Med.* 1997;157:913–919.

7. Jim LK, Gee JP. Adverse effects of drugs on the liver. In: Young LY, Koda-Kimble MA (eds). *Applied Therapeutics: The Clinical Use of Drugs.* Vancouver, Wash: Applied Therapeutics, Inc.; 1995:26.1–26.17.

8. Kachel DL, Moyer TP, Martin WJ 2nd. Amiodarone-induced injury of human pulmonary artery endothelial cells: protection by alpha-tocopherol. *J Pharmacol Exp Ther.* 1990;254:1107–1112.

AMOXICILLIN

1. Tinozzi S, Venegoni A. Effect of bromelain on serum and tissue levels of amoxicillin. *Drugs Exp Clin Res.* 1978;4:39–44.

2. Luerti M, Vignali M. Influence of bromelain on penetration of antibiotics in uterus, salpinx and ovary. *Drugs Exp Clin Res.* 1978;4:45–48.

ANTACIDS

1. Walker JA, Sherman RA, Cody RP. The effect of oral bases on enteral aluminum absorption. *Arch Intern Med.* 1990;150:2037–2039.

2. [No authors listed]. Preliminary findings suggest calcium citrate supplements may raise aluminum levels in blood, urine. *Fam Pract News.* 1992;22:74–75.

Notes

3. Weberg R, Berstad A. Gastrointestinal absorption of aluminium from single doses of aluminium containing antacids in man. *Eur J Clin Invest.* 1986;16:428–432.

4. Nolan CR, Califano JR, Butzin CA. Influence of calcium acetate or calcium citrate on intestinal aluminum absorption. *Kidney Int.* 1990;38:937–941.

5. Slanina P, Frech W, Bernhardson A, et al. Influence of dietary factors on aluminium absorption and retention in the brain and bone of rats. *Acta Pharmacol Toxicol (Copenh).* 1985;56:331–336.

6. Russell RM, Golner BB, Krasinski SD, et al. Effect of antacid and H_2 receptor antagonists on the intestinal absorption of folic acid. *J Lab Clin Med.* 1988;112:458–463.

7. Sturniolo GC, Montino MC, Rossetto L, et al. Inhibition of gastric acid secretion reduces zinc absorption in man. *J Am Coll Nutr.* 1991;4:372–375.

8. Spencer H, Kramer L. Antacid-induced calcium loss. *Arch Intern Med.* 1983;143:657–659.

9. Lotz M, Zisman E, Bartter FC. Evidence for a phosphorus-depletion syndrome in man. *N Engl J Med.* 1968;278:409–415.

10. Hallberg L, Brune M, Erlandsson M, et al. Calcium: effect of different amounts on nonheme- and heme-iron absorption in humans. *Am J Clin Nutr.* 1991;53:112–119.

11. Cook JD, Dassenko SA, Whittaker P. Calcium supplementation: effect on iron absorption. *Am J Clin Nutr.* 1991;53:106–111.

12. Dawson-Hughes B, Seligson FH, Hughes VA. Effects of calcium carbonate and hydroxyapatite on zinc and iron retention in postmenopausal women. *Am J Clin Nutr.* 1986;44:83–88.

13. Read MH, Medeiros D, Bendel R, et al. Mineral supplementation practices of adults in seven western states. *Nutr Res.* 1986;6:375–383.

14. Argiratos V, Samman S. The effect of calcium carbonate and calcium citrate on the absorption of zinc in healthy female subjects. *Eur J Clin Nutr.* 1994;48:198–204.

15. Lewis NM, Marcus MS, Behling AR, et al. Calcium supplements and milk: effects on acid-base balance and on retention of calcium, magnesium, and phosphorus. *Am J Clin Nutr.* 1989;49:527–533.

16. Andon MB, Ilich JZ, Tzagournis MA, et al. Magnesium balance in adolescent females consuming a low- or high-calcium diet. *Am J Clin Nutr.* 1996;63:950–953.

Notes

17. Seaborn CD, Stoecker BJ. Effects of antacid or ascorbic acid on tissue accumulation and urinary excretion of [51]chromium. *Nutr Res.* 1990;10:1401–1407.

18. Freeland-Graves JH, Lin PH. Plasma uptake of manganese as affected by oral loads of manganese, calcium, milk, phosphorus, copper, and zinc. *J Am Coll Nutr.* 1991;10:38–43.

19. Davidsson L, Cederblad A, Lonnerdal B, et al. The effect of individual dietary components on manganese absorption in humans. *Am J Clin Nutr.* 1991;54:1065–1070.

20. Hallberg L, Brune M, Erlandsson M, et al. Calcium: effect of different amounts on nonheme- and heme-iron absorption in humans. *Am J Clin Nutr.* 1991;53:112–119.

21. Cook JD, Dassenko SA, Whittaker P. Calcium supplementation: effect on iron absorption. *Am J Clin Nutr.* 1991;53:106–111.

22. Dawson-Hughes B, Seligson FH, Hughes VA. Effects of calcium carbonate and hydroxyapatite on zinc and iron retention in postmenopausal women. *Am J Clin Nutr.* 1986;44:83–88.

23. Read MH, Medeiros D, Bendel R, et al. Mineral supplementation practices of adults in seven western states. *Nutr Res.* 1986;6:375–383.

24. Sokoll LJ, Dawson-Hughes B. Calcium supplementation and plasma ferritin concentrations in premenopausal women. *Am J Clin Nutr.* 1992;56:1045–1048.

25. Cook JD, Dassenko SA, Whittaker P. Calcium supplementation: effect on iron absorption. *Am J Clin Nutr.* 1991;53:106–111.

26. Argiratos V, Samman S. The effect of calcium carbonate and calcium citrate on the absorption of zinc in healthy female subjects. *Eur J Clin Nutr.* 1994;48:198–204.

27. Dawson-Hughes B, Seligson FH, Hughes VA. Effects of calcium carbonate and hydroxyapatite on zinc and iron retention in postmenopausal women. *Am J Clin Nutr.* 1986;44:83–88.

28. Spencer H, Kramer L, Norris C, et al. Effect of calcium and phosphorus on zinc metabolism in man. *Am J Clin Nutr.* 1984;40:1213–1218.

29. Lewis NM, Marcus MS, Behling AR, et al. Calcium supplements and milk: effects on acid-base balance and on retention of calcium, magnesium, and phosphorus. *Am J Clin Nutr.* 1989;49:527–533.

30. Andon MB, Ilich JZ, Tzagournis MA, et al. Magnesium balance in adolescent females consuming a low- or high-calcium diet. *Am J Clin Nutr.* 1996;63:950–953.

ANTHRACYCLINES

1. Mortensen SA, Leth A, Agner E, et al. Dose-related decrease of serum coenzyme Q10 during treatment with HMG-CoA reductase inhibitors. *Mol Aspects Med*. 1997;18(suppl):S137–S144.

2. Ghirlanda G, Oradei A, Manto A, et al. Evidence of plasma CoQ10-lowering effect by HMG-CoA reductase inhibitors: a double-blind, placebo-controlled study. *J Clin Pharmacol*. 1993;33:226–229.

3. Folkers K, Liu M, Watanabe T, et al., Inhibition by adriamycin of the mitochondrial biosynthesis of coenzyme Q10 and implication for the cardiotoxicity of adriamycin in cancer patients. *Biochem Biophys Res Commun*. 1977;77:1536–1542.

4. Kishi T, Watanabe T, Folkers K. Bioenergetics in clinical medicine: prevention by forms of coenzyme Q of the inhibition by adriamycin of coenzyme Q10-enzymes in mitochondria of the myocardium. *Proc Natl Acad Sci U S A*. 1976;73:4653–4656.

5. Iwamoto Y, Hansen IL, Porter TH, et al. Inhibition of coenzyme Q10-enzymes, succinoxidase and NADH-oxidase, by adriamycin and other quinones having antitumor activity. *Biochem Biophys Res Commun*. 1974;58:633–638.

6. Ohhara H, Kanaide H, Nakamura M. A protective effect of coenzyme Q10 on the adriamycin-induced cardiotoxicity in the isolated perfused rat heart. *J Mol Cell Cardiol*. 1981;13:741–752.

7. Folkers K, Choe JY, Combs AB. Rescue by coenzyme Q10 from electrocardiographic abnormalities caused by the toxicity of adriamycin in the rat. *Proc Natl Acad Sci USA*. 1978;75:5178–5180.

8. Combs AB, Choe JY, Truong DH, et al. Reduction by coenzyme Q10 of the acute toxicity of adriamycin in mice. *Res Commun Chem Pathol Pharmacol*. 1977;18:565–568.

9. Usui T, lshikura H, lzumi Y, et al. Possible prevention from the progression of cardiotoxicity in adriamycin-treated rabbits by coenzyme Q10. *Toxicol Lett*. 1982;12:75–82.

10. Domae N, Sawada H, Matsuyama E, et al. Cardiomyopathy and other chronic toxic effects induced in rabbits by doxorubicin and possible prevention by coenzyme Q10. *Cancer Treat Rep*. 1981;65:79–91.

11. Cortes EP, Gupta M, Chou C, et al., Adriamycin cardiotoxicity: early detection by systolic time interval and possible prevention by coenzyme Q10. *Cancer Treat Rep*. 1978;62:887–891.

Notes

12. Lenzhofer R, Magometschnigg D, Dudczak R, et al. Indication of reduced doxorubicin-induced cardiac toxicity by additional treatment with antioxidative substances. *Experientia.* 1983;39:62–64.

13. Mimnaugh EG, Siddik ZH, Drew R, et al. The effects of alpha-tocopherol on the toxicity, disposition, and metabolism of adriamycin in mice. *Toxicol Appl Pharmacol.* 1979;49:119–126.

14. Hermansen K, Wassermann K. The effect of vitamin E and selenium on doxorubicin (Adriamycin) induced delayed toxicity in mice. *Acta Pharmacol Toxicol (Copenh).* 1986;58:31–37.

15. Wang YM, Madanat FF, Kimball JC, et al., Effect of vitamin E against adriamycin-induced toxicity in rabbits. *Cancer Res.* 1980;40:1022–1027.

16. Milei J, Boveris A, Llesuy S, et al. Amelioration of adriamycin-induced cardiotoxicity in rabbits by prenylamine and vitamins A and E. *Am Heart J.* 1986;111:95–102.

17. Herman EH, Ferrans VJ. Influence of vitamin E and ICRF-187 on chronic doxorubicin cardiotoxicity in miniature swine. *Lab Invest.* 1983;49:69–77.

18. Shinozawa S, Gomita Y, Araki Y. Effect of high dose alpha-tocopherol and alpha-tocopherol acetate pretreatment on adriamycin (doxorubicin) induced toxicity and tissue distribution. *Physiol Chem Phys Med NMR.* 1988;20:329–335.

19. Van Vleet JF, Ferrans VJ. Evaluation of vitamin E and selenium protection against chronic adriamycin toxicity in rabbits. *Cancer Treat Rep.* 1980;64:315–317.

20. Breed JG, Zimmerman AN, Dormans JA, et al. Failure of the antioxidant vitamin E to protect against adriamycin-induced cardiotoxicity in the rabbit. *Cancer Res.* 1980;40:2033–2038.

21. Van Vleet JF, Ferrans VJ, Weirich WE. Cardiac disease induced by chronic adriamycin administration in dogs and an evaluation of vitamin E and selenium as cardioprotectants. *Am J Pathol.* 1980;99:13–42.

22. Lenzhofer R, Ganzinger U, Rameis H, et al. Acute cardiac toxicity in patients after doxorubicin treatment and the effect of combined tocopherol and nifedipine pretreatment. *J Cancer Res Clin Oncol.* 1983;106:143–147.

23. Weitzman SA, Lorell F, Carey RW, et al. Prospective study of tocopherol prophylaxis for anthracycline cardiac toxicity. *Curr Ther Res.* 1980;28:682–686.

Notes

24. Legha SS, Wang YM, Mackay B, et al. Clinical and pharmacologic investigation of the effects of alpha-tocopherol on adriamycin cardiotoxicity *Ann N Y Acad Sci.* 1982;393:411–418.

25. Wood LA. Possible prevention of adriamycin-induced alopecia by tocopherol [letter]. *N Engl J Med.* 1985;312:1060.

26. Legha SS, Wang YM, Mackay B, et al. Clinical and pharmacologic investigation of the effects of alpha-tocopherol on adriamycin cardiotoxicity *Ann N Y Acad Sci.* 1982;393:411–418.

27. Martin-Jimenez M, Diaz-Rubio E, Gonzalez Larriba JL, et al. Failure of high-dose tocopherol to prevent alopecia induced by doxorubicin. *N Engl J Med.* 1986;315:894–895.

28. Perez JE, Macchiavelli M, Leone BA, et al. High-dose alpha-tocopherol as a preventive of doxorubicin-induced alopecia. *Cancer Treat Rep.* 1986;70:1213–1214.

29. Ludwig CU, Stoll HR, Obrist R, et al. Prevention of cytotoxic drug induced skin ulcers with dimethyl sulfoxide (DMSO) and alpha-tocopherole. *Eur J Cancer Clin Oncol.* 1987;23:327–329.

30. Hermansen K, Wassermann K. The effect of vitamin E and selenium on doxorubicin (Adriamycin) induced delayed toxicity in mice. *Acta Pharmacol Toxicol (Copenh).* 1986;58:31–37.

31. Van Vleet JF, Ferrans VJ. Evaluation of vitamin E and selenium protection against chronic adriamycin toxicity in rabbits. *Cancer Treat Rep.* 1980;64:315–317.

32. Dimitrov NV, Hay MB, Siew S, et al. Abrogation of adriamycin-induced cardiotoxicity by selenium in rabbits. *Am J Pathol.* 1987;126:376–383.

33. Lenzhofer R, Magometschnigg D, Dudczak R, et al. Indication of reduced doxorubicin-induced cardiac toxicity by additional treatment with antioxidative substances. *Experientia.* 1983;39:62–64.

34. Yoda Y, Nakazawa M, Abe T, et al. Prevention of doxorubicin myocardial toxicity in mice by reduced glutathione. *Cancer Res.* 1986;46:2551–2556.

35. Dorr RT. Cytoprotective agents for anthracyclines. *Semin Oncol.* 1996;23(4 suppl 8):23–34.

36. Shimpo K, Nagatsu T, Yamada K, et al. Ascorbic acid and adriamycin toxicity. *Am J Clin Nutr.* 1991;54:1298S–1301S.

37. Fujita K, Shinpo K, Yamada K, et al., Reduction of adriamycin toxicity by ascorbate in mice and guinea pigs. *Cancer Res.* 1982;42:309–316.

38. Hajarizadeh H, Lebredo L, Barrie R, et al. Protective effect of doxorubicin in vitamin C or dimethyl sulfoxide against skin ulceration in the pig. *Ann Surg Oncol.* 1994;1:411–414.

39. Doroshow JH, Locker GY, Ifrim I, et al. Prevention of doxorubicin cardiac toxicity in the mouse by N-acetylcysteine. *J Clin Invest.* 1981;68:1053–1064.

40. Unverferth DV, Leier CV, Balcerzak SP, et al. Usefulness of a free radical scavenger in preventing doxorubicin-induced heart failure in dogs. *Am J Cardiol.* 1985;56:157–161.

41. Unverferth DV, Jagadeesh JM, Unverferth BJ, et al. Attempt to prevent doxorubicin-induced acute human myocardial morphologic damage with acetylcysteine. *J Natl Cancer Inst.* 1983;71:917–920.

42. Myers C, Bonow R, Palmeri S, et al. A randomized controlled trial assessing the prevention of doxorubicin cardiomyopathy by N-acetylcysteine. *Semin Oncol.* 1983;10(1 suppl 1):53–55.

ANTIBIOTICS

1. Colombel JF, Cortot A, Neut C, et al. Yoghurt with *Bifidobacterium longum* reduces erythromycin-induced gastrointestinal effects. *Lancet.* 1987;2:43.

2. Elmer GW, Surawicz CM, McFarland LV. Biotherapeutic agents. A neglected modality for the treatment and prevention of selected intestinal and vaginal infections. *JAMA.* 1996;275:870–876.

3. McFarland LV, Surawicz CM, Greenberg RN, et al. Prevention of beta-lactam-associated diarrhea by *Saccharomyces boulardii* compared with placebo. *Am J Gastroenterol.* 1995;90:439–448.

4. Pothoulakis C, Kelly CP, Joshi MA, et al. *Saccharomyces boulardii* inhibits *Clostridium difficile* toxin A binding and enterotoxicity in rat ileum. *Gastroenterology.* 1993;104:1108–1115.

5. Surawicz CM, Elmer GW, Speelman P, et al. Prevention of antibiotic-associated diarrhea by *Saccharomyces boulardii*: a prospective study. *Gastroenterology.* 1989;96:981–988.

6. Bleichner G, Blehaut H, Mentec H, et al. Saccharomyces boulardii prevents diarrhea in critically ill tube-fed patients. A multicenter, randomized, double-blind placebo-controlled trial. *Intensive Care Med.* 1997;23:517–523.

7. Izadnia F, Wong CT, Kocoshis SA. Brewer's yeast and *Saccharomyces boulardii* both attenuate Clostridium difficile-induced colonic secretion in the rat. *Dig Dis Sci.* 1998;43:2055–2060.

8. Kollaritsch H, Holst H, Grobara P, et al. Prevention of traveler's diarrhea with *Saccharomyces boulardii*. Results of a placebo controlled double-blind study [translated from German]. *Fortschr Med*. 1993;111:152–156.

9. Lewis SJ, Potts LF, Barry RE. The lack of therapeutic effect of *Saccharomyces boulardii* in the prevention of antibiotic related diarrhea in elderly patients. *J Infect*. 1998;36:171–174.

10. Cohen H, Scott SD, Mackie IJ, et al. The development of hypoprothrombinaemia following antibiotic therapy in malnourished patients with low serum vitamin K1 levels. *Br J Haematol*. 1988;68:63–66.

11. Lipsky JJ. Nutritional sources of vitamin K. *Mayo Clin Proc*. 1994;69:462–466.

ANTICONVULSANT AGENTS

1. Arenz A, Klein M, Fiehe K. Occurrence of neurotoxic 4'-O-methylpyridoxine in *Ginkgo biloba* leaves, ginkgo medications and Japanese ginkgo food. *Planta Med*. 1996;62:548–551.

2. Mizuno N, Kawakami K, Morita E. Competitive inhibition between 4'-substituted pyridoxine analogues and pyridoxal for pyridoxal kinase from mouse brain. *J Nutr Sci Vitaminol (Tokyo)*. 1980;26:535–543.

3. Wada K, Ishigaki S, Ueda K, et al. An antivitamin B6, 4'-methoxypyridoxine, from the seed of *Ginkgo biloba* L. *Chem Pharm Bull (Tokyo)*. 1985;33:3555–3557.

4. Yagi M, Wada K, Sakata M, et al. Studies on the constituents of edible and medicinal plants. IV. Determination of 4-O-methylpyridoxine in serum of the patient with gin-nan food poisoning [in Japanese; English abstract]. *Yakugaku Zasshi*. 1993;113:596–599.

5. Arenz A, Klein M, Fiehe K. Occurrence of neurotoxic 4'-O-methylpyridoxine in *Ginkgo biloba* leaves, ginkgo medications and Japanese ginkgo food. *Planta Med*. 1996;62:548–551.

6. *A to Z Drug Facts* [book on CD-ROM]. 2nd ed. St. Louis, Mo: Facts and Comparisons; 2000.

7. Takanaga H, Ohnishi A, Murakami H, et al. Relationship between time after intake of grapefruit juice and the effect on pharmacokinetics and pharmacodynamics of nisoldipine in healthy subjects. *Clin Pharmacol Ther*. 2000;67:201–214.

8. Monostory K, Vereczkey L, Levai F, et al. Ipriflavone as an inhibitor of human cytochrome P450 enzymes. *Br J Pharmacol*. 1998;123:605–610.

9. Almeida JC, Grimsley EW. Coma from the health food store: interaction between kava and alprazolam. *Ann Intern Med.* 1996;125:940–941.

10. Bourgeois BF, Dodson WE, Ferrendelli JA. Interactions between primidone, carbamazepine, and nicotinamide. *Neurology.* 1982;32:1122–1126.

11. Bourgeois BF, Dodson WE, Ferrendelli JA. Interactions between primidone, carbamazepine, and nicotinamide. *Neurology.* 1982;32:1122–1126.

12. Nau H, Tzimas G, Mondry M, et al. Antiepileptic drugs alter endogenous retinoid concentrations: a possible mechanism of teratogenesis of anticonvulsant therapy. *Life Sci.* 1995;57:53–60.

13. Inoue F, Walsh RJ. Folate supplements and phenytoin-salicylate interaction. *Neurology.* 1983;33:115–116.

14. Krause KH, Bonjour JP, Berlit P, et al. Biotin status of epileptics. *Ann N Y Acad Sci.* 1985;447:297–313.

15. Said HM, Redha R, Nylander W. Biotin transport in the human intestine: inhibition by anticonvulsant drugs. *Am J Clin Nutr.* 1989;49:127–131.

16. Ono H, Sakamoto A, Eguchi T, et al. Plasma total homocysteine concentrations in epileptic patients taking anticonvulsants. *Metabolism.* 1997;46:959–962.

17. Lewis DP, Van Dyke DC, Stumbo PJ, et al. Drug and environmental factors associated with adverse pregnancy outcomes. Part I: Antiepileptic drugs, contraceptives, smoking, and folate. *Ann Pharmacother.* 1998;32:802–817.

18. Kishi T, Fujita N, Eguchi T, et al. Mechanism for reduction of serum folate by antiepileptic drugs during prolonged therapy. *J Neurol Sci.* 1997;145:109–112.

19. Reynolds EH. Mental effects of anticonvulsants, and folic acid metabolism. *Brain.* 1968;91:197–214.

20. Hendel J, Dam M, Gram L, et al. The effects of carbamazepine and valproate on folate metabolism. *Acta Neurol Scand.* 1984;69:226–231.

21. Berg MJ, Stumbo PJ, Chenard CA, et al. Folic acid improves phenytoin pharmacokinetics. *J Am Diet Assoc.* 1995;95:352–356.

22. Lewis DP, Van Dyke DC, Willhite LA, et al. Phenytoin-folic acid interaction. *Ann Pharmacother.* 1995;29:726–735.

23. Kishi T, Fujita N, Eguchi T, et al. Mechanism for reduction of serum folate by antiepileptic drugs during prolonged therapy. *J Neurol Sci.* 1997;145:109–112.

24. Berg MJ, Stumbo PJ, Chenard CA, et al. Folic acid improves phenytoin pharmacokinetics. *J Am Diet Assoc.* 1995;95:352–56.

25. Lewis DP, Van Dyke DC, Stumbo PJ, et al. Drug and environmental factors associated with adverse pregnancy outcomes. Part I: Antiepileptic drugs, contraceptives, smoking, and folate. *Ann Pharmacother.* 1998;32:802–817.

26. Wahl TO, Gobuty AH, Lukert BP. Long-term anticonvulsant therapy and intestinal calcium absorption. *Clin Pharmacol Ther.* 1981;30:506–512.

27. Weinstein RS, Bryce GF, Sappington LJ, et al. Decreased serum ionized calcium and normal vitamin D metabolite levels with anticonvulsant drug treatment. *J Clin Endocrinol Metab.* 1984;58:1003–1009.

28. Weinstein RS, Bryce GF, Sappington LJ, et al. Decreased serum ionized calcium and normal vitamin D metabolite levels with anticonvulsant drug treatment. *J Clin Endocrinol Metab.* 1984;58:1003–1009.

29. Carter BL, Garnett WR, Pellock JM, et al. Effect of antacids on phenytoin bioavailability. *Ther Drug Monit.* 1981;3:333–340.

30. McElnay JC, Uprichard G, Collier PS. The effect of activated dimethicone and a proprietary antacid preparation containing this agent on the absorption of phenytoin. *Br J Clin Pharmacol.* 1982;13:501–505.

31. De Vivo DC, Bohan TP, Coulter DL, et al. L-carnitine supplementation in childhood epilepsy: current perspectives. *Epilepsia.* 1998;39:1216–1225.

32. Coulter DL. Carnitine deficiency: a possible mechanism for valproate hepatotoxicity [letter]. *Lancet.* 1984;1:689.

33. Ater SB., et al. A developmental center population treated with VPA and L-carnitine. In: Update 1993: inborn errors of metabolism in the patient with epilepsy. Sigma-Tau Pharmaceuticals; 1993.

34. Dreifuss FE, Langer DH. Hepatic considerations in the use of antiepileptic drugs. *Epilepsia.* 1987;28(suppl 2):S23–S29.

35. Ater SB., et al. A developmental center population treated with VPA and L-carnitine. In: Update 1993: inborn errors of metabolism in the patient with epilepsy. Sigma-Tau Pharmaceuticals; 1993.

36. Freeman JM, Vining EP, Cost S, et al. Does carnitine administration improve the symptoms attributed to anticonvulsant medications? A double-blinded, crossover study. *Pediatrics.* 1994;93:893–895.

37. De Vivo DC, Bohan TP, Coulter DL, et al. L-carnitine supplementation in childhood epilepsy: current perspectives. *Epilepsia.* 1998;39:1216–1225.

Notes

38. Hahn TJ, Hendin BA, Scharp CR, et al. Effect of chronic anticonvulsant therapy on serum 25-hydroxycalciferol levels in adults. *N Engl J Med.* 1972;287:900–904.

39. Hahn TJ, Hendin BA, Scharp CR, et al. Effect of chronic anticonvulsant therapy on serum 25-hydroxycalciferol levels in adults. *N Engl J Med.* 1972;287:900–904.

40. Jubiz W, Haussler MR, McCain TA, et al. Plasma 1,25-dihydroxyvitamin D levels in patients receiving anticonvulsant drugs. *J Clin Endocrinol Metab.* 1977;44:617–621.

41. Brodie MJ, Boobis AR, Dollery CT, et al. Rifampicin and vitamin D metabolism. *Clin Pharmacol Ther.* 1980;27:810–814.

42. Williams C, Netzloff M, Folkerts L, et al. Vitamin D metabolism and anticonvulsant therapy: effect of sunshine on incidence of osteomalacia. *South Med J.* 1984;77:834–836, 842.

43. Cornelissen M, Steegers-Theunissen R, Kollee, L, et al. Increased incidence of neonatal vitamin K deficiency resulting from maternal anticonvulsant therapy. *Am J Obstet Gynecol.* 1993;168:923–928.

44. Cornelissen M, Steegers-Theunissen R, Kollee L, et al. Supplementation of vitamin K in pregnant women receiving anticonvulsant therapy prevents neonatal vitamin K deficiency. *Am J Obstet Gynecol.* 1993;168:884–888.

ANTIDIABETIC AGENTS

1. Monostory K, Vereczkey L, Levai F, et al. Ipriflavone as an inhibitor of human cytochrome P450 enzymes. *Br J Pharmacol.* 1998;123:605–610.

2. *A to Z Drug Facts* [book on CD-ROM]. 2nd ed. St. Louis, Mo: Facts and Comparisons; 2000.

3. Anderson RA, Cheng N, Bryden NA, et al. Elevated intakes of supplemental chromium improve glucose and insulin variables in individuals with type 2 diabetes. *Diabetes.* 1997;46:1786–1791.

4. Ravina A, Slezack L. Chromium in the treatment of clinical diabetes mellitus [translated from Hebrew]. *Harefuah.* 1993;125:142–145.

5. Jovanovic L, Gutierrez M, Peterson CM. Chromium supplementation for women with gestational diabetes mellitus. *J Trace Elem Exp Med.* 1999;12:91–97.

6. Ravina A, Slezak L, Mirsky N, et al. Reversal of corticosteroid-induced diabetes mellitus with supplemental chromium. *Diabet Med.* 1999;16:164–167.

7. Ravina A, Slezak L, Mirsky N, et al. Control of steroid-induced diabetes with supplemental chromium. *J Trace Elem Exp Med.* 1999;12:375–378.

8. Rabinowitz MB, Gonick HC, Levin SR, et al. Effects of chromium and yeast supplements on carbohydrate and lipid metabolism in diabetic men. *Diabetes Care.* 1983;6:319–327.

9. Trow LG, Lewis J, Greenwood RH, et al. Lack of effect of dietary chromium supplementation on glucose tolerance, plasma insulin and lipoprotein levels in patients with type 2 diabetes. *Int J Vitam Nutr Res.* 2000;70:14–18.

10. Sotaniemi EA, Haapakoski E, Rautio A. Ginseng therapy in non-insulin–dependent diabetic patients. *Diabetes Care.* 1995;18:1373–1375.

11. Vuksan V, Sievenpiper JL, Koo VY, et al. American ginseng (*Panax quinquefolius* L) reduces postprandial glycemia in nondiabetic subjects and subjects with type 2 diabetes mellitus. *Arch Intern Med.* 2000;160:1009–1013.

12. Elamin A, Tuvemo T. Magnesium and insulin-dependent diabetes mellitus. *Diabetes Res Clin Pract.* 1990;10:203–209.

13. Tosiello L. Hypomagnesemia and diabetes mellitus. *Arch Intern Med.* 1996;156:1143–1148.

14. Zuccaro P, Pacifici R, Pichini S, et al. Influence of antacids on the bioavailability of glibenclamide. *Drugs Exp Clin Res.* 1989;15:165–169.

15. Kivisto KT, Neuvonen PJ. Effect of magnesium hydroxide on the absorption and efficacy of tolbutamide and chlorpropamide. *Eur J Clin Pharmacol.* 1992;42:675–679.

16. Shamberger RJ. The insulin-like effects of vanadium. *J Adv Med.* 1996;9:121–131.

17. Shamberger RJ. The insulin-like effects of vanadium. *J Adv Med.* 1996;9:121–131.

18. Halberstam M, Cohen N, Shlimovich P, et al. Oral vanadyl sulfate improves insulin sensitivity in NIDDM but not in obese nondiabetic subjects. *Diabetes.* 1996;45:659–666.

19. Domingo JL, Gomez M, Llobet JM, et al. Oral vanadium administration to streptozotocin-diabetic rats has marked negative effects side-effects which are independent of the form of vanadium used. *Toxicology.* 1991;66:279–287.

20. Domingo JL. Vanadium: a review of the reproductive and developmental toxicity. *Reprod Toxicol.* 1996;10:175–182.

Notes

21. Paolisso G, D'Amore A, Giugliano D, et al. Pharmacologic doses of vitamin E improve insulin action in healthy subjects and non-insulin-dependent diabetic patients. *Am J Clin Nutr*. 1993;57:650–656.

22. Paolisso G, D'Amore A, Giugliano D, et al. Pharmacologic doses of vitamin E improve insulin action in healthy subjects and non-insulin-dependent diabetic patients. *Am J Clin Nutr*. 1993;57:650–656.

23. Brinker F. *Herb Contraindications and Drug Interactions: with Appendices Addressing Specific Conditions and Medicines*. 2nd ed. Sandy, Ore: Eclectic Medical Publications; 1998.

24. Yaniv Z, Dafni A, Friedman J, et al. Plants used for the treatment of diabetes in Israel. *J Ethnopharmacol*. 1987;19:145–151.

25. Teixeira CC, Pinto LP, Kessler FH, et al. The effect of *Syzygium cumini* (L.) skeels on post-prandial blood glucose levels in non-diabetic rats and rats with streptozotocin-induced diabetes mellitus. *J Ethnopharmacol*. 1997;56:209–213.

26. Bever BO, Zahnd GR. Plants with oral hypoglycaemic action. *Q J Crude Drug Res*. 1979;17:139–196.

27. Mathew PT, Augusti KT. Hypoglycaemic effects of onion, *Allium cepa* Linn. on diabetes mellitus—a preliminary report. *Indian J Physiol Pharmacol*. 1975;19:213–217.

28. Manickam M, Ramanathan M, Jahromi MA, et al. Antihyperglycemic activity of phenolics from *Pterocarpus marsupium*. *J Nat Prod*. 1997;60:609–610.

29. Ahmad F, Khalid P, Khan MM, et al. Insulin like activity in (-) epicatechin. *Acta Diabetol Lat*. 1989;26:291–300.

30. Stern E. Successful use of *Atriplex halimus* in the treatment of type 2 diabetic patients. A preliminary study. Unpublished study conducted at the Zamenhoff Medical Center, Tel Aviv, Israel, 1989.

31. Earon G, Stern E, Lavosky H. Successful use of *Atriplex halimus* in the treatment of type 2 diabetic patients. Controlled clinical research report on the subject of Atriplex. Unpublished study conducted at the Hebrew University, Jerusalem; 1989.

32. Khan AK, Akhtar S, Mahtab H. Treatment of diabetes mellitus with *Coccinia indica*. *Br Med J*. 1980;280:1044.

33. Welihinda J, Karunanayake EH, Sheriff MH, et al. Effect of *Momordica charantia* on the glucose tolerance in maturity onset diabetes. *J Ethnopharmacol*. 1986;17:277–282.

34. Akhtar MS. Trial of *Momordica charantia* Linn (Karela) powder in patients with maturity-onset diabetes. *JPMA J Pak Med Assoc.* 1982;32:106–107.

35. Leatherdale BA, Panesar RK, Singh G, et al. Improvement in glucose tolerance due to *Momordica charantia* (karela). *Br Med J (Clin Res Ed)* 1981;282:1823–1824.

36. Boden G, Chen X, Ruiz J, et al. Effects of vanadyl sulfate on carbohydrate and lipid metabolism in patients with non-insulin-dependent diabetes mellitus. *Metabolism.* 1996;45:1130–1135.

37. Halberstam M, Cohen N, Shlimovich P, et al. Oral vanadyl sulfate improves insulin sensitivity in NIDDM but not in obese nondiabetic subjects. *Diabetes.* 1996;45:659–666

38. Anderson RA, Cheng N, Bryden NA, et al. Elevated intakes of supplemental chromium improve glucose and insulin variables in individuals with type 2 diabetes. *Diabetes.* 1997;46:1786–1791.

39. Ravina A, Slezack L. Chromium in the treatment of clinical diabetes mellitus [translated from Hebrew]. *Harefuah.* 1993;125:142–145.

40. Jovanovic L, Gutierrez M, Peterson CM. Chromium supplementation for women with gestational diabetes mellitus. *J Trace Elem Exp Med.* 1999;12:91–97.

41. Rabinowitz MB, Gonick HC, Levin SR, et al. Effects of chromium and yeast supplements on carbohydrate and lipid metabolism in diabetic men. *Diabetes Care.* 1983;6:319–327.

42. Cignarella A, Nastasi M, Cavalli E, et al. Novel lipid-lowering properties of *Vaccinium myrtillus L.* leaves, a traditional antidiabetic treatment, in several models of rat dyslipidaemia: a comparison with ciprofibrate. *Thromb Res.* 1996;84:311–322.

43. Mingrone G, Greco AV, Capristo E, et al. L-carnitine improves glucose disposal in type 2 diabetic patients. *J Am Coll Nutr.* 1999;18:77–82.

44. Jacob S, Ruus P, Hermann R, et al. Oral administration of RAC-alpha-lipoic acid modulates insulin sensitivity in patients with type-2 diabetes mellitus: a placebo-controlled pilot trial. *Free Radic Biol Med.* 1999;27:309–314.

45. Al-Awadi FM, Gumaa KA. Studies on the activity of individual plants of an antidiabetic plant mixture. *Acta Diabetol Lat.* 1987;24:37–41.

46. Adams JF, Clark JS, Ireland JT, et al. Malabsorption of vitamin B12 and intrinsic factor secretion during biguanide therapy. *Diabetologia.* 1983;24:16–18.

Notes

47. Bauman WA, Shaw S, Jayatilleke E, et al. Increased intake of calcium reverses vitamin B12 malabsorption induced by metformin. *Diabetes Care*. 2000;23:1227–1231.

48. Schafer G. Some new aspects on the interaction of hypoglycemia-producing biguanides with biological membranes. *Biochem Pharmacol*. 1976;25:2015–2024.

49. Carmel R, Rosenberg AH, Lau KS, et al. Vitamin B12 uptake by human small bowel homogenate and its enhancement by intrinsic factor. *Gastroenterology*. 1969;56:548–555.

50. Mortensen SA, Leth A, Agner E, et al. Dose-related decrease of serum coenzyme Q10 during treatment with HMG-CoA reductase inhibitors. *Mol Aspects Med*. 1997;18(suppl):S137–S144.

51. Ghirlanda G, Oradei A, Manto A, et al. Evidence of plasma CoQ10-lowering effect by HMG-CoA reductase inhibitors: a double-blind, placebo-controlled study. *J Clin Pharmacol*. 1993;33:226–229.

52. Kishi T, Kishi H, Watanabe T, et al. Bioenergetics in clinical medicine. XI. Studies on Coenzyme Q and diabetes mellitus. *J Med*. 1976;7:307–321.

53. Adams JF, Clark JS, Ireland JT, et al. Malabsorption of vitamin B12 and intrinsic factor secretion during biguanide therapy. *Diabetologia*. 1983;24:16–18.

ANTIHYPERTENSIVE AGENTS

1. Mortensen SA, Leth A, Agner E, et al. Dose-related decrease of serum coenzyme Q10 during treatment with HMG-CoA reductase inhibitors. *Mol Aspects Med*. 1997;18(suppl):S137–S144.

2. Ghirlanda G, Oradei A, Manto A, et al. Evidence of plasma CoQ10-lowering effect by HMG-CoA reductase inhibitors: a double-blind, placebo-controlled study. *J Clin Pharmacol*. 1993;33:226–229.

3. Mortensen SA, Vadhanavikit S, Muratsu K, et al. Coenzyme Q10: clinical benefits with biochemical correlates suggesting a scientific breakthrough in the management of chronic heart failure. *Int J Tissue React*. 1990;12:155–162.

4. Kishi H, Kishi T, Folkers K. Bioenergetics in clinical medicine. III. Inhibition of coenzyme Q10-enzymes by clinically used anti-hypertensive drugs. *Res Commun Chem Pathol Pharmacol*. 1975;12:533–540.

Notes

ANTIPSYCHOTIC AGENTS

1. Schelosky L, Raffauf C, Jendroska K, et al. Kava and dopamine antagonism [letter]. *J Neurol Neurosurg Psychiatry.* 1995;58:639–640.

2. Schelosky L, Raffauf C, Jendroska K, et al. Kava and dopamine antagonism [letter]. *J Neurol Neurosurg Psychiatry.* 1995;58:639–640.

3. Almeida JC, Grimsley EW. Coma from the health food store: interaction between kava and alprazolam. *Ann Intern Med.* 1996;125:940–941.

4. Mosnik DM, Spring B, Rogers K, et al. Tardive dyskinesia exacerbated after ingestion of phenylalanine by schizophrenic patients. *Neuropsychopharmacology.* 1997;16:136–146.

5. Gardos G, Cole JO, Mathews JD, et al. The acute effects of a loading dose of phenylalanine in unipolar depressed patients with and without tardive dyskinesia. *Neuropsychopharmacology.* 1992;6:241–247.

6. De Smet PA, Touw DJ. Safety of St. John's wort [letter]. *Lancet.* 2000;355:575–576.

7. Brinker F. *Herb Contraindications and Drug Interactions: with Appendices Addressing Specific Conditions and Medicines.* 2nd ed. Sandy, Ore: Eclectic Medical Publications; 1998.

8. Mortensen SA, Leth A, Agner E, et al. Dose-related decrease of serum coenzyme Q10 during treatment with HMG-CoA reductase inhibitors. *Mol Aspects Med.* 1997;18(suppl):S137–S144.

9. Ghirlanda G, Oradei A, Manto A, et al. Evidence of plasma CoQ10-lowering effect by HMG-CoA reductase inhibitors: a double-blind, placebo-controlled study. *J Clin Pharmacol.* 1993;33:226–229.

10. Kishi T, Makino K, Okamoto T, et al. Inhibition of myocardial respiration by psychotherapeutic drugs and prevention by coenzyme Q. *Biomed Clin Aspects Coenzyme Q.* 1980;2:139–157.

11. Mortensen SA, Vadhanavikit S, Muratsu K, et al. Coenzyme Q10: clinical benefits with biochemical correlates suggesting a scientific breakthrough in the management of chronic heart failure. *Int J Tissue React.* 1990;12:155–162.

12. Folkers K. Basic chemical research on coenzyme Q10 and integrated clinical research on therapy of diseases. In: Lenaz G, ed. *Coenzyme Q: Biochemistry, Bioenergetics, and Clinical Applications of Ubiquinone.* New York, NY: Wiley; 1985.

13. Liu P, Luo HC, Shen YC, et al. Combined use of Ginkgo biloba extracts on the efficacy and adverse reactions of various antipsychotics [translated from Chinese]. *Chin J Clin Pharmacol.* 1997;13:193–198.

14. Palasciano G, Portincasa P, Palmieri V, et al. The effect of silymarin on plasma levels of malon-dialdehyde in patients receiving long-term treatment with psychotropic drugs. *Curr Ther Res*. 1994;55:537–545.

15. Soares KV, McGrath JJ. The treatment of tardive dyskinesia—a systematic review and meta-analysis. *Schizophr Res*. 1999;39:1–18.

16. Barak Y, Swartz M, Shamir E, et al. Vitamin E (alpha-tocopherol) in the treatment of tardive dyskinesia: a statistical meta-analysis. *Ann Clin Psychiatry*. 1998;10:101–105.

17. Boomershine KH, Shelton PS, Boomershine JE. Vitamin E in the treatment of tardive dyskinesia. *Ann Pharmacother*. 1999;33:1195–1202.

18. Gupta S, Mosnik D, Black DW, et al. Tardive dyskinesia: review of treatments past, present, and future. *Ann Clin Psychiatry*. 1999;11:257–266.

19. Adler LA, Edson R, Lavori P, et al. Long-term treatment effects of vitamin E for tardive dyskinesia. *Biol Psychiatry*. 1998;43:868–872.

20. Adler LA, Edson R, Lavori P, et al. Long-term treatment effects of vitamin E for tardive dyskinesia. *Biol Psychiatry*. 1998;43:868–872.

AZOLE ANTIFUNGAL AGENTS

1. *A to Z Drug Facts* [book on CD-ROM]. 2nd ed. St. Louis, Mo: Facts and Comparisons; 2000.

2. *A to Z Drug Facts* [book on CD-ROM]. 2nd ed. St. Louis, Mo: Facts and Comparisons; 2000.

3. Takanaga H, Ohnishi A, Murakami H, et al. Relationship between time after intake of grapefruit juice and the effect on pharmacokinetics and pharmacodynamics of nisoldipine in healthy subjects. *Clin Pharmacol Ther*. 2000;67:201–214.

BENZODIAZEPINES

1. *A to Z Drug Facts* [book on CD-ROM]. 2nd ed. St. Louis, Mo: Facts and Comparisons; 2000.

2. Takanaga H, Ohnishi A, Murakami H, et al. Relationship between time after intake of grapefruit juice and the effect on pharmacokinetics and pharmacodynamics of nisoldipine in healthy subjects. *Clin Pharmacol Ther*. 2000;67:201–214.

3. Almeida JC, Grimsley EW. Coma from the health food store: interaction between kava and alprazolam. *Ann Intern Med*. 1996;125:940–941.

Notes

4. Jussofie A, Schmiz A, Hiemke C. Kavapyrone enriched extract from *Piper methysticum* as modulator of the GABA binding site in different regions of rat brain. *Psychopharmacology (Berl).* 1994;116:469–474.

5. Boonen G, Haberlein H. Influence of genuine kavapyrone enantiomers of the GABA-A binding site. *Planta Med.* 1998;64:504–506.

6. Boonen G, Ferger B, Kuschinsky K,et al. In vivo effects of the kavapyrones (+)-dihydromethysticin and (+/-)-kavain on dopamine, 3,4-dihydroxyphenylacetic acid, serotonin and 5-hydroxyindoleacetic acid levels in striatal and cortical brain regions. *Planta Med.* 1998;64:507–510.

7. Garfinkel D, Zisapel N, Wainstein J, et al. Facilitation of benzodiazepine discontinuation by melatonin: a new clinical approach. *Arch Intern Med.* 1999;159:2456–2460.

BETA-BLOCKERS

1. Kirch W, Schafer-Korting M, Axthelm T, et al. Interaction of atenolol with furosemide and calcium and aluminum salts. *Clin Pharmacol Ther.* 1981;4:429–435.

2. Roeback JR Jr, Hla KM, Chambless LE, et al. Effects of chromium supplementation on serum high-density lipoprotein cholesterol levels in men taking beta-blockers. A randomized, controlled trial. *Ann Intern Med.* 1991;115:917–924.

3. Mortensen SA, Leth A, Agner E, et al. Dose-related decrease of serum coenzyme Q10 during treatment with HMG-CoA reductase inhibitors. *Mol Aspects Med.* 1997;18(suppl):S137–S144.

4. Ghirlanda G, Oradei A, Manto A, et al. Evidence of plasma CoQ10-lowering effect by HMG-CoA reductase inhibitors: a double-blind, placebo-controlled study. *J Clin Pharmacol.* 1993;33:226–229.

5. Mortensen SA, Vadhanavikit S, Muratsu K, et al. Coenzyme Q10: clinical benefits with biochemical correlates suggesting a scientific breakthrough in the management of chronic heart failure. *Int J Tissue React.* 1990;12:155–162.

6. Kishi T, Watanabe T, Folkers K. Bioenergetics in clinical medicine XV. Inhibition of coenzyme Q10-enzymes by clinically used adrenergic blockers of beta-receptors. *Res Commun Chem Pathol Pharmacol.* 1977;17:157–164.

7. Kishi H, Kishi T, Folkers K. Bioenergetics in clinical medicine. III. Inhibition of coenzyme Q10-enzymes by clinically used anti-hypertensive drugs. *Res Commun Chem Pathol Pharmacol.* 1975;12:533–540.

Notes

8. Hamada M, Kazatain Y, Ochi T, et al. Correlation between serum CoQ10 level and myocardial contractility in hypertensive patients. *Biomed Clin Aspects Coenzyme Q.* 1984;4:263–270.

9. Kishi H, Kishi T, Folkers K. Bioenergetics in clinical medicine. III. Inhibition of coenzyme Q10-enzymes by clinically used anti-hypertensive drugs. *Res Commun Chem Pathol Pharmacol.* 1975;12:533–540.

BILE ACID SEQUESTRANTS

1. Hoppner K, Lampi B. Bioavailability of folate following ingestion of cholestyramine in the rat. *Int J Vitam Nutr Res.* 1991;61:130–134.

2. West RJ, Lloyd JK. The effect of cholestyramine on intestinal absorption. *Gut.* 1975;16:93–98.

3. West RJ, Lloyd JK. The effect of cholestyramine on intestinal absorption. *Gut.* 1975;16:93–98.

4. Hoppner K, Lampi B. Bioavailability of folate following ingestion of cholestyramine in the rat. *Int J Vitam Nutr Res.* 1991;61:130–134.

5. West RJ, Lloyd JK. The effect of cholestyramine on intestinal absorption. *Gut.* 1975;16:93–98.

6. West RJ, Lloyd JK. The effect of cholestyramine on intestinal absorption. *Gut.* 1975;16:93–98.

BISPHOSPHONATES

1. Fleisch H. Experimental basis for the use of bisphosphonates in Paget's disease of bone. *Clin Orthop.* 1987;217:72–78.

BROMOCRIPTINE (PARLODEL)

1. Jarry H, Leonhardt S, Wuttke W. Agnus castus as a dopaminergic active principle in Mastodynon® N [in German; English abstract]. *Z Phytother.* 1991;12:77–82.

2. Jarry H, Leonhardt S, Gorkow C, et al. In vitro prolactin but not LH and FSH release is inhibited by compounds in extracts of Agnus castus: direct evidence for a dopaminergic principle by the dopamine receptor assay. *Exp Clin Endocrinol.* 1994;102:448–454.

3. Milewicz A, Gejdel E, Sworen H, et al. *Vitex agnus castus* extract in the treatment of luteal phase defects due to latent hyperprolactinemia. Results of a randomized placebo-controlled double-blind study [translated from German]. *Arzneimittelforschung.* 1993;43:752–756.

Notes

4. Sliutz G, Speiser P, Schultz AM, et al. *Agnus castus* extracts inhibit prolactin secretion of rat pituitary cells. *Horm Metab Res*. 1993;25:253–255.

5. Winterhoff H. Influences on thyroid and ovary function [translated from German]. *Z Phytother*. 1993;14:83–94.

6. Wuttke W. Dopaminergic compounds in *Vitex agnus castus*. In: Lowe D ed. *Phytopharmaka: Forschung und klinische Anwendung*. Darmstadt, Germany: Steinkopff; 1996:81–91.

CALCIUM-CHANNEL BLOCKERS

1. Guadagnino V, Greengart A, Hollander G, et al. Treatment of severe left ventricular dysfunction with calcium chloride in patients receiving verapamil. *J Clin Pharmacol*. 1987;27:407–409.

2. Salerno DM, Anderson B, Sharkey PJ, et al. Intravenous verapamil for treatment of multifocal atrial tachycardia with and without calcium pretreatment. *Ann Intern Med*. 1987;107:623–628.

3. Luscher TF, Noll G, Sturmer T, et al. Calcium gluconate in severe verapamil intoxication. *N Engl J Med*. 1994;330:718–720.

4. Orr GM, Bodansky HJ, Dymond DS, et al. Fatal verapamil overdose. *Lancet*. 1982;2:1218–1219.

5. Bar-Or D, Gasiel Y. Calcium and calciferol antagonize effect of verapamil in atrial fibrillation. *Br Med J (Clin Res Ed)*. 1981;282:1585–1586.

6. *A to Z Drug Facts* [book on CD-ROM]. 2nd ed. St. Louis, Mo: Facts and Comparisons; 2000.

7. Takanaga H, Ohnishi A, Murakami H, et al. Relationship between time after intake of grapefruit juice and the effect on pharmacokinetics and pharmacodynamics of nisoldipine in healthy subjects. *Clin Pharmacol Ther*. 2000;67:201–214.

CARBAMAZEPINE

1. Arenz A, Klein M, Fiehe K. Occurrence of neurotoxic 4'-O-methylpyridoxine in *Ginkgo biloba* leaves, ginkgo medications and Japanese ginkgo food. *Planta Med*. 1996;62:548–551.

2. Mizuno N, Kawakami K, Morita E. Competitive inhibition between 4'-substituted pyridoxine analogues and pyridoxal for pyridoxal kinase from mouse brain. *J Nutr Sci Vitaminol (Tokyo)*. 1980;26:535–543.

3. Wada K, Ishigaki S, Ueda K, et al. An antivitamin B6, 4'-methoxypyridoxine, from the seed of *Ginkgo biloba* L. *Chem Pharm Bull (Tokyo)*. 1985;33:3555–3557.

4. Yagi M, Wada K, Sakata M, et al. Studies on the constituents of edible and medicinal plants. IV. Determination of 4-O-methylpyridoxine in serum of the patient with gin-nan food poisoning [in Japanese; English abstract]. *Yakugaku Zasshi*. 1993;113:596–599.

5. Arenz A, Klein M, Fiehe K. Occurrence of neurotoxic 4'-O-methylpyridoxine in *Ginkgo biloba* leaves, ginkgo medications and Japanese ginkgo food. *Planta Med*. 1996;62:548–551.

6. *A to Z Drug Facts* [book on CD-ROM]. 2nd ed. St. Louis, Mo: Facts and Comparisons; 2000.

7. Takanaga H, Ohnishi A, Murakami H, et al. Relationship between time after intake of grapefruit juice and the effect on pharmacokinetics and pharmacodynamics of nisoldipine in healthy subjects. *Clin Pharmacol Ther*. 2000;67:201–214.

8. Monostory K, Vereczkey L, Levai F, et al. Ipriflavone as an inhibitor of human cytochrome P450 enzymes. *Br J Pharmacol*. 1998;123:605–610.

9. Almeida JC, Grimsley EW. Coma from the health food store: interaction between kava and alprazolam. *Ann Intern Med*. 1996;125:940–941.

10. Bourgeois BF, Dodson WE, Ferrendelli JA. Interactions between primidone, carbamazepine, and nicotinamide. *Neurology*. 1982;32:1122–1126.

11. Bourgeois BF, Dodson WE, Ferrendelli JA. Interactions between primidone, carbamazepine, and nicotinamide. *Neurology*. 1982;32:1122–1126.

12. Krause KH, Bonjour JP, Berlit P, et al. Biotin status of epileptics. *Ann N Y Acad Sci*. 1985;447:297–313.

13. Said HM, Redha R, Nylander W. Biotin transport in the human intestine: inhibition by anticonvulsant drugs. *Am J Clin Nutr*. 1989;49:127–131.

14. Kishi T, Fujita N, Eguchi T, et al. Mechanism for reduction of serum folate by antiepileptic drugs during prolonged therapy. *J Neurol Sci*. 1997;145:109–112.

15. Kishi T, Fujita N, Eguchi T, et al. Mechanism for reduction of serum folate by antiepileptic drugs during prolonged therapy. *J Neurol Sci*. 1997;145:109–112.

16. Reynolds EH. Mental effects of anticonvulsants, and folic acid metabolism. *Brain*. 1968;91:197–214.

17. Berg MJ, Stumbo PJ, Chenard CA, et al. Folic acid improves phenytoin pharmacokinetics. *J Am Diet Assoc.* 1995;95:352–56.

18. Lewis DP, Van Dyke DC, Willhite LA, et al. Phenytoin-folic acid interaction. *Ann Pharmacother.* 1995;29:726–735.

19. Lewis DP, Van Dyke DC, Stumbo PJ, et al. Drug and environmental factors associated with adverse pregnancy outcomes. Part I: Antiepileptic drugs, contraceptives, smoking, and folate. *Ann Pharmacother.* 1998;32:802–817.

20. Ono H, Sakamoto A, Eguchi T, et al. Plasma total homocysteine concentrations in epileptic patients taking anticonvulsants. *Metabolism.* 1997;46:959–962.

21. Lewis DP, Van Dyke DC, Stumbo PJ, et al. Drug and environmental factors associated with adverse pregnancy outcomes. Part I: Antiepileptic drugs, contraceptives, smoking, and folate. *Ann Pharmacother.* 1998;32:802–817.

22. Wahl TO, Gobuty AH, Lukert BP. Long-term anticonvulsant therapy and intestinal calcium absorption. *Clin Pharmacol Ther.* 1981;30:506–512.

23. Weinstein RS, Bryce GF, Sappington LJ, et al. Decreased serum ionized calcium and normal vitamin D metabolite levels with anticonvulsant drug treatment. *J Clin Endocrinol Metab.* 1984;58:1003–1009.

24. Weinstein RS, Bryce GF, Sappington LJ, et al. Decreased serum ionized calcium and normal vitamin D metabolite levels with anticonvulsant drug treatment. *J Clin Endocrinol Metab.* 1984;58:1003–1009.

25. Carter BL, Garnett WR, Pellock JM, et al. Effect of antacids on phenytoin bioavailability. *Ther Drug Monit.* 1981;3:333–340.

26. McElnay JC, Uprichard G, Collier PS. The effect of activated dimethicone and a proprietary antacid preparation containing this agent on the absorption of phenytoin. *Br J Clin Pharmacol.* 1982;13:501–505.

27. De Vivo DC, Bohan TP, Coulter DL, et al. L-carnitine supplementation in childhood epilepsy: current perspectives. *Epilepsia.* 1998;39:1216–1225.

28. Coulter DL. Carnitine deficiency: a possible mechanism for valproate hepatotoxicity [letter]. *Lancet.* 1984;1:689.

29. Ater SB. et al. A developmental center population treated with VPA and L-carnitine. In: Update: inborn errors of metabolism in the patient with epilepsy. Sigma-Tau Pharmaceuticals; 1993.

30. Dreifuss FE, Langer DH. Hepatic considerations in the use of antiepileptic drugs. *Epilepsia.* 1987;28(suppl 2):S23–S29.

Notes

31. Ater SB, et al. A developmental center population treated with VPA and L-carnitine. In: Update: inborn errors of metabolism in the patient with epilepsy. Sigma-Tau Pharmaceuticals; 1993.

32. Freeman JM, Vining EP, Cost S, et al. Does carnitine administration improve the symptoms attributed to anticonvulsant medications? A double-blinded, crossover study. *Pediatrics*. 1994;93:893–895.

33. De Vivo DC, Bohan TP, Coulter DL, et al. L-carnitine supplementation in childhood epilepsy: current perspectives. *Epilepsia*. 1998;39:1216–1225.

34. Hahn TJ, Hendin BA, Scharp CR, et al. Effect of chronic anticonvulsant therapy on serum 25-hydroxycalciferol levels in adults. *N Engl J Med*. 1972;287:900–904.

35. Hahn TJ, Hendin BA, Scharp CR, et al. Effect of chronic anticonvulsant therapy on serum 25-hydroxycalciferol levels in adults. *N Engl J Med*. 1972;287:900–904.

36. Jubiz W, Haussler MR, McCain TA, et al. Plasma 1,25-dihydroxyvitamin D levels in patients receiving anticonvulsant drugs. *J Clin Endocrinol Metab*. 1977;44:617–621.

37. Brodie MJ, Boobis AR, Dollery CT, et al. Rifampicin and vitamin D metabolism. *Clin Pharmacol Ther*. 1980;27:810–814.

38. Williams C, Netzloff M, Folkerts L, et al. Vitamin D metabolism and anticonvulsant therapy: effect of sunshine on incidence of osteomalacia. *South Med J*. 1984;77:834–836, 842.

39. Cornelissen M, Steegers-Theunissen R, Kollee, L, et al. Increased incidence of neonatal vitamin K deficiency resulting from maternal anticonvulsant therapy. *Am J Obstet Gynecol*. 1993;168:923–928.

40. Cornelissen M, Steegers-Theunissen R, Kollee L, et al. Supplementation of vitamin K in pregnant women receiving anticonvulsant therapy prevents neonatal vitamin K deficiency. *Am J Obstet Gynecol*. 1993;168:884–888.

CEPHALOSPORINS

1. Cohen H, Scott SD, Mackie IJ, et al. The development of hypoprothrombinaemia following antibiotic therapy in malnourished patients with low serum vitamin K1 levels. *Br J Haematol*. 1988;68:63–66.

2. Lipsky JJ. Nutritional sources of vitamin K. *Mayo Clin Proc*. 1994;69:462–466.

3. Cohen H, Scott SD, Mackie IJ, et al. The development of hypoprothrombinaemia following antibiotic therapy in malnourished patients with low serum vitamin K1 levels. *Br J Haematol*. 1988;68:63–66.

4. Shearer MJ, Bechtold H, Andrassy K, et al. Mechanism of cephalosporin-induced hypoprothrombinemia: relation to cephalosporin side chain, vitamin K metabolism, and vitamin K status. *J Clin Pharmacol*. 1988;28:88–95.

5. Goss TF, Walawander CA, Grasela TH Jr, et al. Prospective evaluation of risk factors for antibiotic-associated bleeding in critically ill patients. *Pharmacotherapy*. 1992;12:283–291.

6. Allison PM, Mummah-Schendal LL, Kindberg CG, et. al. Effects of a vitamin K-deficient diet and antibiotics in normal human volunteers. *J Lab Clin Med*. 1987;110:180–188.

CISPLATIN

1. Sommer S, Thorling EB, Jakobsen A, et al. Can bismuth decrease the kidney toxic effect of cis-platinum? *Eur J Cancer Clin Oncol*. 1989;25:1903–1904.

2. Zhang JG, Lindup WE. Role of mitochondria in cisplatin-induced oxidative damage exhibited by rat renal cortical slices. *Biochem Pharmacol*. 1993;45:2215–2222.

3. Tedeschi M, DE Cesare A, Oriana S, et al. The role of glutathione in combination with cisplatin in the treatment of ovarian cancer. *Cancer Treat Rev*. 1991;18:253–259.

4. Di Re F, Bohm S, Oriana S, et al. High-dose cisplatin and cyclophosphamide with glutathione in the treatment of advanced ovarian cancer. *Ann Oncol*. 1993;4:55–61.

5. Plaxe S, Freddo J, Kim S, et al. Phase I trial of cisplatin in combination with glutathione *Gynecol Oncol*. 1994;55:82–86.

6. Di Re F, Bohm S, Oriana S, et al. High-dose cisplatin and cyclophosphamide with glutathione in the treatment of advanced ovarian cancer. *Ann Oncol*. 1993;4:55–61.

7. Parnis FX, Coleman RE, Harper PG, et al. A randomised double-blind placebo controlled clinical trial assessing the tolerability and efficacy of glutathione as an adjuvant to escalating doses of cisplatin in the treatment of advanced ovarian cancer. *Eur J Cancer*. 1995;31A:1721.

8. Bianchetti MG, Kanaka C, Ridolfi-Luthy A, et al. Chronic renal magnesium loss, hypocalciuria and mild hypokalaemic metabolic alkalosis

after cisplatin. *Pediatr Nephrol.* 1990;4:219–222.

9. Vogelzang NJ, Torkelson JL, Kennedy BJ. Hypomagnesemia, renal dysfunction, and Raynaud's phenomenon in patients treated with cisplatin, vinblastine, and bleomycin. *Cancer.* 1985;56:2765–2770.

10. Icli F, Karaoguz H, Dincol D, et al. Severe vascular toxicity associated with cisplatin-based chemotherapy. *Cancer.* 1993;72:587–593.

11. Vogelzang NJ, Torkelson JL, Kennedy BJ. Hypomagnesemia, renal dysfunction, and Raynaud's phenomenon in patients treated with cisplatin, vinblastine, and bleomycin. *Cancer.* 1985;56:2765–2770.

12. Willox JC, McAllister EJ, Sangster G, et al. Effects of magnesium supplementation in testicular cancer patients receiving cis-platin: a randomised trial. *Br J Cancer.* 1986;54:19–23.

13. Rodriguez M, Solanki DL, Whang R. Refractory potassium repletion due to cisplatin-induced magnesium depletion. *Arch Intern Med.* 1989;149:2592–2594.

14. Whang R, Whang DD, Ryan MP. Refractory potassium repletion. A consequence of magnesium deficiency. *Arch Intern Med.* 1992;152:40–45.

15. Hu YJ, Chen Y, Zhang YQ, et al. The protective role of selenium on the toxicity of cisplatin-contained chemotherapy regimen in cancer patients. *Biol Trace Elem Res.* 1997;56:331–341.

16. Satoh M, Naganuma A, Imura N. Deficiency of selenium intake enhances manifestation of renal toxicity of cis-diamminedichloroplatinum in mice. *Toxicol Lett.* 1987;38:155–160.

17. Satoh M, Naganuma A, Imura N. Effect of coadministration of selenite on the toxicity and antitumor activity of cis-diamminedichloroplatinum (II) given repeatedly to mice. *Cancer Chemother Pharmacol.* 1992;30:439–443.

18. Ohkawa K, Tsukada Y, Dohzono H, et al. The effects of co-administration of selenium and cis-platin (CDDP) on CDDP-induced toxicity and antitumour activity. *Br J Cancer.* 1988;58:38–41.

19. Baldew GS, McVie JG, van der Valk MA, et al. Selective reduction of cis-diamminedichloroplatinum(II) nephrotoxicity by ebselen. *Cancer Res.* 1990;50:7031–7036.

20. Berry JP, Pauwells C, Tlouzeau S, et al. Effect of selenium in combination with cis-diamminedichloroplatinum(II) in the treatment of murine fibrosarcoma. *Cancer Res.* 1984;44:2864–2868.

Notes

21. Satoh M, Naganuma A, Imura N. Effect of coadministration of selenite on the toxicity and antitumor activity of cis-diamminedichloroplatinum (II) given repeatedly to mice. *Cancer Chemother Pharmacol.* 1992;30:439–443.

22. Sugihara K, Gemba M. Modification of cisplatin toxicity by antioxidants. *Jpn J Pharmacol.* 1986;40:353–355.

23. Bogin E, Marom M, Levi Y. Changes in serum, liver and kidneys of cisplatin-treated rats; effects of antioxidants. *Eur J Clin Chem Clin Biochem.* 1994;32:843–851.

24. Wadleigh RG, Redman RS, Graham ML, et al. Vitamin E in the treatment of chemotherapy-induced mucositis *Am J Med.* 1992;92:481–484.

25. Lopez I, Goudou C, Ribrag V, et al. Therapy of mucositis with vitamin E during administration of neutropenic antineoplastic agents [translated from French]. *Ann Med Interne (Paris).* 1994;145:405–408.

26. Gaedeke J, Fels LM, Bokemeyer C, et al. Cisplatin nephrotoxicity and protection by silibinin. *Nephrol Dial Transplant.* 1996;11:55–62.

27. Gemba M, Fukuishi N. Amelioration by ascorbic acid of cisplatin-induced injury in cultured renal epithelial cells. *Contrib Nephrol.* 1991;95:138–142.

28. Appenroth D, Winnefeld J, Schroter H, et al. Beneficial effect of acetylcysteine on cisplatin nephrotoxicity in rats. *J Appl Toxicol.* 1993;13:189–192.

29. Inselmann G, Blohmer A, Kottny W, et al. Modification of cisplatin-induced renal p-aminohippurate uptake alteration and lipid peroxidation by thiols, *Ginkgo biloba* extract, deferoxamine and torbafylline. *Nephron.* 1995;70,425–429.

CLONIDINE

1. *Review of Natural Products.* St. Louis, Mo: Facts and Comparisons; 1993: Yohimbe monograph.

2. *Review of Natural Products.* St. Louis, Mo: Facts and Comparisons; 1999:Yohimbe monograph.

3. Goldstein DS, Grossman E, Listwak S, et al. Sympathetic reactivity during a yohimbine challenge test in essential hypertension. *Hypertension.* 1991;18(5 suppl 3):III40–III48.

Notes

4. Hoffmann BB, Lefkowitz RJ. Catecholamines, sympathomimetic drugs, and adrenergic receptor antagonists. In: Hardman JG, Limbird LE, eds. *Goodman & Gilman's The Pharmacological Basis of Therapeutics*. 9th ed. New York, NY: McGraw-Hill, Health Professions Division; 1996:100–248.

5. Charney DS, Heninger GR, Sternberg DE. Assessment of alpha 2 adrenergic autoreceptor function in humans: effects of oral yohimbine. *Life Sci*. 1982;30:2033–2041.

6. De Smet PA, Smeets OS. Potential risks of health food products containing yohimbe extracts. *BMJ*. 1994;309:958.

COLCHICINE

1. Webb DI, Chodos RB, Mahar CQ, et al. Mechanism of vitamin B12 malabsorption in patients receiving colchicine. *N Engl J Med*. 1968;279:845–850.

CORTICOSTEROIDS (GLUCOCORTICOIDS)

1. Tamura Y, Nishikawa T, Yamada K, et al. Effects of glycyrrhetinic acid and its derivatives on delta-4-5-alpha- and 5-beta-reductase in rat liver. *Arzneimittelforschung*. 1979;29:647–649.

2. Chen MF, Shimada F, Kato H, et al. Effect of glycyrrhizin on the pharmacokinetics of prednisolone following low dosage of prednisolone hemisuccinate. *Endocrinol Jpn*. 1990;37:331–341.

3. Kumagai A, Nanaboshi M, Asanuma Y, et al. Effects of glycyrrhizin on thymolytic and immunosuppressive action of cortisone. *Endocrinol Jpn*. 1967;14:39–42.

4. Chen MF, Shimada F, Kato H, et al. Effect of glycyrrhizin on the pharmacokinetics of prednisolone following low dosage of prednisolone hemisuccinate. *Endocrinol Jpn*. 1990;37:331–341.

5. Tamura Y, Nishikawa T, Yamada K, et al. Effects of glycyrrhetinic acid and its derivatives on delta-4-5-alpha- and 5-beta-reductase in rat liver. *Arzneimittelforschung*. 1979;29:647–649.

6. Shintani, Murase H, Tsukagoshi H, et al. Glycyrrhizin (licorice)-induced hypokalemic myopathy. Report of 2 cases and review of the literature. *Eur Neurol*. 1992;32:44–51.

7. Blachley JD, Knochel JP. Tobacco chewer's hypokalemia: licorice revisited. *N Engl J Med*. 1980;302:784–785.

8. Ravina A, Slezak L, Mirsky N, et al. Control of steroid-induced diabetes with supplemental chromium. *J Trace Elem Exp Med*. 1999;12:375–378.

9. Anderson RA, Cheng N, Bryden NA, et al. Elevated intakes of supplemental chromium improve glucose and insulin variables in individuals with type 2 diabetes. *Diabetes*. 1997;46:1786–1791.

10. Ravina A, Slezack L. Chromium in the treatment of clinical diabetes mellitus [translated from Hebrew]. *Harefuah*. 1993;125:142–145.

11. Jovanovic L, Gutierrez M, Peterson CM. Chromium supplementation for women with gestational diabetes mellitus. *J Trace Elem Exp Med*. 1999;12:91–97.

12. Buckley LM, Leib ES, Cartularo KS, et al. Calcium and vitamin D_3 supplementation prevents bone loss in the spine secondary to low-dose corticosteroids in patients with rheumatoid arthritis. A randomized, double-blind, placebo-controlled trial. *Ann Intern Med*. 1996;125:961–968.

13. Homik J, Suarez-Almazor ME; Shea B, et al. Calcium and vitamin D for corticosteroid-induced osteoporosis. *Cochrane Database Syst Rev*. 2000;30:1–9.

14. Reid IR, Ibbertson HK. Calcium supplements in the prevention of steroid-induced osteoporosis. *Am J Clin Nutr*. 1986;44:287–290.

15. Adachi JD, Bensen WG, Bianchi F, et al. Vitamin D and calcium in the prevention of corticosteroid induced osteoporosis: a 3 year followup. *J Rheumatol*. 1996;23:995–1000.

16. Robinzon B, Cutolo M. Should dehydroepiandrosterone replacement therapy be provided with glucocorticoids? *Rheumatology*. 1999;38:488–495.

17. van Vollenhoven RF, Park JL, Genovese MC, et al. A double-blind, placebo-controlled, clinical trial of dehydroepiandrosterone in severe systemic lupus erythematosus. *Lupus*. 1999;8:181–187.

18. Davis RH, Parker WL, Murdoch DP. *Aloe vera* as a biologically active vehicle for hydrocortisone acetate. *J Am Podiatr Med Assoc*. 1991;81:1–9.

19. Teelucksingh S, Mackie AD, Burt D, et al. Potentiation of hydrocortisone activity in skin by glycyrrhetinic acid. *Lancet*. 1990;335:1060–1063.

20. Davis RH, Parker WL, Murdoch DP. *Aloe vera* as a biologically active vehicle for hydrocortisone acetate. *J Am Podiatr Med Assoc*. 1991;81:1–9.

21. Teelucksingh S, Mackie AD, Burt D, et al. Potentiation of hydrocortisone activity in skin by glycyrrhetinic acid. *Lancet*. 1990;335:1060–1063.

Notes

CYCLOSPORINE

1. *A to Z Drug Facts* [book on CD-ROM]. 2nd ed. St. Louis, Mo: Facts and Comparisons; 2000.

2. Takanaga H, Ohnishi A, Murakami H, et al. Relationship between time after intake of grapefruit juice and the effect on pharmacokinetics and pharmacodynamics of nisoldipine in healthy subjects. *Clin Pharmacol Ther*. 2000;67:201–214.

3. Ernst E. Second thoughts about safety of St. John's wort. *Lancet*. 1999;354:2014–2016.

4. Guengerich FP. Cytochrome P-450 3A4: regulation and role in drug metabolism. *Annu Rev Pharmacol Toxicol*. 1999;39:1–17.

5. Ruschitzka F, Meier PJ, Turina M, et al. Acute heart transplant rejection due to Saint John's wort [letter]. *Lancet*. 2000;355:548–549.

6. Breidenbach T, Hoffmann MW, Becker T, et al. Drug interaction of St John's wort with cyclosporin. *Lancet*. 2000;355:1912.

DIGOXIN

1. Perez Gutierrez RM, Laguna GY, Walkowski A. Diuretic activity of Mexican equisetum. *J Ethnopharmacol*. 1985;14:269–272.

2. Walker BR, Edwards CR. Licorice-induced hypertension and syndromes of apparent mineralocorticoid excess. *Endocrinol Metab Clin North Am*. 1994;23:359–377.

3. Epstein MT, Espiner EA, Donald RA, et al. Liquorice toxicity and the renin-angiotensin-aldosterone axis in man. *Br Med J*. 1977;1:209–210.

4. Wash LK, Bernard JD. Licorice-induced pseudoaldosteronism. *Am J Hosp Pharm*. 1975;32:73–74.

5. de Klerk GJ, Nieuwenhuis MG, Beutler JJ. Hypokalemia and hypertension associated with use of liquorice flavoured chewing gum. *BMJ*. 1997;314:731–732.

6. Corsi FM, Galgani S, Gasparini C, et al. Acute hypokalemic myopathy due to chronic licorice ingestion: report of a case. *Ital J Neurol Sci*. 1983;4:493–497.

7. Walker BR, Edwards CR. Licorice-induced hypertension and syndromes of apparent mineralocorticoid excess. *Endocrinol Metab Clin North Am*. 1994;23:359–377.

8. Epstein MT, Espiner EA, Donald RA, et al. Liquorice toxicity and the renin-angiotensin-aldosterone axis in man. *Br Med J*. 1977;1:209–210.

9. Blachley JD, Knochel JP. Tobacco chewer's hypokalemia: licorice revisited. *N Engl J Med.* 1980;302:784–785.

10. McRae S. Elevated serum digoxin levels in a patient taking digoxin and Siberian ginseng. *Can Med Assoc J.* 1996;155:293–295.

11. Maurer A. Interaction of St. John's wort extract with phenprocoumon. *Eur J Clin Pharmacol.* 1999;55:A22.

12. Yue QY, Bergquist C, Gerden B. Safety of St. John's wort [letter]. *Lancet.* 2000;355:576–577.

13. Kupfer S, Kosovsky JD. Effects of cardiac glycosides on renal tubular transport of calcium, magnesium, inorganic phosphate, and glucose in the dog. *J Clin Invest.* 1965;44:1132–1143.

14. Whang R, Oei TO, Watanabe A. Frequency of hypomagnesemia in hospitalized patients receiving digitalis. *Arch Intern Med.* 1985;145:655–656.

15. Toffaletti J. Electrolytes, divalent cations, and blood gases (magnesium). *Anal Chem.* 1991;63:192R–194R.

16. Landauer JA. Magnesium deficiency and digitalis toxicity [letter]. *JAMA.* 1984;251:730.

17. Cohen L, Kitzes R. Magnesium sulfate and digitalis-toxic arrhythmias. *JAMA.* 1983;249:2808–2810.

18. Brown DD, Juhl RP. Decreased bioavailability of digoxin due to antacids and kaolin-pectin. *N Engl J Med.* 1976;295;1034–1037.

ESTROGEN

1. King DS, Sharp RL, Vukovich MD, et al. Effect of oral androstenedione on serum testosterone and adaptations to resistance training in young men: a randomized controlled trial. *JAMA.* 1999;281:2020–2028.

2. Leder, BZ;, Longcope C, Caitlin DH, et al. Oral androstenedione administration and serum testosterone concentrations in young men. *JAMA.* 2000;283:779–782.

3. Ballantyne CS, Phillips SM, MacDonald JR, et al. The acute effects of androstenedione supplementation in healthy young males. *Can J Appl Physiol.* 2000;25:68–78.

4. Nielsen FH, Hunt CD, Mullen LM, et al. Effect of dietary boron on mineral, estrogen, and testosterone metabolism in postmenopausal women. *FASEB J.* 1987;1:394–397.

Notes

5. Naghii MR, Samman S. The effect of boron supplementation on its urinary excretion and selected cardiovascular risk factors in healthy male subjects. *Biol Trace Elem Res.* 1997;56:273–286.

6. Wilbur P. The phyto-oestrogen debate. *Eur J Herbal Med.* 1996;2:20–26.

7. Hirata JD, Swiersz LM, Zell B, et al. Does dong quai have estrogenic effects in postmenopausal women? A double-blind, placebo-controlled trial. *Fertil Steril.* 1997;68:981–986.

8. *A to Z Drug Facts* [book on CD-ROM]. 2nd ed. St. Louis, Mo: Facts and Comparisons; 2000.

9. Takanaga H, Ohnishi A, Murakami H, et al. Relationship between time after intake of grapefruit juice and the effect on pharmacokinetics and pharmacodynamics of nisoldipine in healthy subjects. *Clin Pharmacol Ther.* 2000;67:201–214.

10. Choi YK, Han IK, Yoon HK. Ipriflavone for the treatment of osteoporosis. *Osteoporos Int.* 1997;7(suppl 3):S174–S178.

11. de Aloysio D, Gambacciani M, Altieri P, et al. Bone density changes in postmenopausal women with the administration of ipriflavone alone or in association with low-dose ERT. *Gynecol Endocrinol.* 1997;11:289–293.

12. Gambacciani M, Ciaponi M, Cappagli B, et al. Effects of combined low dose of the isoflavone derivative ipriflavone and estrogen replacement on bone mineral density and metabolism in postmenopausal women. *Maturitas.* 1997;28:75–81.

13. Melis GB, Paoletti AM, Bartolini R, et al. Ipriflavone and low doses of estrogens in the prevention of bone mineral loss in climacterium. *Bone Miner.* 1992;19(suppl 1):S49–S56.

14. Nozaki M, Hashimoto K, Inoue Y, et al. Treatment of bone loss in oophorectomized women with a combination of ipriflavone and conjugated equine estrogen. *Int J Gynaecol Obstet.* 1998;62:69–75.

15. Petilli M, Fiorelli G, Benevenuti S, et al. Interactions between ipriflavone and the estrogen receptor. *Calcif Tissue Int.* 1995;56:160–165.

16. Cecchini MG, Fleisch H, Muhibauer RC. Ipriflavone inhibits bone resorption in intact and ovariectomized rats. *Calcif Tissue Int.* 1997;61(suppl 1):S9–S11.

17. Osteoporosis Prevention, Diagnosis, and Therapy. National Institutes of Health. Consensus Development Conference Statement. March 27–29, 2000.

18. Seelig MS. Interrelationship of magnesium and estrogen in cardiovascular and bone disorders, eclampsia, migraine, and premenstrual syndrome. *J Am Coll Nutr.* 1993;12:442–458.

Notes

19. Blum M, Kitai E, Ariel Y, et al. Oral contraceptive lowers serum magnesium [translated from Hebrew]. *Harefuah.* 1991;121:363–364.

20. Blum M, Kitai E, Ariel Y, et al. Oral contraceptive lowers serum magnesium [translated from Hebrew]. *Harefuah.* 1991;121:363–364.

ETHAMBUTOL

1. Solecki TJ, Aviv A, Bogden JD. Effect of a chelating drug on balance and tissue distribution of four essential metals. *Toxicology.* 1984;31:207–216.

ETOPOSIDE

1. Baker RK, Brandt TL, Siegel D, et al. Inhibition of DNA topoisomerase II-alpha activity by hypericin [abstract]. *Proc Am Assoc Cancer Res.* 1998;39:422.

2. Peebles KA. Catalytic inhibition of DNA topoisomerase IIa by hypericin, a naphthodianthrone from St. John's wort (*Hypericum perforatum*). *Biochem Pharmacol.* Not yet published.

FLUOROQUINOLONES

1. Zhu M, Wong PY, Li RC. Effect of oral administration of fennel (*Foeniculum vulgare*) on ciprofloxacin absorption and disposition in the rat. *J Pharm Pharmacol.* 1999;51:1391–1396.

2. Neuvonen PJ, Kivisto KT, Lehto P. Interference of dairy products with the absorption of ciprofloxacin. *Clin Pharmacol Ther.* 1991;50(5 pt 1): 498–502.

3. Minami R, Inotsume N, Nakano M, et al. Effect of milk on absorption of norfloxacin in healthy volunteers. *J Clin Pharmacol.* 1993;33:1238–1240.

4. Lehto P, Kivisto KT. Different effects of products containing metal ions on the absorption of lomefloxacin. *Clin Pharmacol Ther.* 1994;56:477–482.

5. Dudley MN, Marchbanks CR, Flor SC, et al. The effect of food or milk on the absorption kinetics of ofloxacin. *Eur J Clin Pharmacol.* 1991;41:569–571.

6. Flor S, Guay DR, Opsahl JA, et al. Effects of magnesium-aluminum hydroxide and calcium carbonate antacids on bioavailability of ofloxacin. *Antimicrob Agents Chemother.* 1990;34:2436–2438.

Notes

7. Polk RE, Healy DP, Sahai J, et al. Effect of ferrous sulfate and multivitamins with zinc on absorption of ciprofloxacin in normal volunteers. *Antimicrob Agents Chemother.* 1989;33:1841–1844.

8. Kara M, Hasinoff BB, McKay DW, et al. Clinical and chemical interactions between iron preparations and ciprofloxacin. *Br J Clin Pharmacol.* 1991;31:257.

9. Lomaestro BM, Bailie GR. Quinolone-cation interactions: a review. *DICP.* 1991;25:1249–1258.

10. Campbell NR, Kara M, Hasinoff BB, et al. Norfloxacin interaction with antacids and minerals. *Br J Clin Pharmacol.* 1992;33:115–116.

11. Lehto P, Kivisto KT, Neuvonen PJ. The effect of ferrous sulphate on the absorption of norfloxacin, ciprofloxacin and ofloxacin. *Br J Clin Pharmacol.* 1994;37:82–85.

12. Lehto P, Kivisto KT. Different effects of products containing metal ions on the absorption of lomefloxacin. *Clin Pharmacol Ther.* 1994;56:477–482.

13. Polk RE, Healy DP, Sahai J, et al. Effect of ferrous sulfate and multivitamins with zinc on absorption of ciprofloxacin in normal volunteers. *Antimicrob Agents Chemother.* 1989;33:1841–1844.

14. Campbell NR, Kara M, Hasinoff BB, et al. Norfloxacin interaction with antacids and minerals. *Br J Clin Pharmacol.* 1992;33:115–116.

15. Lomaestro BM, Bailie GR. Quinolone-cation interactions: a review. *DICP.* 1991;25:1249–1258.

16. Nix DE, Wilton JH, Ronald B, et al. Inhibition of norfloxacin absorption by antacids. *Antimicrob Agents Chemother.* 1990;34:432–435.

17. Grasela TH Jr, Schentag JJ, Sedman AJ, et al. Inhibition of enoxacin absorption by antacids or ranitidine. *Antimicrob Agents Chemother.* 1989;33:615–617.

18. Shimada J, Shiba K, Oguma T, et al. Effect of antacid on absorption of the quinolone lomefloxacin. *Antimicrob Agents Chemother.* 1992;36:1219–1224.

19. Teng R, Dogolo LC, Willavize SA, et al. Effect of Maalox and omeprazole on the bioavailability of trovafloxacin. *J Antimicrob Chemother.* 1997;39(suppl B):93–97.

20. Shiba K, Sakamoto M, Nakazawa Y, et al. Effects of antacid on absorption and excretion of new quinolones. *Drugs.* 1995;49(suppl 2):360–361.

H₂ ANTAGONISTS

1. Bachmann KA, Sullivan TJ, Jauregui L, et al. Drug interactions of H2-receptor antagonists. *Scand J Gastroenterol.* 1994;29(suppl 206):14–19.

2. Russell RM, Golner BB, Krasinski SD, et al. Effect of antacid and H₂ receptor antagonists on the intestinal absorption of folic acid. *J Lab Clin Med.* 1988;112:458–463.

3. Streeter AM, Goulston KJ, Bathur FA, et al. Cimetidine and malabsorption of cobalamin. *Dig Dis Sci.* 1982;27:13–16.

4. Salom IL, Silvis SE, Doscherholmen A. Effect of cimetidine on the absorption of vitamin B12. *Scand J Gastroenterol.* 1982;17:129–131.

5. Belaiche J, Zittoun J, Marquet J, et al. Effect of ranitidine on secretion of gastric intrinsic factor and absorption of vitamin B 12 [translated from French]. *Gastroenterol Clin Biol.* 1983;7:381–384.

6. Salom IL, Silvis SE, Doscherholmen A. Effect of cimetidine on the absorption of vitamin B12. *Scand J Gastroenterol.* 1982;17:129–131.

7. Bengoa JM, Bolt MJ, Rosenberg IH. Hepatic vitamin D 25-hydroxylase inhibition by cimetidine and isoniazid. *J Lab Clin Med.* 1984;104:546–552.

8. [No authors listed]. Cimetidine inhibits the hepatic hydroxylation of vitamin D. *Nutr Rev.* 1985;43:184–185.

9. Odes HS, Fraser GM, Krugliak P, et al. Effect of cimetidine on hepatic vitamin D metabolism in humans. *Digestion.* 1990;46:61–64.

10. Sturniolo GC, Montino MC, Rossetto L, et al. Inhibition of gastric acid secretion reduces zinc absorption in man. *J Am Coll Nutr.* 1991;4:372–375.

11. Champagne ET. Low gastric hydrochloric acid secretion and mineral bioavailability. *Adv Exp Med Biol.* 1989;249:173–184.

HEPARIN

1. Gadkari JV, Joshi VD. Effect of ingestion of raw garlic on serum cholesterol level, clotting time and fibrinolytic activity in normal subjects. *J Postgrad Med.* 1991;37:128–131.

2. Burnham BE. Garlic as a possible risk for postoperative bleeding. *Plast Reconstr Surg.* 1995;95:213.

Notes

3. Sunter WH. Warfarin and garlic. *Pharm J.* 1991;246:722.

4. Rosenblatt M, Mindel J. Spontaneous hyphema associated with ingestion of *Ginkgo biloba* extract [letter]. *N Engl J Med.* 1997;336:1108.

5. Rowin J, Lewis SL. Spontaneous bilateral subdural hematomas with chronic *Ginkgo biloba* ingestion. *Neurology.* 1996;46:1775–1776.

6. Vale S. Subarachnoid hemorrhage associated with *Ginkgo biloba* [letter]. *Lancet.* 1998;352:36.

7. Rowin J, Lewis SL. Spontaneous bilateral subdural hematomas with chronic *Ginkgo biloba* ingestion. *Neurology.* 1996;46:1775–1776.

8. van den Besselaar AM. Phosphatidylethanolamine and phosphatidylserine synergistically promote heparin's anticoagulant effect. *Blood Coagul Fibriniolysis.* 1995;6:239–244.

9. Arruzazabala ML, Mas R, Molina V, et al. Effect of policosanol on platelet aggregation in type II hypercholesterolemic patients. *Int J Tissue React.* 1998;20:119–124.

10. Arruzazabala ML, Mas R, Molina V, et al. Effect of policosanol on platelet aggregation in type II hypercholesterolemic patients. *Int J Tissue React.* 1998;20:119–124.

11. Arruzazabala ML, Valdes S, Mas R, et al. Effect of policosanol successive dose increases on platelet aggregation in healthy volunteers. *Pharmacol Res.* 1996;34:181–185.

12. Arruzazabala ML, Valdes S, Mas R, et al. Comparative study of policosanol, aspirin and the combination therapy policosanol-aspirin on platelet aggregation in healthy volunteers. *Pharmacol Res.* 1997; Oct;36:293–297.

13. Owen CA Jr, Tyce GM, Flock EV, et al. Heparin-ascorbic acid antagonism. *Mayo Clin Proc.* 1970;45:140–145.

14. Aarskog D, Aksnes L, Markestad T, et al. Heparin induced inhibition of 1,25-dihydroxyvitamin D formation. *Am J Obstet Gynecol.* 1984;148:1141–1142.

15. Haram K, Hervig T, Thordarson H, et al. Osteopenia caused by heparin treatment in pregnancy. *Acta Obstet Gynecol Scand.* 1993;72:674–675.

16. Haram K, Hervig T, Thordarson H, et al. Osteopenia caused by heparin treatment in pregnancy. *Acta Obstet Gynecol Scand.* 1993;72:674–675.

17. Wise PH, Hall AJ. Heparin-induced osteopenia in pregnancy. *BMJ.* 1980;281:110–111.

Notes

INFLUENZA VACCINE

1. Scaglione F, Cattaneo G, Alessandria M, et al. Efficacy and safety of the standardised ginseng extract G115 for potentiating vaccination against the influenza syndrome and protection against the common cold. *Drugs Exp Clin Res*. 1996;22:65–72.

ISONIAZID

1. Ishii N, Nishihara Y. Pellagra encephalopathy among tuberculous patients: its relation to isoniazid therapy. *J Neurol Neurosurg Psychiatry*. 1985;48:628–634.

2. Shibata K, Marugami M, Kondo T. In vivo inhibition of kynurenine aminotransferase activity by isonicotinic acid hydrazide in rats. *Biosci Biotechnol Biochem*. 1996;60:874–876.

3. DiLorenzo PA. Pellagra-like syndrome associated with isoniazid therapy. *Acta Derm Venereol*. 1967;47:318–322.

4. Shibata K, Marugami M, Kondo T. In vivo inhibition of kynurenine aminotransferase activity by isonicotinic acid hydrazide in rats. *Biosci Biotechnol Biochem*. 1996;60:874–876.

5. Snider DE Jr. Pyridoxine supplementation during isoniazid therapy. *Tubercle*. 1980;61:191–196.

6. Biehl JP, Vilter RW. Effect of isoniazid on vitamin B6 metabolism; its possible significance in producing isoniazid neuritis. *Proc Soc Exp Biol Med*. 1954;85:389–392.

7. Heller CA, Friedman PA. Pyridoxine deficiency and peripheral neuropathy associated with long-term phenelzine therapy. *Am J Med*. 1983;75:887–888.

8. Snider DE Jr. Pyridoxine supplementation during isoniazid therapy. *Tubercle*. 1980;61:191–196.

9. Snider DE Jr. Pyridoxine supplementation during isoniazid therapy. *Tubercle*. 1980;61:191–196.

10. Brodie, MJ, Boobis AR, Hillyard CJ, et al. Effect of isoniazid on vitamin D metabolism and hepatic monooxygenase activity. *Clin Pharmacol Ther*. 1981;30:363–367.

11. Bengoa JM, Bolt MJ, Rosenberg IH. Hepatic vitamin D 25-hydroxylase inhibition by cimetidine and isoniazid. *J Lab Clin Med*. 1984;104:546–552.

Notes

12. Brodie, MJ, Boobis AR, Hillyard CJ, et al. Effect of isoniazid on vitamin D metabolism and hepatic monooxygenase activity. *Clin Pharmacol Ther.* 1981;30:363–367.

13. Williams SE, Wardman AG, Taylor GA, et al. Long term study of the effect of rifampicin and isoniazid on vitamin D metabolism. *Tubercle.* 1985;66:49–54.

14. Perry W, Erooga MA, Brown J, et al. Calcium metabolism during rifampicin and isoniazid therapy for tuberculosis. *J R Soc Med.* 1982;75:533–536.

ITRACONAZOLE

1. *A to Z Drug Facts* [book on CD-ROM]. 2nd ed. St. Louis, Mo: Facts and Comparisons; 2000.

2. *A to Z Drug Facts* [book on CD-ROM]. 2nd ed. St. Louis, Mo: Facts and Comparisons; 2000.

3. Takanaga H, Ohnishi A, Murakami H, et al. Relationship between time after intake of grapefruit juice and the effect on pharmacokinetics and pharmacodynamics of nisoldipine in healthy subjects. *Clin Pharmacol Ther.* 2000;67:201–214.

LEVODOPA

1. Sternberg EM, Van Woert MH, Young SN, et al. Development of a scleroderma-like illness during therapy with L-5-hydroxytryptophan and carbidopa. *N Engl J Med.* 1980;303:782–787.

2. Joly P, et al. Development of pseudobullous morphea and scleroderma-like illness during therapy with L-5-hydroxytryptophan and carbidopa. *J Am Acad Dermatol.* 1991;25:332–333.

3. Auffranc JC, Berbis P, Fabre JF, et al. Sclerodermiform and poikilodermal syndrome observed during treatment with carbidopa and 5-hydroxytryptophan [translated from French]. *Ann Dermatol Venereol.* 1985;112:691–692.

4. Robertson DR, Higginson I, Macklin BS, et al. The influence of protein containing meals on the pharmacokinetics of levodopa in healthy volunteers. *Br J Clin Pharmacol.* 1991;31:413–417.

5. Campbell NR, Hasinoff BB. Iron supplements: a common cause of drug interactions. *Br J Clin Pharmacol.* 1991;31:251–255.

6. Schelosky L, Raffauf C, Jendroska K, et al. Kava and dopamine antagonism [letter]. *J Neurol Neurosurg Psychiatry.* 1995;58:639–640.

7. Schelosky L, Raffauf C, Jendroska K, et al. Kava and dopamine antagonism [letter]. *J Neurol Neurosurg Psychiatry.* 1995;58:639–640.

8. Leon AS, Spiegel HE, Thomas G, et al. Pyridoxine antagonism of levodopa in parkinsonism. *JAMA.* 1971;218:1924–1927.

9. Yahr MD, Duvoisin RC. Pyridoxine and levodopa in the treatment of Parkinsonism. *JAMA.* 1972;220:861.

10. Liu X, Lamango N, Charlton C. L-dopa depletes S-adenosylmethionine and increases S-adenosyl homocysteine: Relationship to the wearing off effects. *Soc Neurosci.* 1998;24:1469.

11. Bottiglieri T, Hyland K, Reynolds EH. The clinical potential in ademetionine (S-adenosylmethionine) in neurological disorders. *Drugs.* 1994;48:137–152.

12. Carrieri PB, Indaco A, Gentile S, et al. S-adenosylmethionine treatment of depression in patients with Parkinson's disease: a double-blind, crossover study versus placebo. *Curr Ther Res.* 1990;48:154–160.

13. Liu X, Lamango N, Charlton C. L-dopa depletes S-adenosylmethionine and increases S-adenosyl homocysteine: Relationship to the wearing off effects. *Soc Neurosci.* 1998;24:1469.

LEVODOPA/CARBIDOPA

1. Sternberg EM, Van Woert MH, Young SN, et al. Development of a scleroderma-like illness during therapy with L-5-hydroxytryptophan and carbidopa. *N Engl J Med.* 1980;303:782–787.

2. Joly P, et al. Development of pseudobullous morphea and scleroderma-like illness during therapy with L-5-hydroxytryptophan and carbidopa. *J Am Acad Dermatol.* 1991;25:332–333.

3. Auffranc JC, Berbis P, Fabre JF, et al. Sclerodermiform and poikilodermal syndrome observed during treatment with carbidopa and 5-hydroxytryptophan [translated from French]. *Ann Dermatol Venereol.* 1985;112:691–692.

4. Robertson DR, Higginson I, Macklin BS, et al. The influence of protein containing meals on the pharmacokinetics of levodopa in healthy volunteers. *Br J Clin Pharmacol.* 1991;31:413–417.

5. Campbell NR, Hasinoff BB. Iron supplements: a common cause of drug interactions. *Br J Clin Pharmacol.* 1991;31:251–255.

6. Schelosky L, Raffauf C, Jendroska K, et al. Kava and dopamine antagonism [letter]. *J Neurol Neurosurg Psychiatry.* 1995;58:639–640.

Notes

7. Schelosky L, Raffauf C, Jendroska K, et al. Kava and dopamine antagonism [letter]. *J Neurol Neurosurg Psychiatry.* 1995;58:639–640.

8. Liu X, Lamango N, Charlton C. L-dopa depletes S-adenosylmethionine and increases S-adenosyl homocysteine: Relationship to the wearing off effects. *Soc Neurosci.* 1998;24:1469.

9. Bottiglieri T, Hyland K, Reynolds EH. The clinical potential in ademetionine (S-adenosylmethionine) in neurological disorders. *Drugs.* 1994;48:137–152.

10. Carrieri PB, Indaco A, Gentile S, et al. S-adenosylmethionine treatment of depression in patients with Parkinson's disease: a double-blind, crossover study versus placebo. *Curr Ther Res.* 1990;48:154–160.

11. Liu X, Lamango N, Charlton C. L-dopa depletes S-adenosylmethionine and increases S-adenosyl homocysteine: Relationship to the wearing off effects. *Soc Neurosci.* 1998;24:1469.

LOOP DIURETICS

1. Walker BR, Edwards CR. Licorice-induced hypertension and syndromes of apparent mineralocorticoid excess. *Endocrinol Metab Clin North Am.* 1994;23:359–377.

2. Epstein MT, Espiner EA, Donald RA, et al. Liquorice toxicity and the renin-angiotensin-aldosterone axis in man. *Br Med J.* 1977;1:209–210.

3. Wash LK, Bernard JD. Licorice-induced pseudoaldosteronism. *Am J Hosp Pharm.* 1975;32:73–74.

4. de Klerk GJ, Nieuwenhuis MG, Beutler JJ. Hypokalemia and hypertension associated with use of liquorice flavoured chewing gum. *BMJ.* 1997;314:731–732.

5. Corsi FM, Galgani S, Gasparini C, et al. Acute hypokalemic myopathy due to chronic licorice ingestion: report of a case. *Ital J Neurol Sci.* 1983;4:493–497.

6. Blachley JD, Knochel JP. Tobacco chewer's hypokalemia: licorice revisited. *N Engl J Med.* 1980;302:784–785.

7. al-Ghamdi SM, Cameron EC, and Sutton RA. Magnesium deficiency: pathophysiologic and clinical overview. *Am J Kidney Dis.* 1994;24:737–752.

8. Dorup I. Magnesium and potassium deficiency. Its diagnosis, occurrence and treatment in diuretic therapy and its consequences for growth, protein synthesis and growth factors. *Acta Physiol Scand Suppl.* 1994;618:1–55.

9. Martin BJ, Milligan K. Diuretic-associated hypomagnesemia in the elderly. *Arch Intern Med.* 1987;147:1768–1771.

10. Whang R, Whang DD, Ryan MP. Refractory potassium repletion. A consequence of magnesium deficiency. *Arch Intern Med.* 1992;152:40–45.

11. Seligmann H, Halkin H, Rauchfleisch S, et al. Thiamine deficiency in patients with congestive heart failure receiving long-term furosemide therapy: a pilot study. *Am J Med.* 1991;91:151–155.

12. Brady JA, Rock CL, Horneffer MR. Thiamin status, diuretic medications, and the management of congestive heart failure. *J Am Diet Assoc.* 1995;95:541–544.

13. Seligmann H, Halkin H, Rauchfleisch S, et al. Thiamine deficiency in patients with congestive heart failure receiving long-term furosemide therapy: a pilot study. *Am J Med.* 1991;91:151–155.

14. Shimon I, Almog S, Vered Z, et al. Improved left ventricular function after thiamine supplementation in patients with congestive heart failure receiving long-term furosemide therapy. *Am J Med.* 1995;98:485–490.

MAO INHIBITORS

1. Shader RI, Greenblatt DJ. Phenelzine and the dream machine— ramblings and reflections. *J Clin Psychopharmacol.* 1985;5:65.

2. Jones BD, Runikis AM. Interaction of ginseng with phenelzine. *J Clin Psychopharmacol.* 1987;7:201–202.

3. Jones BD, Runikis AM. Interaction of ginseng with phenelzine. *J Clin Psychopharmacol.* 1987;7:201–202.

4. Oura H, Hiai S, Nakashima S, et al. Stimulating effect of roots of *Panax ginseng* C.A. Meyer on the incorporation of labeled precursors into rat liver RNA. *Chem Pharm Bull (Tokyo).* 1971;19:453–459.

5. Baldwin CA, Anderson LA, Phillipson JD. What pharmacists should know about ginseng. *Pharm J.* 1986;237:583–586.

6. Blumenthal M, ed. *The Complete German Commission E Monographs, Therapeutic Guide to Herbal Medicines.* Boston, Mass: Integrative Medicine Communications;1998.

7. Dingemanse J, Guentert T, Gieschke R, et al. Modification of the cardiovascular effects of ephedrine by the reversible monoamine oxidase A-inhibitor moclobemide. *J Cardiovasc Pharmacol.* 1996;28:856–861.

Notes

8. Iruela LM, Minguex L, Merino J, et al. Toxic interaction of S-adenosylmethionine and clomipramine [letter]. *Am J Psychiatry.* 1993;150:522.

9. Brinker F. Interactions of pharmaceutical and botanical medicines. *J Naturopath Med.* 1997;7:14–20.

10. Demott K. St. John's wort tied to serotonin syndrome. *Clin Psychiatry News.* 1998;26:28.

11. Gordon JB. SSRIs and St. John's wort: possible toxicity? [letter]. *Am Fam Physician.* 1998;57:950, 953.

12. Heller CA, Friedman PA. Pyridoxine deficiency and peripheral neuropathy associated with long-term phenelzine therapy. *Am J Med.* 1983;75:887–888.

METHOTREXATE

1. *A to Z Drug Facts* [book on CD-ROM]. 2nd ed. St. Louis, Mo: Facts and Comparisons; 2000.

2. Tracy TS, Krohn K, Jones DR, et al. The effects of a salicylate, ibuprofen, and naproxen on the disposition of methotrexate in patients with rheumatoid arthritis. *Eur J Clin Pharmacol.* 1992;42:121–125.

3. Morgan SL, Baggott JE, Vaughn WH, et al. Supplementation with folic acid during methotrexate therapy for rheumatoid arthritis. A double-blind, placebo-controlled trial. *Ann Intern Med.* 1994;121:833–841.

4. Duhra P. Treatment of gastrointestinal symptoms associated with methotrexate therapy for psoriasis. *J Am Acad Dermatol.* 1993;28:466–469.

5. Hunt PG, Rose CD, McIlvain-Simpson G, et al. The effects of daily intake of folic acid on the efficacy of methotrexate therapy in children with juvenile rheumatoid arthritis. A controlled study. *J Rheumatol.* 1997;24:2230–2232.

6. Morgan SL, Baggott JE, Vaughn WH, et al. Supplementation with folic acid during methotrexate therapy for rheumatoid arthritis. A double-blind, placebo-controlled trial. *Ann Intern Med.* 1994;121:833–841.

7. Duhra P. Treatment of gastrointestinal symptoms associated with methotrexate therapy for psoriasis. *J Am Acad Dermatol.* 1993;28:466–469.

8. Hunt PG, Rose CD, McIlvain-Simpson G, et al. The effects of daily intake of folic acid on the efficacy of methotrexate therapy in children with juvenile rheumatoid arthritis. A controlled study. *J Rheumatol.* 1997;24:2230–2232.

METHYLDOPA (ALDOCLOR, ALDOMET)

1. Campbell N, Paddock V, Sundaram R. Alteration of methyldopa absorption, metabolism, and blood pressure control caused by ferrous sulfate and ferrous gluconate. *Clin Pharmacol Ther.* 1988;43:381–386.

2. Campbell NR, Hasinoff BB. Iron supplements: a common cause of drug interactions. *Br J Clin Pharmacol.* 1991;31:251–255.

NITROFURANTOIN

1. Naggar VF, Khalil SA. Effect of magnesium trisilicate on nitrofurantoin absorption. *Clin Pharmacol Ther.* 1979;25:857–863.

2. Mannisto P. The effect of crystal size, gastric content and emptying rate on the absorption of nitrofurantoin in healthy human volunteers. *Int J Clin Pharmacol Biopharm.* 1978;16:223–228.

NITROGLYCERIN (NTG)

1. Ghio S, de Servi S, Perotti R, et al. Different susceptibility to the development of nitroglycerin tolerance in the arterial and venous circulation in humans. Effects of N-acetylcysteine administration. *Circulation.* 1992;86:798–802.

2. May DC, Popma JJ, Black WH, et al. In vivo induction and reversal of nitroglycerin tolerance in human coronary arteries. *N Engl J Med.* 1987;317:805–809.

3. Hogan JC, Lewis MJ, Henderson AH. N-acetylcysteine fails to attenuate haemodynamic tolerance to glycerol trinitrate in healthy volunteers. *Br J Clin Pharmacol.* 1989;28:421–426.

4. Hogan JC, Lewis MJ, Henderson AH. Chronic administration of N-acetylcysteine fails to prevent nitrate tolerance in patients with stable angina pectoris. *Br J Clin Pharmacol.* 1990;30:573–577.

5. Iversen HK. N-acetylcysteine enhances nitroglycerin-induced headache and cranial arterial responses. *Clin Pharmacol Ther.* 1992;52:125–133.

6. Ardissino D, Merlini PA, Savonitto S, et al. Effect of transdermal nitroglycerin or N-acetyl cysteine, or both, in the long-term treatment of unstable angina pectoris. *J Am Coll Cardiol.* 1997;29:941–947.

7. Watanabe H, Kakihana M, Ohtsuka S, et al. Randomized, double-blind, placebo-controlled study of the preventive effect of supplemental oral vitamin C on attenuation of development of nitrate tolerance. *J Am Coll Cardiol.* 1998;31:1323–1329.

8. Bassenge E, Fink N, Skatchkov M, et al. Dietary supplement with vitamin C prevents nitrate tolerance. *J Clin Invest.* 1998;31:67–71.

9. Bassenge E, Fink N, Skatchkov M, et al. Dietary supplement with vitamin C prevents nitrate tolerance. *J Clin Invest.* 1998;31:67–71.

10. Watanabe H, Kakihana M, Ohtsuka S, et al. Randomized, double-blind, placebo-controlled study of the preventive effect of supplemental oral vitamin C on attenuation of development of nitrate tolerance. *J Am Coll Cardiol.* 1998;31:1323–1329.

NITROUS OXIDE

1. Ermens AA, Refsum H, Rupreht J, et al. Monitoring cobalamin inactivation during nitrous oxide anesthesia by determination of homocysteine and folate plasma and urine. *Clin Pharmacol Ther.* 1991;49:385–393.

2. Flippo TS, Holder WD Jr. Neurologic degeneration associated with nitrous oxide anesthesia in patients with vitamin B12 deficiency. *Arch Surg.* 1993;128:1391–1395.

3. Amos RJ, Amess JA, Hinds CJ, et al. Investigations into the effect of nitrous oxide anesthesia on folate metabolism in patients receiving intensive care. *Chemioterapia.* 1985;4:393–399.

4. Amos RJ, Amess JA, Hinds CJ, et al. Incidence and pathogenesis of acute megaloblastic bone-marrow change in patients receiving intensive care. *Lancet.* 1982;2:835–838.

5. Flippo TS, Holder WD Jr. Neurologic degeneration associated with nitrous oxide anesthesia in patients with vitamin B12 deficiency. *Arch Surg.* 1993;128:1391–1395.

6. Amos RJ, Amess JA, Hinds CJ, et al. Incidence and pathogenesis of acute megaloblastic bone-marrow change in patients receiving intensive care. *Lancet.* 1982;2:835–838.

7. Flippo TS, Holder WD Jr. Neurologic degeneration associated with nitrous oxide anesthesia in patients with vitamin B12 deficiency. *Arch Surg.* 1993;128:1391–1395.

8. Nunn JF, Chanarin I, Tanner AG, et al. Megaloblastic bone marrow changes after repeated nitrous oxide anesthesia. Reversal with folinic acid. *Br J Anaesth.* 1986;58:1469–1470.

9. Amos RJ, Amess JA, Hinds CJ, et al. Investigations into the effect of nitrous oxide anesthesia on folate metabolism in patients receiving intensive care. *Chemioterapia.* 1985;4:393–399.

10. Koblin DD, Tomerson BW, Waldman FM, et al. Effect of nitrous oxide on folate and vitamin B12 metabolism in patients. *Anesth Analg. 1990;*71:610–617.

NONSTEROIDAL ANTI-INFLAMMATORY DRUGS (NSAIDs)

1. *AHFS Drug Information.* Bethesda, Md: American Society of Health-System Pharmacists; 2000:2306–2307.

2. Collier HO, Butt NM, McDonald-Gibson WJ, et al. Extract of feverfew inhibits prostaglandin biosynthesis. *Lancet.* 1980;2:922–923.

3. Sumner H, Salan U, Knight DW, et al. Inhibition of 5-lipoxygenase and cyclo-oxygenase in leukocytes by feverfew. Involvement of sesquiterpene lactones and other components. *Biochem Pharmacol.* 1992;43:2313–2320.

4. Williams CA, Hoult JR, Harborne JB, et al. A biologically active lipophilic flavonol from *Tanacetum parthenium. Phytochemistry.* 1995;38:267–270.

5. Gadkari JV, Joshi VD. Effect of ingestion of raw garlic on serum cholesterol level, clotting time and fibrinolytic activity in normal subjects. *J Postgrad Med.* 1991;37:128-131.

6. Burnham BE. Garlic as a possible risk for postoperative bleeding. *Plast Reconstr Surg.* 1995;95:213.

7. Rosenblatt M, Mindel J. Spontaneous hyphema associated with ingestion of *Ginkgo biloba* extract [letter]. *N Engl J Med.* 1997;336:1108.

8. Arruzazabala ML, Mas R, Molina V, et al. Effect of policosanol on platelet aggregation in type II hypercholesterolemic patients. *Int J Tissue React.* 1998;20:119–124.

9. Arruzazabala ML, Mas R, Molina V, et al. Effect of policosanol on platelet aggregation in type II hypercholesterolemic patients. *Int J Tissue React.* 1998;20:119–124.

10. Arruzazabala ML, Valdes S, Mas R, et al. Effect of policosanol successive dose increases on platelet aggregation in healthy volunteers. *Pharmacol Res.* 1996;34:181–185.

11. Arruzazabala ML, Valdes S, Mas R, et al. Comparative study of policosanol, aspirin and the combination therapy policosanol-aspirin on platelet aggregation in healthy volunteers. *Pharmacol Res.* 1997;36:293–297.

12. *A to Z Drug Facts* [book on CD-ROM]. 2nd ed. St. Louis, Mo: Facts and Comparisons; 2000.

Notes

13. Liede KE, Haukka JK, Saxen LM, et al. Increased tendency towards gingival bleeding caused by joint effect of alpha-tocopherol supplementation and acetylsalicylic acid. *Ann Med.* 1998;30:542–546.

14. Leppala JM, Virtamo J, Fogelholm R, et al. Controlled trial of alpha-tocopherol and beta-carotene supplements on stroke incidence and mortality in male smokers. *Arterioscler Thromb Vasc Biol.* 2000;20:230–235.

15. Abdel Salam OM, Moszik G, and Szolcsanyi J. Studies on the effect of intragastric capsaicin on gastric ulcer and on the prostacyclin-induced cytoprotection in rats. *Pharmacol Res.* 1995;32:209–215.

16. Holzer P, Pabst MA, Lippe IT. Intragastric capsaicin protects against aspirin-induced lesion formation and bleeding in the rat gastric mucosa. *Gastroenterology.* 1989;96:1425–1433.

17. Yeoh KG, Kang JY, Yap I, et al. Chili protects against aspirin-induced gastroduodenal mucosal injury in humans. *Dig Dis Sci.* 1995;40:580–583.

18. Yeoh KG, Kang JY, Yap I, et al. Chili protects against aspirin-induced gastroduodenal mucosal injury in humans. *Dig Dis Sci.* 1995;40:580–583.

19. Abdel Salam OM, Moszik G, and Szolcsanyi J. Studies on the effect of intragastric capsaicin on gastric ulcer and on the prostacyclin-induced cytoprotection in rats. *Pharmacol Res.* 1995;32:209–215.

20. Holzer P, Pabst MA, Lippe IT. Intragastric capsaicin protects against aspirin-induced lesion formation and bleeding in the rat gastric mucosa. *Gastroenterology.* 1989;96:1425–1433.

21. Yeoh KG, Kang JY, Yap I, et al. Chili protects against aspirin-induced gastroduodenal mucosal injury in humans. *Dig Dis Sci.* 1995;40:580–583.

22. Playford RJ, Floyd DN, Macdonald CE, et al. Bovine colostrum is a health food supplement which prevents NSAID induced gut damage. *Gut.* 1999;44:653–658.

23. Baggott JE, Morgan SL, Ha T, et al. Inhibition of folate-dependent enzymes by non-steroidal anti-inflammatory drugs. *Biochem J.* 1992;282:197–202.

24. Baum CL, Selhub J, Rosenberg IH. Antifolate actions of sulfasalazine on intact lymphocytes. *J Lab Clin Med.* 1981;97:779–784.

25. Selhub J, Dhar GJ, Rosenberg IH. Inhibition of folate enzymes by sulfasalazine. *J Clin Invest.* 1979;61:221–224.

26. Krogh Jensen M, Ekelund S, Svendsen L. Folate and homocysteine status and haemolysis in patients treated with sulfasalazine for arthritis. *Scand J Clin Lab Invest.* 1996;56:421–429.

Notes

27. Lawrence VA, Loewenstein JE, Eichner ER. Aspirin and folate binding: in vivo and in vitro studies of serum binding and urinary excretion of endogenous folate. *J Lab Clin Med*. 1984;103:944–948.

28. Rees WD, Rhodes J, Wright JE, et al. Effect of deglycyrrhizinated liquorice on gastric mucosal damage by aspirin. *Scand J Gastroenterol*. 1979;14:605–607.

29. Das N, Nebioglu S. Vitamin C aspirin interactions in laboratory animals. *J Clin Pharm Ther*. 1992;17:343–346.

30. Molloy TP, Wilson CW. Protein-binding of ascorbic acid 2. Interaction with acetylsalicylic acid. *Int J Vitam Nutr Res*. 1980;50:387–392.

31. Sahud MA, Cohen RJ. Effect of aspirin ingestion on ascorbic-acid levels in rheumatoid arthritis. *Lancet*. 1971;1:937–938.

ORAL CONTRACEPTIVES (OCs, BIRTH CONTROL PILLS)

1. King DS, Sharp RL, Vukovich MD, et al. Effect of oral androstenedione on serum testosterone and adaptations to resistance training in young men: a randomized controlled trial. *JAMA*. 1999;281:2020–2028.

2. Leder, BZ;, Longcope C, Caitlin DH, et al. Oral androstenedione administration and serum testosterone concentrations in young men. *JAMA*. 2000;283:779–782.

3. Ballantyne CS, Phillips SM, MacDonald JR, et al. The acute effects of androstenedione supplementation in healthy young males. *Can J Appl Physiol*. 2000;25:68–78.

4. Milne DB, Johnson PE. Assessment of copper status: effect of age and gender on reference ranges in healthy adults. *Clin Chem*. 1993;39:883–887.

5. Newhouse IJ, Clement DB, Lai C. Effects of iron supplementation and discontinuation on serum copper, zinc, calcium, and magnesium levels in women. *Med Sci Sports Exerc*. 1993;25:562–571.

6. Berg G, Kohlmeier L, Brenner H. Effect of oral contraceptive progestins on serum copper concentration. *Eur J Clin Nutr*. 1998;52:711–715.

7. Reunanen A, Knekt P, Marniemi J, et al. Serum calcium, magnesium, copper and zinc and the risk of cardiovascular death. *Eur J Clin Nutr*. 1996;50:431–437.

8. Salonen JT, Salonen R, Korpela H, et al. Serum copper and the risk of acute myocardial infarction: a prospective population study in men in eastern Finland. *Am J Epidemiol*. 1991;134:268–276.

Notes

9. Bernardi M, D'Intino PE, Trevisani F, et al. Effects of prolonged ingestion of graded doses of licorice by healthy volunteers. *Life Sci.* 1994;55:863–872.

10. Wash LK, Bernard JD. Licorice-induced pseudoaldosteronism. *Am J Hosp Pharm.* 1975;32:73–74.

11. Stewart PM, Wallace AM, Valentino R, et al. Mineralocorticoid activity of liquorice: 11-beta-hydroxysteroid dehydrogenase deficiency comes of age. *Lancet.* 1987;2:821–824.

12. Walker BR, Edwards CR. Licorice-induced hypertension and syndromes of apparent mineralocorticoid excess. *Endocrinol Metab Clin North Am.* 1994;23:359–377.

13. de Klerk GJ, Nieuwenhuis MG, Beutler JJ. Hypokalemia and hypertension associated with use of liquorice flavoured chewing gum. *BMJ.* 1997;314:731–732.

14. Kim DH, Jin YH, Park JB, et al. Silymarin and its components are inhibitors of beta-glucuronidase. *Biol Pharm Bull.* 1994;17:443–445.

15. Jobst KA, McIntyre M, St. George D, et al. Safety of St. John's wort (*Hypericum perforatum*). *Lancet.* 2000:355:575.

16. Mooij PN, Thomas CM, Doesburg WH, et al. Multivitamin supplementation in oral contraceptive users. *Contraception.* 1991;44:277–288.

17. Steegers-Theunissen RP, Van Rossum JM, Steegers EA, et al. Sub-50 oral contraceptives affect folate kinetics. *Gynecol Obstet Invest.* 1993;36:230–233.

18. Green TJ, Houghton LA, Donovan U, et al. Oral contraceptives did not affect biochemical folate indexes and homocysteine concentrations in adolescent females. *J Am Diet Assoc.* 1998;98:49–55.

19. Steegers-Theunissen RP, Van Rossum JM, Steegers EA, et al. Sub-50 oral contraceptives affect folate kinetics. *Gynecol Obstet Invest.* 1993;36:230–233.

20. Seelig MS. Interrelationship of magnesium and estrogen in cardiovascular and bone disorders, eclampsia, migraine, and premenstrual syndrome. *J Am Coll Nutr.* 1993;12:442–458.

21. Blum M, Kitai E, Ariel Y, et al. Oral contraceptive lowers serum magnesium [translated from Hebrew]. *Harefuah.* 1991;121:363–364.

22. Martini MC, Dancisak BB, Haggans CJ, et al. Effects of soy intake on sex hormone metabolism in premenopausal women. *Nutr Cancer.* 1999;34:133–139.

Notes

23. Webb JL. Nutritional effects of oral contraceptive use: a review. *J Reprod Med.* 1980;25:150–156.

24. Larsson-Cohn U. Oral contraceptives and vitamins: a review. *Am J Obstet Gynecol.* 1975;121:84–90.

25. Wynn V. Vitamins and oral contraceptive use. *Lancet.* 1975;1:561–564.

26. Amatayakul K, Uttaravichai C, Singkamani R, et al. Vitamin metabolism and the effects of multivitamin supplementation in oral contraceptive users. *Contraception.* 1984;30:179–196.

27. Masse PG, van den Berg H, Duguay C, et al. Early effect of a low dose (30 g) ethinyl estradiol-containing Triphasil on vitamin B6 status. A follow-up study on six menstrual cycles. *Int J Vitam Nutr Res.* 1996;66:46–54.

28. van der Vange N, van der Berg H, Kloosterboet HJ, et al. Effects of seven low-dose combined contraceptives on vitamin B6 status. *Contraception.* 1989;40:377–384.

29. Kant AK, Block G. Dietary vitamin B-6 intake and food sources in the US population: NHANES II, 1976–1980. *Am J Clin Nutr.* 1990;52:707–716.

30. Green TJ, Houghton LA, Donovan U, et al. Oral contraceptives did not affect biochemical folate indexes and homocysteine concentrations in adolescent females. *J Am Diet Assoc.* 1998;98:49–55.

31. Steegers-Theunissen RP, Van Rossum JM, Steegers EA, et al. Sub-50 oral contraceptives affect folate kinetics. *Gynecol Obstet Invest.* 1993;36:230–233.

32. Hjelt K, Brynskov J, Hippe E, et al. Oral contraceptives and the cobalamin (vitamin B12) metabolism. *Acta Obstet Gynecol Scand.* 1985;64:59–63.

33. Rivers JM, Devine M. Plasma ascorbic acid concentrations and oral contraceptives. *Am J Clin Nutr.* 1972;25:684–689.

34. Webb JL. Nutritional effects of oral contraceptive use: a review. *J Reprod Med.* 1980;25:150–156.

35. Larsson-Cohn U. Oral contraceptives and vitamins: a review. *Am J Obstet Gynecol.* 1975;121:84–90.

36 Wynn V. Vitamins and oral contraceptive use. *Lancet.* 1975;1:561–564.

37. Briggs M, Briggs M. Vitamin C requirements and oral contraceptives. *Nature.* 1972;238:277.

38. Webb JL. Nutritional effects of oral contraceptive use: a review. *J Reprod Med.* 1980;25:150–156.

39. Larsson-Cohn U. Oral contraceptives and vitamins: a review. *Am J Obstet Gynecol*. 1975;121:84–90.

40. Wynn V. Vitamins and oral contraceptive use. *Lancet*. 1975;1:561–564.

41. Webb JL. Nutritional effects of oral contraceptive use: a review. *J Reprod Med*. 1980;25:150–156.

42. Rivers JM, Devine M. Plasma ascorbic acid concentrations and oral contraceptives. *Am J Clin Nutr*. 1972;25:684–689.

43. Briggs M, Briggs M. Vitamin C requirements and oral contraceptives. *Nature*. 1972;238:277.

44. Seelig MS. Increased need for magnesium with the use of combined oestrogen and calcium for osteoporosis treatment. *Magnes Res*. 1990;3:197–215.

45. Blum M, Kitai E, Ariel Y, et al. Oral contraceptive lowers serum magnesium [translated from Hebrew]. *Harefuah*. 1991;121:363–364.

PENICILLAMINE

1. Osman MA, Patel RB, Schuna A, et al. Reduction in oral penicillamine absorption by food, antacid, and ferrous sulfate. *Clin Pharmacol Ther*. 1983;33:465–470.

2. Osman MA, Patel RB, Schuna A, et al. Reduction in oral penicillamine absorption by food, antacid, and ferrous sulfate. *Clin Pharmacol Ther*. 1983;33:465–470.

3. Rumsby PC, Shepherd DM. The effect of penicillamine on vitamin B6 function in man. *Biochem Pharmacol*. 1981;30:3051–3053.

4. Kant AK, Block G. Dietary vitamin B-6 intake and food sources in the US population: NHANES II, 1976–1980. *Am J Clin Nutr*. 1990;52:707–716.

5. van der Wielen RP, de Groot LC, van Staveren WA. Dietary intake of water soluble vitamins in elderly people living in a Western society (1980–1993). *Nutr Res*. 1994;14:605–638.

6. Albertson AM, Tobelmann RC, Engstrom A, et al. Nutrient intakes of 2- to 10-year-old American children: 10-year trends. *J Am Diet Assoc*. 1992;92:1492–1496.

PENTOXIFYLLINE

1. Gadkari JV, Joshi VD. Effect of ingestion of raw garlic on serum cholesterol level, clotting time and fibrinolytic activity in normal subjects. *J Postgrad Med*. 1991;37:128-131.

2. Burnham BE. Garlic as a possible risk for postoperative bleeding. *Plast Reconstr Surg.* 1995;95:213.

3. Chung KF, Dent G, McCusker M, et al. Effect of a ginkgolide mixture (BN 52063) in antagonising skin and platelet responses to platelet activating factor in man. *Lancet.* 1987;1:248-251.

4. Rosenblatt M, Mindel J. Spontaneous hyphema associated with ingestion of Ginkgo biloba extract [letter]. *N Engl J Med.* 1997;336:1108.

5. Rowin J, Lewis SL. Spontaneous bilateral subdural hematomas with chronic Ginkgo biloba ingestion. *Neurology.* 1996;46:1775-1776.

6. Vale S. Subarachnoid hemorrhage associated with Ginkgo biloba [letter]. *Lancet.* 1998;352:36.

PHENOBARBITAL

1. Arenz A, Klein M, Fiehe K. Occurrence of neurotoxic 4'-O-methylpyridoxine in *Ginkgo biloba* leaves, ginkgo medications and Japanese ginkgo food. *Planta Med.* 1996;62:548–551.

2. Mizuno N, Kawakami K, Morita E. Competitive inhibition between 4'-substituted pyridoxine analogues and pyridoxal for pyridoxal kinase from mouse brain. *J Nutr Sci Vitaminol (Tokyo).* 1980;26:535–543.

3. Wada K, Ishigaki S, Ueda K, et al. An antivitamin B6, 4'-methoxypyridoxine, from the seed of *Ginkgo biloba* L. *Chem Pharm Bull (Tokyo).* 1985;33:3555–3557.

4. Yagi M, Wada K, Sakata M, et al. Studies on the constituents of edible and medicinal plants. IV. Determination of 4-O-methylpyridoxine in serum of the patient with gin-nan food poisoning [in Japanese; English abstract]. *Yakugaku Zasshi.* 1993;113:596–599.

5. Arenz A, Klein M, Fiehe K. Occurrence of neurotoxic 4'-O-methylpyridoxine in *Ginkgo biloba* leaves, ginkgo medications and Japanese ginkgo food. *Planta Med.* 1996;62:548–551.

6. Almeida JC, Grimsley EW. Coma from the health food store: interaction between kava and alprazolam. *Ann Intern Med.* 1996;125:940–941.

7. Bourgeois BF, Dodson WE, Ferrendelli JA. Interactions between primidone, carbamazepine, and nicotinamide. *Neurology.* 1982;32:1122–1126.

8. Bourgeois BF, Dodson WE, Ferrendelli JA. Interactions between primidone, carbamazepine, and nicotinamide. *Neurology.* 1982;32:1122–1126.

Notes

9. Krause KH, Bonjour JP, Berlit P, et al. Biotin status of epileptics. *Ann N Y Acad Sci*. 1985;447:297–313.

10. Said HM, Redha R, Nylander W. Biotin transport in the human intestine: inhibition by anticonvulsant drugs. *Am J Clin Nutr*. 1989;49:127–131.

11. Kishi T, Fujita N, Eguchi T, et al. Mechanism for reduction of serum folate by antiepileptic drugs during prolonged therapy. *J Neurol Sci*. 1997;145:109–112.

12. Kishi T, Fujita N, Eguchi T, et al. Mechanism for reduction of serum folate by antiepileptic drugs during prolonged therapy. *J Neurol Sci*. 1997;145:109–112.

13. Reynolds EH. Mental effects of anticonvulsants, and folic acid metabolism. *Brain*. 1968;91:197–214.

14. Berg MJ, Stumbo PJ, Chenard CA, et al. Folic acid improves phenytoin pharmacokinetics. *J Am Diet Assoc*. 1995;95:352–356.

15. Lewis DP, Van Dyke DC, Willhite LA, et al. Phenytoin-folic acid interaction. *Ann Pharmacother*. 1995;29:726–735.

16. Kishi T, Fujita N, Eguchi T, et al. Mechanism for reduction of serum folate by antiepileptic drugs during prolonged therapy. *J Neurol Sci*. 1997;145:109–112.

17. Lewis DP, Van Dyke DC, Stumbo PJ, et al. Drug and environmental factors associated with adverse pregnancy outcomes. Part I: Antiepileptic drugs, contraceptives, smoking, and folate. *Ann Pharmacother*. 1998;32:802–817.

18. Ono H, Sakamoto A, Eguchi T, et al. Plasma total homocysteine concentrations in epileptic patients taking anticonvulsants. *Metabolism*. 1997;46:959–962.

19. Lewis DP, Van Dyke DC, Stumbo PJ, et al. Drug and environmental factors associated with adverse pregnancy outcomes. Part I: Antiepileptic drugs, contraceptives, smoking, and folate. *Ann Pharmacother*. 1998;32:802–817.

20. Wahl TO, Gobuty AH, Lukert BP. Long-term anticonvulsant therapy and intestinal calcium absorption. *Clin Pharmacol Ther*. 1981;30:506–512.

21. Weinstein RS, Bryce GF, Sappington LJ, et al. Decreased serum ionized calcium and normal vitamin D metabolite levels with anticonvulsant drug treatment. *J Clin Endocrinol Metab*. 1984;58:1003–1009.

22. Weinstein RS, Bryce GF, Sappington LJ, et al. Decreased serum ionized calcium and normal vitamin D metabolite levels with anticonvulsant drug treatment. *J Clin Endocrinol Metab*. 1984;58:1003–1009.

Notes

23. Carter BL, Garnett WR, Pellock JM, et al. Effect of antacids on phenytoin bioavailability. *Ther Drug Monit.* 1981;3:333–340.

24. McElnay JC, Uprichard G, Collier PS. The effect of activated dimethicone and a proprietary antacid preparation containing this agent on the absorption of phenytoin. *Br J Clin Pharmacol.* 1982;13:501–505.

25. De Vivo DC, Bohan TP, Coulter DL, et al. L-carnitine supplementation in childhood epilepsy: current perspectives. *Epilepsia.* 1998;39:1216–1225.

26. Coulter DL. Carnitine deficiency: a possible mechanism for valproate hepatotoxicity [letter]. *Lancet.* 1984;1:689.

27. Ater SB, et al. A developmental center population treated with VPA and L-carnitine. In: Update 1993: inborn errors of metabolism in the patient with epilepsy. Sigma-Tau Pharmaceuticals; 1993.

28. Dreifuss FE, Langer DH. Hepatic considerations in the use of antiepileptic drugs. *Epilepsia.* 1987;28(suppl 2):S23–S29.

29. Ater SB, et al. A developmental center population treated with VPA and L-carnitine. In: Update 1993: inborn errors of metabolism in the patient with epilepsy. Sigma-Tau Pharmaceuticals; 1993.

30. Freeman JM, Vining EP, Cost S, et al. Does carnitine administration improve the symptoms attributed to anticonvulsant medications? A double-blinded, crossover study. *Pediatrics.* 1994;93:893–895.

31. De Vivo DC, Bohan TP, Coulter DL, et al. L-carnitine supplementation in childhood epilepsy: current perspectives. *Epilepsia.* 1998;39:1216–1225.

32. Hahn TJ, Hendin BA, Scharp CR, et al. Effect of chronic anticonvulsant therapy on serum 25-hydroxycalciferol levels in adults. *N Engl J Med.* 1972;287:900–904.

33. Hahn TJ, Hendin BA, Scharp CR, et al. Effect of chronic anticonvulsant therapy on serum 25-hydroxycalciferol levels in adults. *N Engl J Med.* 1972;287:900–904.

34. Jubiz W, Haussler MR, McCain TA, et al. Plasma 1,25-dihydroxyvitamin D levels in patients receiving anticonvulsant drugs. *J Clin Endocrinol Metab.* 1977;44:617–621.

35. Brodie MJ, Boobis AR, Dollery CT, et al. Rifampicin and vitamin D metabolism. *Clin Pharmacol Ther.* 1980;27:810–814.

36. Williams C, Netzloff M, Folkerts L, et al. Vitamin D metabolism and anticonvulsant therapy: effect of sunshine on incidence of osteomalacia. *South Med J.* 1984;77:834–836, 842.

Notes

37. Cornelissen M, Steegers-Theunissen R, Kollee L, et al. Increased incidence of neonatal vitamin K deficiency resulting from maternal anticonvulsant therapy. *Am J Obstet Gynecol.* 1993;168:923–928.

38. Cornelissen M, Steegers-Theunissen R, Kollee L, et al. Supplementation of vitamin K in pregnant women receiving anticonvulsant therapy prevents neonatal vitamin K deficiency. *Am J Obstet Gynecol.* 1993;168:884–888.

PHENYTOIN

1. Arenz A, Klein M, Fiehe K. Occurrence of neurotoxic 4'-O-methylpyridoxine in *Ginkgo biloba* leaves, ginkgo medications and Japanese ginkgo food. *Planta Med.* 1996;62:548–551.

2. Mizuno N, Kawakami K, Morita E. Competitive inhibition between 4'-substituted pyridoxine analogues and pyridoxal for pyridoxal kinase from mouse brain. *J Nutr Sci Vitaminol (Tokyo).* 1980;26:535–543.

3. Wada K, Ishigaki S, Ueda K, et al. An antivitamin B6, 4'-methoxypyridoxine, from the seed of *Ginkgo biloba* L. *Chem Pharm Bull (Tokyo).* 1985;33:3555–3557.

4. Yagi M, Wada K, Sakata M, et al. Studies on the constituents of edible and medicinal plants. IV. Determination of 4-O-methylpyridoxine in serum of the patient with gin-nan food poisoning [in Japanese; English abstract]. *Yakugaku Zasshi.* 1993;113:596–599.

5. Arenz A, Klein M, Fiehe K. Occurrence of neurotoxic 4'-O-methylpyridoxine in *Ginkgo biloba* leaves, ginkgo medications and Japanese ginkgo food. *Planta Med.* 1996;62:548–551.

6. Monostory K, Vereczkey L, Levai F, et al. Ipriflavone as an inhibitor of human cytochrome P450 enzymes. *Br J Pharmacol.* 1998;123:605–610.

7. Almeida JC, Grimsley EW. Coma from the health food store: interaction between kava and alprazolam. *Ann Intern Med.* 1996;125:940–941.

8. Inoue F, Walsh RJ. Folate supplements and phenytoin-salicylate interaction. *Neurology.* 1983;33:115–116.

9. Krause KH, Bonjour JP, Berlit P, et al. Biotin status of epileptics. *Ann N Y Acad Sci.* 1985;447:297–313.

10. Said HM, Redha R, Nylander W. Biotin transport in the human intestine: inhibition by anticonvulsant drugs. *Am J Clin Nutr.* 1989;49:127–131.

11. Kishi T, Fujita N, Eguchi T, et al. Mechanism for reduction of serum folate by antiepileptic drugs during prolonged therapy. *J Neurol Sci.* 1997;145:109–112.

Notes

12. Reynolds EH. Mental effects of anticonvulsants, and folic acid metabolism. *Brain*. 1968;91:197–214.

13. Hendel J, Dam M, Gram L, et al. The effects of carbamazepine and valproate on folate metabolism. *Acta Neurol Scand*. 1984;69:226–231.

14. Berg MJ, Stumbo PJ, Chenard CA, et al. Folic acid improves phenytoin pharmacokinetics. *J Am Diet Assoc*. 1995;95:352–56.

15. Lewis DP, Van Dyke DC, Willhite LA, et al. Phenytoin-folic acid interaction. *Ann Pharmacother*. 1995;29:726–735.

16. Lewis DP, Van Dyke DC, Stumbo PJ, et al. Drug and environmental factors associated with adverse pregnancy outcomes. Part I: Antiepileptic drugs, contraceptives, smoking, and folate. *Ann Pharmacother*. 1998;32:802–817.

17. Ono H, Sakamoto A, Eguchi T, et al. Plasma total homocysteine concentrations in epileptic patients taking anticonvulsants. *Metabolism*. 1997;46:959–962.

18. Lewis DP, Van Dyke DC, Stumbo PJ, et al. Drug and environmental factors associated with adverse pregnancy outcomes. Part I: Antiepileptic drugs, contraceptives, smoking, and folate. *Ann Pharmacother*. 1998;32:802–817.

19. Berg MJ, Stumbo PJ, Chenard CA, et al. Folic acid improves phenytoin pharmacokinetics. *J Am Diet Assoc*. 1995;95:352–56.

20. Lewis DP, Van Dyke DC, Willhite LA, et al. Phenytoin-folic acid interaction. *Ann Pharmacother*. 1995;29:726–735.

21. Kishi T, Fujita N, Eguchi T, et al. Mechanism for reduction of serum folate by antiepileptic drugs during prolonged therapy. *J Neurol Sci*. 1997;145:109–112

22. Berg MJ, Stumbo PJ, Chenard CA, et al. Folic acid improves phenytoin pharmacokinetics. *J Am Diet Assoc*. 1995;95:352–56.

23. Lewis DP, Van Dyke DC, Stumbo PJ, et al. Drug and environmental factors associated with adverse pregnancy outcomes. Part I: Antiepileptic drugs, contraceptives, smoking, and folate. *Ann Pharmacother*. 1998;32:802–817.

24. Wahl TO, Gobuty AH, Lukert BP. Long-term anticonvulsant therapy and intestinal calcium absorption. *Clin Pharmacol Ther*. 1981;30:506–512.

25. Weinstein RS, Bryce GF, Sappington LJ, et al. Decreased serum ionized calcium and normal vitamin D metabolite levels with anticonvulsant drug treatment. *J Clin Endocrinol Metab*. 1984;58:1003–1009.

Notes

26. Weinstein RS, Bryce GF, Sappington LJ, et al. Decreased serum ionized calcium and normal vitamin D metabolite levels with anticonvulsant drug treatment. *J Clin Endocrinol Metab.* 1984;58:1003–1009.

27. Carter BL, Garnett WR, Pellock JM, et al. Effect of antacids on phenytoin bioavailability. *Ther Drug Monit.* 1981;3:333–340.

28. McElnay JC, Uprichard G, Collier PS. The effect of activated dimethicone and a proprietary antacid preparation containing this agent on the absorption of phenytoin. *Br J Clin Pharmacol.* 1982;13:501–505.

29. De Vivo DC, Bohan TP, Coulter DL, et al. L-carnitine supplementation in childhood epilepsy: current perspectives. *Epilepsia.* 1998;39:1216–1225.

30. Coulter DL. Carnitine deficiency: a possible mechanism for valproate hepatotoxicity [letter]. *Lancet.* 1984;1:689.

31. Ater SB, et al. A developmental center population treated with VPA and L-carnitine. In: Update 1993: inborn errors of metabolism in the patient with epilepsy. Sigma-Tau Pharmaceuticals; 1993.

32. Dreifuss FE, Langer DH. Hepatic considerations in the use of antiepileptic drugs. *Epilepsia.* 1987;28(suppl 2):S23–S29.

33. Ater SB, et al. A developmental center population treated with VPA and L-carnitine. In: Update 1993: inborn errors of metabolism in the patient with epilepsy. Sigma-Tau Pharmaceuticals; 1993.

34. Freeman JM, Vining EP, Cost S, et al. Does carnitine administration improve the symptoms attributed to anticonvulsant medications? A double-blinded, crossover study. *Pediatrics.* 1994;93:893–895.

35. De Vivo DC, Bohan TP, Coulter DL, et al. L-carnitine supplementation in childhood epilepsy: current perspectives. *Epilepsia.* 1998;39:1216–1225.

36. Hahn TJ, Hendin BA, Scharp CR, et al. Effect of chronic anticonvulsant therapy on serum 25-hydroxycalciferol levels in adults. *N Engl J Med.* 1972;287:900–904.

37. Hahn TJ, Hendin BA, Scharp CR, et al. Effect of chronic anticonvulsant therapy on serum 25-hydroxycalciferol levels in adults. *N Engl J Med.* 1972;287:900–904.

38. Jubiz W, Haussler MR, McCain TA, et al. Plasma 1,25-dihydroxyvitamin D levels in patients receiving anticonvulsant drugs. *J Clin Endocrinol Metab.* 1977;44:617–621.

39. Brodie MJ, Boobis AR, Dollery CT, et al. Rifampicin and vitamin D metabolism. *Clin Pharmacol Ther.* 1980;27:810–814.

40. Williams C, Netzloff M, Folkerts L, et al. Vitamin D metabolism and anticonvulsant therapy: effect of sunshine on incidence of osteomalacia. *South Med J*. 1984;77:834–836, 842.

41. Cornelissen M, Steegers-Theunissen R, Kollee L, et al. Increased incidence of neonatal vitamin K deficiency resulting from maternal anticonvulsant therapy. *Am J Obstet Gynecol*. 1993;168:923–928.

42. Cornelissen M, Steegers-Theunissen R, Kollee L, et al. Supplementation of vitamin K in pregnant women receiving anticonvulsant therapy prevents neonatal vitamin K deficiency. *Am J Obstet Gynecol*. 1993;168:884–888.

PRIMIDONE

1. Arenz A, Klein M, Fiehe K. Occurrence of neurotoxic 4'-O-methylpyridoxine in *Ginkgo biloba* leaves, ginkgo medications and Japanese ginkgo food. *Planta Med*. 1996;62:548–551.

2. Mizuno N, Kawakami K, Morita E. Competitive inhibition between 4'-substituted pyridoxine analogues and pyridoxal for pyridoxal kinase from mouse brain. *J Nutr Sci Vitaminol (Tokyo)*. 1980;26:535–543.

3. Wada K, Ishigaki S, Ueda K, et al. An antivitamin B6, 4'-methoxypyridoxine, from the seed of *Ginkgo biloba* L. *Chem Pharm Bull (Tokyo)*. 1985;33:3555–3557.

4. Yagi M, Wada K, Sakata M, et al. Studies on the constituents of edible and medicinal plants. IV. Determination of 4-O-methylpyridoxine in serum of the patient with gin-nan food poisoning [in Japanese; English abstract]. *Yakugaku Zasshi*. 1993;113:596–599.

5. Arenz A, Klein M, Fiehe K. Occurrence of neurotoxic 4'-O-methylpyridoxine in *Ginkgo biloba* leaves, ginkgo medications and Japanese ginkgo food. *Planta Med*. 1996;62:548–551.

6. Almeida JC, Grimsley EW. Coma from the health food store: interaction between kava and alprazolam. *Ann Intern Med*. 1996;125:940–941.

7. Bourgeois BF, Dodson WE, Ferrendelli JA. Interactions between primidone, carbamazepine, and nicotinamide. *Neurology*. 1982;32:1122–1126.

8. Bourgeois BF, Dodson WE, Ferrendelli JA. Interactions between primidone, carbamazepine, and nicotinamide. *Neurology*. 1982;32:1122–1126.

9. Krause KH, Bonjour JP, Berlit P, et al. Biotin status of epileptics. *Ann N Y Acad Sci*. 1985;447:297–313.

Notes

10. Said HM, Redha R, Nylander W. Biotin transport in the human intestine: inhibition by anticonvulsant drugs. *Am J Clin Nutr*. 1989;49:127–131.

11. Kishi T, Fujita N, Eguchi T, et al. Mechanism for reduction of serum folate by antiepileptic drugs during prolonged therapy. *J Neurol Sci*. 1997;145:109–112.

12. Kishi T, Fujita N, Eguchi T, et al. Mechanism for reduction of serum folate by antiepileptic drugs during prolonged therapy. *J Neurol Sci*. 1997;145:109–112.

13. Reynolds EH. Mental effects of anticonvulsants, and folic acid metabolism. *Brain*. 1968;91:197–214.

14. Berg MJ, Stumbo PJ, Chenard CA, et al. Folic acid improves phenytoin pharmacokinetics. *J Am Diet Assoc*. 1995;95:352–356.

15. Lewis DP, Van Dyke DC, Willhite LA, et al. Phenytoin-folic acid interaction. *Ann Pharmacother*. 1995;29:726–735.

16. Lewis DP, Van Dyke DC, Stumbo PJ, et al. Drug and environmental factors associated with adverse pregnancy outcomes. Part I: Antiepileptic drugs, contraceptives, smoking, and folate. *Ann Pharmacother*. 1998;32:802–817.

17. Ono H, Sakamoto A, Eguchi T, et al. Plasma total homocysteine concentrations in epileptic patients taking anticonvulsants. *Metabolism*. 1997;46:959–962.

18. Lewis DP, Van Dyke DC, Stumbo PJ, et al. Drug and environmental factors associated with adverse pregnancy outcomes. Part I: Antiepileptic drugs, contraceptives, smoking, and folate. *Ann Pharmacother*. 1998;32:802–817.

19. Wahl TO, Gobuty AH, Lukert BP. Long-term anticonvulsant therapy and intestinal calcium absorption. *Clin Pharmacol Ther*. 1981;30:506–512.

20. Weinstein RS, Bryce GF, Sappington LJ, et al. Decreased serum ionized calcium and normal vitamin D metabolite levels with anticonvulsant drug treatment. *J Clin Endocrinol Metab*. 1984;58:1003–1009.

21. Weinstein RS, Bryce GF, Sappington LJ, et al. Decreased serum ionized calcium and normal vitamin D metabolite levels with anticonvulsant drug treatment. *J Clin Endocrinol Metab*. 1984;58:1003–1009.

22. Carter BL, Garnett WR, Pellock JM, et al. Effect of antacids on phenytoin bioavailability. *Ther Drug Monit*. 1981;3:333–340.

23. McElnay JC, Uprichard G, Collier PS. The effect of activated dimethicone and a proprietary antacid preparation containing this agent on the absorption of phenytoin. *Br J Clin Pharmacol*. 1982;13:501–505.

Notes

24. De Vivo DC, Bohan TP, Coulter DL, et al. L-carnitine supplementation in childhood epilepsy: current perspectives. *Epilepsia.* 1998;39:1216–1225.

25. Coulter DL. Carnitine deficiency: a possible mechanism for valproate hepatotoxicity [letter]. *Lancet.* 1984;1:689.

26. Ater SB, et al. A developmental center population treated with VPA and L-carnitine. In: Update 1993: inborn errors of metabolism in the patient with epilepsy. Sigma-Tau Pharmaceuticals; 1993.

27. Dreifuss FE, Langer DH. Hepatic considerations in the use of antiepileptic drugs. *Epilepsia.* 1987;28(suppl 2):S23–S29.

28. Ater SB, et al. A developmental center population treated with VPA and L-carnitine. In: Update 1993: inborn errors of metabolism in the patient with epilepsy. Sigma-Tau Pharmaceuticals; 1993.

29. Freeman JM, Vining EP, Cost S, et al. Does carnitine administration improve the symptoms attributed to anticonvulsant medications? A double-blinded, crossover study. *Pediatrics.* 1994;93:893–895.

30. De Vivo DC, Bohan TP, Coulter DL, et al. L-carnitine supplementation in childhood epilepsy: current perspectives. *Epilepsia.* 1998;39:1216–1225.

31. Hahn TJ, Hendin BA, Scharp CR, et al. Effect of chronic anticonvulsant therapy on serum 25-hydroxycalciferol levels in adults. *N Engl J Med.* 1972;287:900–904.

32. Hahn TJ, Hendin BA, Scharp CR, et al. Effect of chronic anticonvulsant therapy on serum 25-hydroxycalciferol levels in adults. *N Engl J Med.* 1972;287:900–904.

33. Jubiz W, Haussler MR, McCain TA, et al. Plasma 1,25-dihydroxyvitamin D levels in patients receiving anticonvulsant drugs. *J Clin Endocrinol Metab.* 1977;44:617–621.

34. Brodie MJ, Boobis AR, Dollery CT, et al. Rifampicin and vitamin D metabolism. *Clin Pharmacol Ther.* 1980;27:810–814.

35. Williams C, Netzloff M, Folkerts L, et al. Vitamin D metabolism and anticonvulsant therapy: effect of sunshine on incidence of osteomalacia. *South Med J.* 1984;77:834–836, 842.

36. Cornelissen M, Steegers-Theunissen R, Kollee L, et al. Increased incidence of neonatal vitamin K deficiency resulting from maternal anticonvulsant therapy. *Am J Obstet Gynecol.* 1993;168:923–928.

37. Cornelissen M, Steegers-Theunissen R, Kollee L, et al. Supplementation of vitamin K in pregnant women receiving anticonvulsant therapy prevents neonatal vitamin K deficiency. *Am J Obstet Gynecol.* 1993;168:884–888.

PROTEASE INHIBITORS

1. *A to Z Drug Facts* [book on CD-ROM]. 2nd ed. St. Louis, Mo: Facts and Comparisons; 2000.

2. Takanaga H, Ohnishi A, Murakami H, et al. Relationship between time after intake of grapefruit juice and the effect on pharmacokinetics and pharmacodynamics of nisoldipine in healthy subjects. *Clin Pharmacol Ther*. 2000;67:201–214.

3. Ernst E. Second thoughts about safety of St. John's wort. *Lancet*. 1999;354:2014–2016.

4. Guengerich FP. Cytochrome P-450 3A4: regulation and role in drug metabolism. *Annu Rev Pharmacol Toxicol*. 1999;39:1–17.

5. Piscitelli SC, Burstein AH, Chaitt D, et al. Indinavir concentrations and St. John's wort. *Lancet*. 2000;355:547–548.

PROTON PUMP INHIBITORS

1. Mirossay A, Mirossay L, Tothova J, et al. Potentiation of hypericin and hypocrellin-induced phototoxicity by omeprazole. *Phytomedicine*. 1999;6:311–317.

2. Werler MM, Shapiro S, Mitchell AA. Periconceptional folic acid exposure and risk of occurrent neural tube defects. *JAMA*. 1993;269:1257–1261.

3. Milunsky A, Jick H, Jick SS, et al. Multivitamin/folic acid supplementation in early pregnancy reduces the prevalence of neural tube defects. *JAMA*. 1989;262:2847–2852.

4. Rimm EB, Willett WC, Hu FB, et al. Folate and vitamin B6 from diet and supplements in relation to risk of coronary heart disease among women. *JAMA*. 1998;279:359–364.

5. Graham IM, Daly LE, Refsum HM, et al. Plasma homocysteine as a risk factor for vascular disease. The European Concerted Action Project. *JAMA*. 1997;277:1775–1781.

6. Moghadasian MH, McManus BM, Frohlich JJ, et al. Homocysteine and coronary artery disease. Clinical evidence and genetic and metabolic background. *Arch Intern Med*. 1997;157:2299–2308.

7. Ubbink JB, van der Merwe A, Vermaak WJ, et al. Hyperhomocysteinemia and the response to vitamin supplementation. *Clin Invest*. 1993;71:993–998.

8. den Heijer M, Brouwer IA, Bos GM, et al. Vitamin supplementation reduces blood homocysteine levels: a controlled trial in patients with venous thrombosis and healthy volunteers. *Arterioscler Thromb Vasc Biol*. 1998;18:356–361.

Notes

9. Ward M, McNulty H, McPartlin J, et al. Plasma homocysteine, a risk factor for cardiovascular disease, is lowered by physiological doses of folic acid. *QJM*. 1997;90:519–524.

10. Oakley GP Jr, Adams MJ, Dickinson CM. More folic acid for everyone, now. *J Nutr*. 1996;126:751S–755S.

11. Werbach MR. *Foundations of Nutritional Medicine: A Sourcebook of Clinical Research*. Tarzana, Calif: Third Line Press; 1997: 55–57.

12. Russell RM, Golner BB, Krasinski SD, et al. Effect of antacid and H_2 receptor antagonists on the intestinal absorption of folic acid. *J Lab Clin Med*. 1988;112:458–463.

13. Streeter AM, Goulston KJ, Bathur FA, et al. Cimetidine and malabsorption of cobalamin. *Dig Dis Sci*. 1982;27:13–16.

14. Aymard JP, Aymard B, Netter P, et al. Haematological adverse effects of histamine H_2-receptor antagonists. *Med Toxicol Adverse Drug Exp*. 1988;3:430–448.

15. Saltzman JR, Kemp JA, Golner BB, et al. Effect of hypochlorhydria due to omeprazole treatment or atrophic gastritis on protein-bound vitamin B12 absorption. *J Am Coll Nutr*. 1994;13:584–591.

16. Marcuard SP, Albernaz L, Khazanie PG. Omeprazole therapy causes malabsorption of cyanocobalamin. *Ann Intern Med*. 1994;120:211–215.

17. Marcuard SP, Albernaz L, Khazanie PG. Omeprazole therapy causes malabsorption of cyanocobalamin. *Ann Intern Med*. 1994;120:211–215.

18. Salom IL, Silvis SE, Doscherholmen A. Effect of cimetidine on the absorption of vitamin B12. *Scand J Gastroenterol*. 1982;17:129–131.

19. Saltzman JR, Kemp JA, Golner BB, et al. Effect of hypochlorhydria due to omeprazole treatment or atrophic gastritis on protein-bound vitamin B12 absorption. *J Am Coll Nutr*. 1994;13:584–591.

20. Sturniolo GC, Montino MC, Rossetto L, et al. Inhibition of gastric acid secretion reduces zinc absorption in man. *J Am Coll Nutr*. 1991;4:372–375.

21. Champagne ET. Low gastric hydrochloric acid secretion and mineral bioavailability. *Adv Exp Med Biol*. 1989;249:173–184.

RIFAMPIN

1. Perry W, Erooga MA, Brown J, et al. Calcium metabolism during rifampicin and isoniazid therapy for tuberculosis. *J R Soc Med*. 1982;75:533–536.

2. Brodie MJ, Boobis AR, Hillyard CJ, et al. Effect of isoniazid on vitamin D metabolism and hepatic monooxygenase activity. *Clin Pharmacol Ther.* 1981;30:363–367.

3. Brodie MJ, Boobis AR, Dollery CT, et al. Rifampicin and vitamin D metabolism. *Clin Pharmacol Ther.* 1980;27:810–814.

4. Williams SE, Wardman AG, Taylor GA, et al. Long term study of the effect of rifampicin and isoniazid on vitamin D metabolism. *Tubercle.* 1985;66:49–54.

SELECTIVE SEROTONIN-REUPTAKE INHIBITORS (SSRIs)

1. Iruela LM, Minguex L, Merino J, et al. Toxic interaction of S-adenosylmethionine and clomipramine [letter]. *Am J Psychiatry.* 1993;150:522.

2. Demott K. St. John's wort tied to serotonin syndrome. *Clin Psychiatry News.* 1998;26:28.

3. Gordon JB. SSRIs and St. John's wort: possible toxicity? [letter]. *Am Fam Physician.* 1998;57:950, 953.

4. Lantz MS, Buchalter E, Giambanco V. St. John's wort and antidepressant drug interactions in the elderly. *J Geriatr Psychiatry Neurol.* 1999;12:7–10.

5. Gordon JB. SSRIs and St. John's wort: possible toxicity? [letter]. *Am Fam Physician.* 1998;57:950, 953.

6. Demott K. St. John's wort tied to serotonin syndrome. *Clin Psychiatry News.* 1998;26:28.

7. Cohen AJ, Bartlik B. *Ginkgo biloba* for antidepressant-induced sexual dysfunction. *J Sex Marital Ther.* 1998;24:139–143.

8. Cohen AJ, Bartlik B. Ginkgo biloba for antidepressant-induced sexual dysfunction. *J Sex Marital Ther.* 1998;24:139–143.

9. McCann B. Botanical could improve sex lives of patients on SSRIs. *Drug Topics.* 1997;141:33.

SPIRONOLACTONE

1. *AHFS Drug Information.* Bethesda, Md: American Society of Health-System Pharmacists; 2000:2306–2307.

2. Stewart PM, Wallace AM, Valentino R, et al. Mineralocorticoid activity of liquorice: 11-beta-hydroxysteroid dehydrogenase deficiency comes of age. *Lancet.* 1987;2:821–824.

3. Walker BR, Edwards CR. Licorice-induced hypertension and syndromes of apparent mineralocorticoid excess. *Endocrinol Metab Clin North Am.* 1994;23:359–377.

4. Wash LK, Bernard JD. Licorice-induced pseudoaldosteronism. *Am J Hosp Pharm.* 1975;32:73–74.

5. Bernardi M, D'Intino PE, Trevisani F, et al. Effects of prolonged ingestion of graded doses of licorice by healthy volunteers. *Life Sci.* 1994;55:863–872.

6. Salassa RM. Inhibition of the "mineralocorticoid" activity of licorice by spironolactone. *J Clin Endocrinol.* 1962;22:1156–1159.

7. Devane J, Ryan MP. The effects of amiloride and triamterene on urinary magnesium excretion in conscious saline-loaded rats. *Br J Pharmacol.* 1981;72:285–289.

8. Tweeddale MG, Ogilvie RI. Antagonism of spironolactone-induced natriuresis by aspirin in man. *N Engl J Med.* 1973;289:198–200.

STATIN DRUGS (HMG-COA REDUCTASE INHIBITORS)

1. Alderman S, Kailas S, Goldfarb S, et al. Cholestatic hepatitis after ingestion of chaparral leaf: confirmation by endoscopic retrograde cholangiopancreatography and liver biopsy. *J Clin Gastroenterol.* 1994;19:242–247.

2. [No authors listed]. From the Centers for Disease Control and Prevention. Chaparral-induced toxic hepatitis—California and Texas, 1992. *JAMA.* 1992;268:3295, 3298.

3. Gordon DW, Rosenthal G, Hart J, et al. Chaparral ingestion. The broadening spectrum of liver injury caused by herbal medications. *JAMA.* 1995;273:489–490.

4. Katz M, Saibil F. Herbal hepatitis: subacute hepatic necrosis secondary to chaparral leaf. *J Clin Gastroenterol.* 1990;12:203–206.

5. Smith BC, Desmond PV. Acute hepatitis induced by ingestion of the herbal medication chaparral [letter]. *Aust N Z J Med.* 1993;23:526.

6. Sheikh NM, Philen RM, Love LA. Chaparral-associated hepatotoxicity. *Arch Intern Med.* 1997;157:913–919.

7. Jim LK, Gee JP. Adverse effects of drugs on the liver. In: Young LY, Koda-Kimble MA (eds). *Applied Therapeutics: The Clinical Use of Drugs.* Vancouver, Wash: Applied Therapeutics, Inc.; 1995:26.1–26.17.

8. *A to Z Drug Facts* [book on CD-ROM]. 2nd ed. St. Louis, Mo: Facts and Comparisons; 2000.

Notes

9. Takanaga H, Ohnishi A, Murakami H, et al. Relationship between time after intake of grapefruit juice and the effect on pharmacokinetics and pharmacodynamics of nisoldipine in healthy subjects. *Clin Pharmacol Ther.* 2000;67:201–214.

10. *A to Z Drug Facts* [book on CD-ROM]. 2nd ed. St. Louis, Mo: Facts and Comparisons; 2000.

11. Jacobson TA, Amorosa LF. Combination therapy with fluvastatin and niacin in hypercholesterolemia: a preliminary report on safety. *Am J Cardiol.* 1994;73:25D–29D.

12. Kashyap ML, Evans R, Simmons PD, et al. New combination niacin/statin formulation shows pronounced effects on major lipoproteins and is well tolerated [abstract]. *J Am Coll Cardiol.* 2000;35(2 suppl A):A326.

13. Mortensen SA, Leth A, Agner E, et al. Dose-related decrease of serum coenzyme Q10 during treatment with HMG-CoA reductase inhibitors. *Mol Aspects Med.* 1997;18(suppl):S137–S144.

14. Ghirlanda G, Oradei A, Manto A, et al. Evidence of plasma CoQ10-lowering effect by HMG-CoA reductase inhibitors: a double-blind, placebo-controlled study. *J Clin Pharmacol.* 1993;33:226–229.

15. Mortensen SA, Vadhanavikit S, Muratsu K, et al. Coenzyme Q10: clinical benefits with biochemical correlates suggesting a scientific breakthrough in the management of chronic heart failure. *Int J Tissue React.* 1990;12:155–162.

16. Mortensen SA, Leth A, Agner E, et al. Dose-related decrease of serum coenzyme Q10 during treatment with HMG-CoA reductase inhibitors. *Mol Aspects Med.* 1997;18(suppl):S137–S144.

17. Ghirlanda G, Oradei A, Manto A, et al. Evidence of plasma CoQ10-lowering effect by HMG-CoA reductase inhibitors: a double-blind, placebo-controlled study. *J Clin Pharmacol.* 1993;33:226–229.

18. Folkers K, Langsjoen P, Willis R, et al. Lovastatin decreases coenzyme Q levels in humans. *Proc Natl Acad Sci USA.* 1990;87:8931–8934.

19. Folkers K, Langsjoen P, Willis R, et al. Lovastatin decreases coenzyme Q levels in humans. *Proc Natl Acad Sci USA.* 1990;87:8931–8934.

20. Bargossi AM, Battino M, Gaddi A, et al. Exogenous CoQ10 preserves plasma ubiquinone levels in patients treated with 3-hydroxy-3-methylglutaryl coenzyme A reductase inhibitors. *Int J Clin Lab Res.* 1994;24:171–176.

Notes

TAMOXIFEN

1. Bracke ME, Depypere HT, Boterberg T, et al. Influence of tangeretin on tamoxifen's therapeutic benefit in mammary cancer. *J Natl Cancer Inst.* 1999;91:354–359.

2. Bracke ME, Depypere HT, Boterberg T, et al. Influence of tangeretin on tamoxifen's therapeutic benefit in mammary cancer. *J Natl Cancer Inst.* 1999;91:354–359.

3. Kenny FS, Pinder SE, Ellis IO, et al. Gamma linolenic acid with tamoxifen as primary therapy in breast cancer. *Int J Cancer.* 2000;85:643–648.

TETRACYCLINES

1. *A to Z Drug Facts* [book on CD-ROM]. 2nd ed. St. Louis, Mo: Facts and Comparisons; 2000.

2. Neuvonen PJ. Interactions with the absorption of tetracyclines. *Drugs.* 1976;11:45–54.

3. Campbell NR, Hasinoff BB. Iron supplements: a common cause of drug interactions. *Br J Clin Pharmacol.* 1991;31:251–255.

4. Mapp RK, McCarthy TJ. The effect of zinc sulphate and of bicitropeptide on tetracycline absorption. *S Afr Med J.* 1976;50:1829–1830.

5. Andersson KE, Bratt L, Dencker H, et al. Inhibition of tetracycline absorption by zinc. *Eur J Clin Pharmacol.* 1976;10:59–62.

6. Heinrich HC, Oppitz KH, Gabbe EE. Inhibition of iron absorption in man by tetracycline [in German]. *Klin Wochenschr.* 1974;52:493–498.

THEOPHYLLINE

1. Bouraoui A, Toumi A, Mustapha HB, et al. Effects of capsicum fruit on theophylline absorption and bioavailability in rabbits. *Drug Nutr Interact.* 1988;5:345–350.

2. Monostory K, Vereczkey L. The effect of ipriflavone and its main metabolites on theophylline biotransformation. *Eur J Drug Metab Pharmacokinet.* 1996;21:61–66.

3. Monostory K, Vereczkey L, Levai F, et al. Ipriflavone as an inhibitor of human cytochrome P450 enzymes. *Br J Pharmacol.* 1998;123:605–610.

4. Takahashi J, Kawakatsu K, Wakayama T, et al. Elevation of serum theophylline levels by ipriflavone in a patient with chronic obstructive pulmonary disease. *Eur J Clin Pharmacol*. 1992;43:207–208.

5. Jobst KA, McIntyre M, St. George D, et al. Safety of St. John's wort (*Hypericum perforatum*). *Lancet*. 2000;355:575.

6. Nebel A, Schneider BJ, Baker RK, et al. Potential metabolic interaction between St. John's wort and theophylline [letter]. *Ann Pharmacother*. 1999;33:502.

7. Nebel A, Schneider BJ, Baker RK, et al. Potential metabolic interaction between St. John's wort and theophylline [letter]. *Ann Pharmacother*. 1999;33:502.

8. Delport R, Ubbink JB, Vermaak WJ, et al. Theophylline increases pyridoxal kinase activity independently from vitamin B6 nutritional status. *Res Commun Chem Pathol Pharmacol*. 1993;79:325–333.

9. Ubbink JB, Delport R, Bissbort S, et al. Relationship between vitamin B-6 status and elevated pyridoxal kinase levels induced by theophylline therapy in humans. *J Nutr*. 1990;120:1352–1359.

10. Shimizu T, Maeda S, Mochizuki H, et al. Theophylline attenuates circulating vitamin B6 levels in children with asthma. *Pharmacology*. 1994;49:392–397.

11. Delport R, Ubbink JB, Vermaak WJ, et al. Theophylline increases pyridoxal kinase activity independently from vitamin B6 nutritional status. *Res Commun Chem Pathol Pharmacol*. 1993;79:325–333.

12. Ubbink JB, Delport R, Bissbort S, et al. Relationship between vitamin B-6 status and elevated pyridoxal kinase levels induced by theophylline therapy in humans. *J Nutr*. 1990;120:1352–1359.

13. Bartel PR, Ubbink JB, Delport R, et al. Vitamin B-6 supplementation and theophylline-related effects in humans. *Am J Clin Nutr*. 1994;60:93–99.

14. Dakshinamurti K, Paulose CS, Viswanathan M. Vitamin B6 and hypertension. *Ann NY Acad Sci*. 1990;585:241–249.

15. Kant AK, Block G. Dietary vitamin B-6 intake and food sources in the US population: NHANES II, 1976–1980. *Am J Clin Nutr*. 1990;52:707–716.

THIAZIDE DIURETICS

1. Riis B, Christiansen C. Actions of thiazide on vitamin D metabolism: a controlled therapeutic trial in normal women early in the postmenopause. *Metabolism*. 1985;34:421–424.

Notes

2. Lemann J, Gray RW, Maierhofer WJ, et al. Hydrochlorothiazide inhibits bone resorption in men despite experimentally elevated serum 1,25-dihydroxyvitamin D concentrations. *Kidney Int.* 1985;28:951–958.

3. Crowe M, Wollner L, Griffiths RA. Hypercalcaemia following vitamin D and thiazide therapy in the elderly. *Practitioner.* 1984;228:312–313.

4. Gora ML, Seth SK, Bay WH, et al. Milk-alkali syndrome associated with use of chlorothiazide and calcium carbonate. *Clin Pharm.* 1989;8:227–229.

5. Shintani, Murase H, Tsukagoshi H, et al. Glycyrrhizin (licorice)-induced hypokalemic myopathy. Report of 2 cases and review of the literature. *Eur Neurol.* 1992;32:44–51.

6. Walker BR, Edwards CR. Licorice-induced hypertension and syndromes of apparent mineralocorticoid excess. *Endocrinol Metab Clin North Am.* 1994;23:359–377.

7. Epstein MT, Espiner EA, Donald RA, et al. Liquorice toxicity and the renin-angiotensin-aldosterone axis in man. *Br Med J.* 1977;1:209–210.

8. Wash LK, Bernard JD. Licorice-induced pseudoaldosteronism. *Am J Hosp Pharm.* 1975;32:73–74.

9. de Klerk GJ, Nieuwenhuis MG, Beutler JJ. Hypokalemia and hypertension associated with use of liquorice flavoured chewing gum. *BMJ.* 1997;314:731–732.

10. Corsi FM, Galgani S, Gasparini C, et al. Acute hypokalemic myopathy due to chronic licorice ingestion: report of a case. *Ital J Neurol Sci.* 1983;4:493–497.

11. Blachley JD, Knochel JP. Tobacco chewer's hypokalemia: licorice revisited. *N Engl J Med.* 1980;302:784–785.

12. al-Ghamdi SM, Cameron EC, and Sutton RA. Magnesium deficiency: pathophysiologic and clinical overview. *Am J Kidney Dis.* 1994;24:737–752.

13. Dorup I. Magnesium and potassium deficiency. Its diagnosis, occurrence and treatment in diuretic therapy and its consequences for growth, protein synthesis and growth factors. *Acta Physiol Scand Suppl.* 1994;618:1–55.

14. Martin BJ, Milligan K. Diuretic-associated hypomagnesemia in the elderly. *Arch Intern Med.* 1987;147:1768–1771.

15. Whang R, Whang DD, Ryan MP. Refractory potassium repletion.A consequence of magnesium deficiency. *Arch Intern Med.* 1992;152:40–45.

16. Reyes AJ, Leary WP, Lockett CJ, et al. Diuretics and zinc. *S Afr Med J.* 1982;62:373–375.

Notes

17. Reyes AJ, Leary WP, Lockett CJ, et al. Diuretics and zinc. *S Afr Med J.* 1982;62:373–375.

18. Reyes AJ, Olhaberry JV, Leary WP, et al. Urinary zinc excretion, diuretics, zinc deficiency and some side-effects of diuretics. *S Afr Med J.* 1983;64:936–941.

THYROID HORMONE

1. Butner LE, Fulco PP, Feldman G. Calcium carbonate-induced hypothyroidism. *Ann Intern Med.* 2000;132:595.

2. Schneyer CR. Calcium carbonate and reduction of levothyroxine efficacy [letter]. *JAMA.* 1998;279:750.

3. Singh N, Singh PN, Hershman JM, et al. Effect of calcium carbonate on the absorption of levothyroxine. *JAMA.* 2000;283:2822–2825.

4. Campbell NR, Hasinoff BB. Iron supplements: a common cause of drug interactions. *Br J Clin Pharmacol.* 1991;31:251–255.

5. Jabbar MA, Larrea J, Shaw RA. Abnormal thyroid function tests in infants with congenital hypothyroidism: the influence of soy-based formula. *J Am Coll Nutr.* 1997;16:280–282.

6. Divi RL, Chang HC, Doerge DR. Anti-thyroid isoflavones from soybean: isolation, characterization, and mechanisms of action. *Biochem Pharmacol.* 1997;54:1087–1096.

7. Chorazy PA, Himelhoch S, Hopwood NJ, et al. Persistent hypothyroidism in an infant receiving a soy formula: case report and review of the literature. *Pediatrics.* 1995;96(1 Pt 1):148–150.

TRAMADOL

1. Mason BJ, Blackburn KH. Possible serotonin syndrome associated with tramadol and sertraline coadministration *Ann Pharmacother.* 1997;31:175–177.

2. Hernandez AF, Montero MN, Pla A, et al. Fatal moclobemide overdose or death caused by serotonin syndrome? *J Forensic Sci.* 1995;40:128–130.

3. Demott K. St. John's wort tied to serotonin syndrome. *Clin Psychiatry News.* 1998;26:28.

4. Gordon JB. SSRIs and St. John's wort: possible toxicity? [letter]. *Am Fam Physician.* 1998;57:950, 953.

5. Iruela LM, Minguex L, Merino J, et al. Toxic interaction of S-adenosylmethionine and clomipramine [letter]. *Am J Psychiatry.* 1993;150:522.

TRIAMTERENE

1. *AHFS Drug Information*. Bethesda, Md: American Society of Health-System Pharmacists; 2000:2306–2307.

2. Stewart PM, Wallace AM, Valentino R, et al. Mineralocorticoid activity of liquorice: 11-beta-hydroxysteroid dehydrogenase deficiency comes of age. *Lancet*. 1987;2:821–824.

3. Walker BR, Edwards CR. Licorice-induced hypertension and syndromes of apparent mineralocorticoid excess. *Endocrinol Metab Clin North Am*. 1994;23:359–377.

4. Wash LK, Bernard JD. Licorice-induced pseudoaldosteronism. *Am J Hosp Pharm*. 1975;32:73–74.

5. Bernardi M, D'Intino PE, Trevisani F, et al. Effects of prolonged ingestion of graded doses of licorice by healthy volunteers. *Life Sci*. 1994;55:863–872.

6. Salassa RM. Inhibition of the "mineralocorticoid" activity of licorice by spironolactone. *J Clin Endocrinol*. 1962;22:1156–1159.

7. Devane J, Ryan MP. The effects of amiloride and triamterene on urinary magnesium excretion in conscious saline-loaded rats. *Br J Pharmacol*. 1981;72:285–289.

8. Lieberman FL, Bateman JR. Megaloblastic anemia possibly induced by triamterene in patients with alcoholic cirrhosis. *Ann Intern Med*. 1968;68:168–173.

9. Mason JB, Zimmerman J, Otradovec CL, et al. Chronic diuretic therapy with moderate doses of triamterene is not associated with folate deficiency. *J Lab Clin Med*. 1991;117:365–369.

10. Lieberman FL, Bateman JR. Megaloblastic anemia possibly induced by triamterene in patients with alcoholic cirrhosis. *Ann Intern Med*. 1968;68:168–173.

TRICYCLIC ANTIDEPRESSANTS

1. Almeida JC, Grimsley EW. Coma from the health food store: interaction between kava and alprazolam. *Ann Intern Med*. 1996;125:940–941.

2. Iruela LM, Minguex L, Merino J, et al. Toxic interaction of S-adenosylmethionine and clomipramine [letter]. *Am J Psychiatry*. 1993;150:522.

3. Lantz MS, Buchalter E, Giambanco V. St. John's wort and antidepressant drug interactions in the elderly. *J Geriatr Psychiatry Neurol*. 1999;12:7–10.

4. Gordon JB. SSRIs and St. John's wort: possible toxicity? [letter]. *Am Fam Physician.* 1998;57:950, 953.

5. Demott K. St. John's wort tied to serotonin syndrome. *Clin Psychiatry News.* 1998;26:28.

6. *A to Z Drug Facts* [book on CD-ROM]. 2nd ed. St. Louis, Mo: Facts and Comparisons; 2000.

7. Takanaga H, Ohnishi A, Murakami H, et al. Relationship between time after intake of grapefruit juice and the effect on pharmacokinetics and pharmacodynamics of nisoldipine in healthy subjects. *Clin Pharmacol Ther.* 2000;67:201–214.

8. Mortensen SA, Leth A, Agner E, et al. Dose-related decrease of serum coenzyme Q10 during treatment with HMG-CoA reductase inhibitors. *Mol Aspects Med.* 1997;18(suppl):S137–S144.

9. Ghirlanda G, Oradei A, Manto A, et al. Evidence of plasma CoQ10-lowering effect by HMG-CoA reductase inhibitors: a double-blind, placebo-controlled study. *J Clin Pharmacol.* 1993;33:226–229.

10. Folkers K. Basic chemical research on coenzyme Q10 and integrated clinical research on therapy of diseases. In: Lenaz G, ed. *Coenzyme Q: Biochemistry, Bioenergetics, and Clinical Applications of Ubiquinone.* New York, NY: Wiley; 1985.

11. Kishi T, Makino K, Okamoto T, et al. Inhibition of myocardial respiration by psychotherapeutic drugs and prevention by coenzyme Q. *Biomed Clin Aspects Coenzyme Q.* 1980;2:139–157.

12. Folkers K. Basic chemical research on coenzyme Q10 and integrated clinical research on therapy of diseases. In: Lenaz G, ed. *Coenzyme Q: Biochemistry, Bioenergetics, and Clinical Applications of Ubiquinone.* New York, NY: Wiley; 1985.

13. Kishi T, Makino K, Okamoto T, et al. Inhibition of myocardial respiration by psychotherapeutic drugs and prevention by coenzyme Q. *Biomed Clin Aspects Coenzyme Q.* 1980;2:139–157.

TRIMETHOPRIM-SULFAMETHOXAZOLE (TMP-SMZ)

1. Vinnicombe HG, Derrick JP. Dihydropteroate synthase from *Streptococcus pneumoniae*: characterization of substrate binding order and sulfonamide inhibition. *Biochem Biophys Res Commun.* 1999;258:752–757.

2. Kahn SB, Fein SA, Brodsky I. Effects of trimethoprim on folate metabolism in man. *Clin Pharmacol Ther.* 1968;9:550–560.

3. Vinnicombe HG, Derrick JP. Dihydropteroate synthase from *Streptococcus pneumoniae*: characterization of substrate binding order and sulfonamide inhibition. *Biochem Biophys Res Commun.* 1999;258:752–757.

4. Degowin RL, Eppes RB, Carson PE, et al. The effects of diaphenylsulfone (DDS) against chloroquine-resistant *Plasmodium falciparum*. *Bull World Health Organ.* 1966;34:671–681.

5. Alappan R, Perazella MA, Buller GK. Hyperkalemia in hospitalized patients treated with trimethoprim-sulfamethoxazole. *Ann Intern Med.* 1996;124:316–320.

6. Kahn SB, Fein SA, Brodsky I. Effects of trimethoprim on folate metabolism in man. *Clin Pharmacol Ther.* 1968;9:550–560.

7. Akerlund B, Tynell E, Bratt G, et al. N-acetylcysteine treatment and the risk of toxic reactions to trimethoprim-sulphamethoxazole in primary Pneumocystis carinii prophylaxis in HIV-infected patients. *J Infect.* 1997;35:143–147.

8. Walmsley SL, Khorasheh S, Singer J, et al. A randomized trial of N-acetylcysteine for prevention of trimethoprim-sulfamethoxazole hypersensitivity reactions in *Pneumocystis carinii* pneumonia prophylaxis (CTN 057). Canadian HIV Trials Network 057 Study Group. *J Acquir Immune Defic Syndr Hum Retrovirol.* 1998;19:498–505.

VALPROIC ACID

1. Arenz A, Klein M, Fiehe K. Occurrence of neurotoxic 4'-O-methylpyridoxine in *Ginkgo biloba* leaves, ginkgo medications and Japanese ginkgo food. *Planta Med.* 1996;62:548–551.

2. Mizuno N, Kawakami K, Morita E. Competitive inhibition between 4'-substituted pyridoxine analogues and pyridoxal for pyridoxal kinase from mouse brain. *J Nutr Sci Vitaminol (Tokyo).* 1980;26:535–543.

3. Wada K, Ishigaki S, Ueda K, et al. An antivitamin B6, 4'-methoxypyridoxine, from the seed of *Ginkgo biloba* L. *Chem Pharm Bull (Tokyo).* 1985;33:3555–3557.

4. Yagi M, Wada K, Sakata M, et al. Studies on the constituents of edible and medicinal plants. IV. Determination of 4-O-methylpyridoxine in serum of the patient with gin-nan food poisoning [in Japanese; English abstract]. *Yakugaku Zasshi.* 1993;113:596–599.

5. Arenz A, Klein M, Fiehe K. Occurrence of neurotoxic 4'-O-methylpyridoxine in *Ginkgo biloba* leaves, ginkgo medications and Japanese ginkgo food. *Planta Med.* 1996;62:548–551.

6. Almeida JC, Grimsley EW. Coma from the health food store: interaction between kava and alprazolam. *Ann Intern Med.* 1996;125:940–941.

7. Nau H, Tzimas G, Mondry M, et al. Antiepileptic drugs alter endogenous retinoid concentrations: a possible mechanism of teratogenesis of anticonvulsant therapy. *Life Sci.* 1995;57:53–60.

8. Krause KH, Bonjour JP, Berlit P, et al. Biotin status of epileptics. *Ann N Y Acad Sci.* 1985;447:297–313.

9. Said HM, Redha R, Nylander W. Biotin transport in the human intestine: inhibition by anticonvulsant drugs. *Am J Clin Nutr.* 1989;49:127–131.

10. Hendel J, Dam M, Gram L, et al. The effects of carbamazepine and valproate on folate metabolism. *Acta Neurol Scand.* 1984;69:226–231.

11. Kishi T, Fujita N, Eguchi T, et al. Mechanism for reduction of serum folate by antiepileptic drugs during prolonged therapy. *J Neurol Sci.* 1997;145:109–112.

12. Reynolds EH. Mental effects of anticonvulsants, and folic acid metabolism. *Brain.* 1968;91:197–214.

13. Berg MJ, Stumbo PJ, Chenard CA, et al. Folic acid improves phenytoin pharmacokinetics. *J Am Diet Assoc.* 1995;95:352–356.

14. Lewis DP, Van Dyke DC, Willhite LA, et al. Phenytoin-folic acid interaction. *Ann Pharmacother.* 1995;29:726–735.

15. Lewis DP, Van Dyke DC, Stumbo PJ, et al. Drug and environmental factors associated with adverse pregnancy outcomes. Part I: Antiepileptic drugs, contraceptives, smoking, and folate. *Ann Pharmacother.* 1998;32:802–817.

16. Ono H, Sakamoto A, Eguchi T, et al. Plasma total homocysteine concentrations in epileptic patients taking anticonvulsants. *Metabolism.* 1997;46:959–962.

17. Lewis DP, Van Dyke DC, Stumbo PJ, et al. Drug and environmental factors associated with adverse pregnancy outcomes. Part I: Antiepileptic drugs, contraceptives, smoking, and folate. *Ann Pharmacother.* 1998;32:802–817.

18. Wahl TO, Gobuty AH, Lukert BP. Long-term anticonvulsant therapy and intestinal calcium absorption. *Clin Pharmacol Ther.* 1981;30:506–512.

19. Weinstein RS, Bryce GF, Sappington LJ, et al. Decreased serum ionized calcium and normal vitamin D metabolite levels with anticonvulsant drug treatment. *J Clin Endocrinol Metab.* 1984;58:1003–1009.

20. Weinstein RS, Bryce GF, Sappington LJ, et al. Decreased serum ionized calcium and normal vitamin D metabolite levels with anticonvulsant drug treatment. *J Clin Endocrinol Metab.* 1984;58:1003–1009.

Notes

21. Carter BL, Garnett WR, Pellock JM, et al. Effect of antacids on phenytoin bioavailability. *Ther Drug Monit.* 1981;3:333–340.

22. McElnay JC, Uprichard G, Collier PS. The effect of activated dimethicone and a proprietary antacid preparation containing this agent on the absorption of phenytoin. *Br J Clin Pharmacol.* 1982;13:501–505.

23. De Vivo DC, Bohan TP, Coulter DL, et al. L-carnitine supplementation in childhood epilepsy: current perspectives. *Epilepsia.* 1998;39:1216–1225.

24. Coulter DL. Carnitine deficiency: a possible mechanism for valproate hepatotoxicity [letter]. *Lancet.* 1984;1:689.

25. Ater SB, et al. A developmental center population treated with VPA and L-carnitine. In: Update 1993: inborn errors of metabolism in the patient with epilepsy. Sigma-Tau Pharmaceuticals; 1993.

26. Dreifuss FE, Langer DH. Hepatic considerations in the use of antiepileptic drugs. *Epilepsia.* 1987;28(suppl 2):S23–S29.

27. Ater SB, et al. A developmental center population treated with VPA and L-carnitine. In: Update 1993: inborn errors of metabolism in the patient with epilepsy. Sigma-Tau Pharmaceuticals; 1993.

28. Freeman JM, Vining EP, Cost S, et al. Does carnitine administration improve the symptoms attributed to anticonvulsant medications? A double-blinded, crossover study. *Pediatrics.* 1994;93:893–895.

29. De Vivo DC, Bohan TP, Coulter DL, et al. L-carnitine supplementation in childhood epilepsy: current perspectives. *Epilepsia.* 1998;39:1216–1225.

30. Hahn TJ, Hendin BA, Scharp CR, et al. Effect of chronic anticonvulsant therapy on serum 25-hydroxycalciferol levels in adults. *N Engl J Med.* 1972;287:900–904.

31. Hahn TJ, Hendin BA, Scharp CR, et al. Effect of chronic anticonvulsant therapy on serum 25-hydroxycalciferol levels in adults. *N Engl J Med.* 1972;287:900–904.

32. Jubiz W, Haussler MR, McCain TA, et al. Plasma 1,25-dihydroxyvitamin D levels in patients receiving anticonvulsant drugs. *J Clin Endocrinol Metab.* 1977;44:617–621.

33. Brodie MJ, Boobis AR, Dollery CT, et al. Rifampicin and vitamin D metabolism. *Clin Pharmacol Ther.* 1980;27:810–814.

34. Williams C, Netzloff M, Folkerts L, et al. Vitamin D metabolism and anticonvulsant therapy: effect of sunshine on incidence of osteomalacia. *South Med J.* 1984;77:834–836, 842.

Notes

35. Cornelissen M, Steegers-Theunissen R, Kollee L, et al. Increased incidence of neonatal vitamin K deficiency resulting from maternal anticonvulsant therapy. *Am J Obstet Gynecol.* 1993;168:923–928.

36. Cornelissen M, Steegers-Theunissen R, Kollee L, et al. Supplementation of vitamin K in pregnant women receiving anticonvulsant therapy prevents neonatal vitamin K deficiency. *Am J Obstet Gynecol.* 1993;168:884–888.

WARFARIN

1. Janetzky K, Morreale AP. Probable interaction between warfarin and ginseng. *Am J Health Syst Pharm.* 1997;54:692–693.

2. Mortensen SA, Leth A, Agner E, et al. Dose-related decrease of serum coenzyme Q10 during treatment with HMG-CoA reductase inhibitors. *Mol Aspects Med.* 1997;18(suppl):S137–S144.

3. Ghirlanda G, Oradei A, Manto A, et al. Evidence of plasma CoQ10-lowering effect by HMG-CoA reductase inhibitors: a double-blind, placebo-controlled study. *J Clin Pharmacol.* 1993;33:226–229.

4. Combs AB, Porter TH, Folkers K. Anticoagulant activity of a naphtoquinone analog of vitamin K and an inhibitor of coenzyme Q10-enzyme systems. *Res Commun Chem Pathol Pharmacol.* 1976;13:109–114.

5. Spigset O. Reduced effect of warfarin caused by ubidecarenone [letter]. *Lancet.* 1994;344:1372–1373.

6. Lo ACT, Chan K, Yeung JHK, et al. The effects of Danshen (*Salvia miltorrhiza*) on pharmacokinetics and pharmacodynamics of warfarin in rats. *Eur J Drug Metab Pharmacokinet.* 1992;17:257–262.

7. Brinker F. *Herb Contraindications and Drug Interactions: with Appendices Addressing Specific Conditions and Medicines.* 2nd ed. Sandy, Ore: Eclectic Medical Publications; 1998.

8. Lo ACT, Chan K, Yeung JHK, et al. The effects of Danshen (*Salvia miltorrhiza*) on pharmacokinetics and pharmacodynamics of warfarin in rats. *Eur J Drug Metab Pharmacokinet.* 1992;17:257–262.

9. Shaw D, Leon C, Kolev S, et al. Traditional remedies and food supplements. A 5-year toxicological study (1991–1995). *Drug Saf.* 1997;17:342–356.

10. Page RL II, Lawrence JD. Potentiation of warfarin by dong quai. *Pharmacotherapy.* 1999;19:870–876.

Notes

11. Heptinstall S, Groenewegen WA, Spangenberg P, et al. Extracts of feverfew may inhibit platelet behavior via neutralization of sulphydryl groups. *J Pharm Pharmacol.* 1987;39:459–465.

12. Makheja AN, Bailey JM. The active principle in feverfew [letter]. *Lancet.* 1981;2:1054.

13. Sumner H, Salan U, Knight DW, et al. Inhibition of 5-lipoxygenase and cyclo-oxygenase in leukocytes by feverfew. Involvement of sesquiterpene lactones and other components. *Biochem Pharmacol.* 1992;43:2313–2320.

14. Groenewegen WA, Heptinstall S. A comparison of the effects of an extract of feverfew and parthenolide, a component of feverfew, on human platelet activity in-vitro. *J Pharm Pharmacol.* 1990;42:553–557.

15. Biggs MJ, Johnson ES, Persaud NP, et al. Platelet aggregation in patients using feverfew for migraine [letter]. *Lancet.* 1982;2:776.

16. Gadkari JV, Joshi VD. Effect of ingestion of raw garlic on serum cholesterol level, clotting time and fibrinolytic activity in normal subjects. *J Postgrad Med.* 1991;37:128–131.

17. Burnham BE. Garlic as a possible risk for postoperative bleeding. *Plast Reconstr Surg.* 1995;95:213.

18. Kiesewetter H, Jung F, Jung EM, et al. Effect of garlic on platelet aggregation in patients with increased risk of juvenile ischemic attack. *Eur J Clin Pharmacol.* 1993;45:333–336.

19. [No authors listed]. The effect of essential oil of garlic on hyperlipemia and platelet aggregation-an analysis of 308 cases. Cooperative Group for Essential Oil of Garlic. *J Tradit Chin Med.* 1986;6:117–120.

20. Bordia A. Effect of garlic on human platelet aggregation in vitro. *Atherosclerosis.* 1978;30:355–360.

21. Rose KD, Croissant PD, Parliament CF, et al. Spontaneous spinal epidural hematoma with associated platelet dysfunction from excessive garlic ingestion: a case report. *Neurosurgery.* 1990;26:880–882.

22. Sunter WH. Warfarin and garlic. *Pharm J.* 1991;246:722.

23. Backon J. Ginger: inhibition of thromboxane synthetase and stimulation of prostacyclin: relevance for medicine and psychiatry. *Med Hypotheses.* 1986;20:271–278.

24. Srivastava KC. Aqueous extracts of onion, garlic and ginger inhibit platelet aggregation and alter arachidonic acid metabolism. *Biomed Biochim Acta.* 1984;43:S335–S346.

25. Bordia A, Verma SK, Srivastava KC. Effect of ginger (*Zingiber officinale* Rosc.) and fenugreek (*Trigonella foenumgraecum L.*) on blood lipids, blood sugar and platelet aggregation in patients with coronary artery disease. *Prostaglandins Leukot Essent Fatty Acids*. 1997;56:379–384.

26. Janssen PL, Meyboom S, van Staveren WA, et al. Consumption of ginger (*Zingiber officinale* roscoe) does not affect ex vivo platelet thromboxane production in humans. *Eur J Clin Nutr*. 1996;50:772–774.

27. Lumb AB. Effect of dried ginger on human platelet function. *Thromb Haemost*. 1994;71:110–111.

28. Chung KF, Dent G, McCusker M, et al. Effect of a ginkgolide mixture (BN 52063) in antagonising skin and platelet responses to platelet activating factor in man. *Lancet*. 1987;1:248–251.

29. Rosenblatt M, Mindel J. Spontaneous hyphema associated with ingestion of *Ginkgo biloba* extract [letter]. *N Engl J Med*. 1997;336:1108.

30. Rowin J, Lewis SL. Spontaneous bilateral subdural hematomas with chronic *Ginkgo biloba* ingestion. *Neurology*. 1996;46:1775–1776.

31. Vale S. Subarachnoid hemorrhage associated with *Ginkgo biloba* [letter]. *Lancet*. 1998;352:36.

32. Matthews MK Jr. Association of *Ginkgo biloba* with intracerebral hemorrhage. *Neurology*. 1998;50:1933–1934.

33. Taylor JR, Wilt VM. Probable antagonism of warfarin by green tea. *Ann Pharmacother*. 1999;33:426–428.

34. Monostory K, Vereczkey L, Levai F, et al. Ipriflavone as an inhibitor of human cytochrome P450 enzymes. *Br J Pharmacol*. 1998;123:605–610.

35. Shaw D, Leon C, Kolev S, et al. Traditional remedies and food supplements. A 5-year toxicological study (1991–1995). *Drug Saf*. 1997;17:342–356.

36. Arruzazabala ML, Mas R, Molina V, et al. Effect of policosanol on platelet aggregation in type II hypercholesterolemic patients. *Int J Tissue React*. 1998;20:119–124.

37. Arruzazabala ML, Mas R, Molina V, et al. Effect of policosanol on platelet aggregation in type II hypercholesterolemic patients. *Int J Tissue React*. 1998;20:119–124.

38. Arruzazabala ML, Valdes S, Mas R, et al. Effect of policosanol successive dose increases on platelet aggregation in healthy volunteers. *Pharmacol Res*. 1996;34:181–185.

Notes

39. Arruzazabala ML, Valdes S, Mas R, et al. Comparative study of policosanol, aspirin and the combination therapy policosanol-aspirin on platelet aggregation in healthy volunteers. *Pharmacol Res.* 1997;36:293–297.

40. Maurer A. Interaction of St. John's wort extract with phenprocoumon. *Eur J Clin Pharmacol.* 1999;55:A22.

41. Jobst KA, McIntyre M, St. George D, et al. Safety of St. John's wort (*Hypericum perforatum*). *Lancet.* 2000:355:575.

42. Johne A, Brockmöller J, Bauer S, et al. Pharmacokinetic interaction of digoxin with an herbal extract from St. John's wort (*Hypericum perforatum*). *Clin Pharmacol Ther.* 1999;66:338–345.

43. Yue QY, Bergquist C, Gerden B. Safety of St. John's wort [letter]. *Lancet.* 2000;355:576–577.

44. Hitzenberger G, Sommer W, Grandt R. Influence of vinpocetine on warfarin-induced inhibition of coagulation. *Int J Clin Pharmacol Ther Toxicol.* 1990;28:323–328.

45. Harris JE. Interaction of dietary factors with oral anticoagulants: review and applications. *J Am Dietet Assoc.* 1995;95:580–584.

46. Harris JE. Interaction of dietary factors with oral anticoagulants: review and applications. *J Am Dietet Assoc.* 1995;95:580–584.

47. Schrogie JJ. Letter: Coagulopathy and fat-soluble vitamins. *JAMA.* 1975;232:19.

48. Rosenthal G. Interaction of ascorbic acid and warfarin [letter]. *JAMA.* 1971;215:1671.

49. Smith EC, Skalski RJ, Johnson GC, et al. Interaction of ascorbic acid and warfarin [letter]. *JAMA.* 1972;221:1166.

50. White JG, Rao GH, Gerrard JM. Effects of nitroblue tetrazolium and vitamin E on platelet ultrastructure, aggregation, and secretion. *Am J Pathol.* 1977;88:387–402.

51. Kim JM, White RH. Effect of vitamin E on the anticoagulant response to warfarin. *Am J Cardiol.* 1996;77:545–546.

52. Corrigan J, Marcus FI. Coagulopathy associated with vitamin E ingestion. *JAMA.* 1974;230:1300–1301.

53. Schrogie JJ. Letter: Coagulopathy and fat-soluble vitamins. *JAMA.* 1975;232:19.

54. Pedersen FM, Hamberg O, Hess K, et al. The effect of dietary vitamin K on warfarin-induced anticoagulation. *J Intern Med.* 1991;229:517–520.

Notes

55. Chow WH, Chow TC, Tse TM, et al. Anticoagulation instability with life-threatening complication after dietary modification. *Postgrad Med J*. 1990;66:855–857.

ZIDOVUDINE (AZT)

1. Semino-Mora MC, Leon-Monzon ME, Dalakas MC. Effect of L-carnitine on the zidovudine-induced destruction of human myotubes. Part I: L-carnitine prevents the myotoxicity of AZT in vitro. *Lab Invest*. 1994;71:102–112.

2. Famularo G, De Simone C, Cifone G. Carnitine stands on its own in HIV infection treatment. *Arch Intern Med*. 1999;159:1143–1144.

3. Moretti S, Alesse E, Di Marzio L, et al. Effect of L-carnitine on human immunodeficiency virus-1 infection–associated apoptosis: a pilot study. *Blood*. 1998;91:3817–3824.

4. Baum MK, Javier JJ, Mantero-Atienza F, et at, Zidovudine-associated adverse reactions in a longitudinal study of asymptomatic HIV-1-infected homosexual males. *J Acquir Immune Defic Syndr*. 1991;4:1218–1226.

5. Mocchegiani E, Veccia S, Ancarani F, et al. Benefit of oral zinc supplementation as an adjunct to zidovudine (AZT) therapy against opportunistic infections in AIDS. *Int J Immunopharmacol*. 1995;17:719–727.

6. Tang AM, Graham NHM, Kirby AJ, et al. Dietary micronutrient intake and risk of progression to acquired immunodeficiency syndrome (AIDS) in human immunodeficiency virus type 1(HIV-1)-infected homosexual men. *Am J Epidemiol*. 1993;138:937–951.

7. Tang AM, Graham NM, Saah AJ. Effects of micronutrient intake on survival in human immunodeficiency virus type 1 infection. *Am J Epidemiol*. 1996;143:1244–1256.

8. Paltiel O, Falutz J, Veilleux M, et al. Clinical correlates of subnormal vitamin B12 levels in patients infected with the human immunodeficiency virus. *Am J Hematol*. 1995;49:318–322.

ZOLPIDEM

1. Elko CJ, Burgess JL, Robertson WO. Zolpidem-associated hallucinations and serotonin reuptake inhibition: a possible interaction. *J Toxicol Clin Toxicol*. 1998;36:195–203.

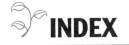

INDEX

Index

E

Index

Index

Index

Index

ABOUT THE AUTHORS

RICHARD HARKNESS, Pharm., FASCP, is a consultant pharmacist and nationally syndicated newspaper columnist, lecturer, and educator with specialties in geriatric practice, lipid therapy, smoking cessation, and evidence-based natural medicine. He is a former columnist for *Drug Topics* and has written continuing education courses and medication counseling guidelines for pharmacists as well as numerous other articles for national publications. He is the author of the following titles in THE NATURAL PHARMACIST™ series: *Reducing Cancer Risk, Preventing Heart Disease*, and *Drug-Herb-Vitamin Interactions Bible*. His other published books include *The Cholestin Breakthrough* (Prima), *Drug Interactions Guide Book, Drug Interactions Handbook*, and *OTC Handbook: What to Recommend & Why*.

STEVEN BRATMAN, M.D., is senior editor for THE NATURAL PHARMACIST™ series. Dr. Bratman is both a strong proponent and vocal critic of alternative treatments, and he believes that alternative medicine has both strengths and weaknesses, just like conventional medicine. This even-handed critique has made him a trusted party on both sides of the debate.

His books include *The Alternative Medicine Sourcebook: A Realistic Evaluation of Alternative Healing Methods, The Alternative Medicine Ratings Guide: An Expert Panel Ranks the Best Alternative Treatments for Over 80 Conditions* (Prima), the professional text *Clinical Evaluation of Medicinal Herbs and Other Therapeutic Natural Products* (Prima), *Health Food Junkies*, and the following titles in THE NATURAL PHARMACIST™ series: *Your Complete Guide to Herbs; Your Complete Guide to Illnesses and Their Natural Remedies; Natural Health Bible, Revised and Expanded 2nd Edition;* and *St. John's Wort and Depression*. He is also co-author of *The Natural Pharmacist: Drug-Herb-Vitamin Interactions Bible*.

Dr. Bratman has published articles in numerous national magazines, including *Yoga Journal, Utne Reader, Bottom-line Health, Delicious, Managed Healthcare*, and the peer-reviewed *Alternative Therapies in Health and Medicine*. He has been a contributor to America Online's Alternative Medicine forum, and he's a background source for numerous health-related Web sites and radio and TV programs.

Dr. Bratman has studied acupuncture, herbology, nutrition, massage, osteopathic manipulation, and body-oriented psychotherapy, and he has worked closely with a wide variety of alternative practitioners.